COMMON DIAGNOSTIC TESTS
Use and Interpretation

**Also Available from
the American College of Physicians:**

American College of Physicians Ethics Manual

Clinical Efficacy Reports
  (evaluations of medical tests and procedures, in
  looseleaf form)

Guide for Adult Immunization

How to Keep Up with the Medical Literature

Implementation of SI Units for Clinical Laboratory Data:
  Style Specifications and Conversion Tables

**Publications Department
American College of Physicians
4200 Pine Street
Philadelphia, PA 19104**

COMMON DIAGNOSTIC TESTS

Use and Interpretation

Harold C. Sox, Jr., MD, FACP
Editor

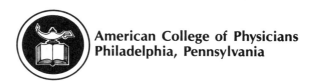

American College of Physicians
Philadelphia, Pennsylvania

First Edition

Printed in the United States of America

Library of Congress Cataloging-in-Publication Data
Main entry under title:

Common diagnostic tests.

    Includes index.
    1. Diagnosis, Laboratory—Handbooks, manuals, etc.
2. Function tests (Medicine)—Handbooks, manuals, etc.
I. Sox, Harold C.
RM38.2.C65   1987   616.07'5   87-1104

Library of Congress Catalog Card No. 87-70148
ISBN 0-943126-03-7

Editorial Advisors:	Edward J. Huth, M.D.
	David B. Nash, M.D.
Consultants:	John M. Eisenberg, M.D.
	Sankey V. Williams, M.D.
Project Coordinator:	Diane M. McCabe
Production Manager:	Kathleen Case

CONTENTS

OTHER DIAGNOSTIC APPLICATIONS

APPENDIXES

Mark D. Aronson, M.D.
Associate Professor of Medicine
Harvard Medical School
Boston, Massachusetts

J. Robert Beck, M.D.
Assistant Professor of Pathology and Community and
    Family Medicine
Departments of Pathology and Community and Family
    Medicine
Dartmouth-Hitchcock Medical Center
Hanover, New Hampshire

Laurence H. Beck, M.D.
Sylvan Eisman Professor of Medicine
University of Pennsylvania School of Medicine
Philadelphia, Pennsylvania

David H. Bor, M.D.
Chief of Infectious Diseases
Cambridge Hospital
Cambridge, Massachusetts

Randall D. Cebul, M.D.
Assistant Professor of Medicine
Henry J. Kaiser Family Foundation Faculty Scholar in
    General Medicine
Department of Medicine
University of Pennsylvania
Philadelphia, Pennsylvania

Robert M. Centor, M.D.
Chief
Division of General Internal Medicine and Primary Care
Medical College of Virginia
Richmond, Virginia

Henry P. Dalton, Ph.D.
Professor of Pathology and Microbiology
Medical College of Virginia
Richmond, Virginia

Robert H. Fletcher, M.D., F.A.C.P.
Professor of Medicine and Epidemiology
The University of North Carolina at Chapel Hill
Chapel Hill, North Carolina

Ary L. Goldberger, M.D.
Assistant Professor of Medicine
Harvard Medical School
Cardiovascular Division
Boston, Massachusetts
and
Beth Israel Hospital
Boston, Massachusetts

Lee Goldman, M.D.
Associate Professor of Medicine
Harvard Medical School
Boston, Massachusetts
and
Assistant Physician-in-Chief
Brigham and Women's Hospital
Boston, Massachusetts

Sheldon Greenfield, M.D.
Professor of Medicine and Public Health
University of California, Los Angeles
Los Angeles, California
and
Co-Director
Rand/UCLA Center for Health Policy Study
Los Angeles, California

Paul F. Griner, M.D., F.A.C.P.
Samuel E. Durand Professor of Medicine
University of Rochester School of Medicine and
    Dentistry
Rochester, New York
and
General Director
Strong Memorial Hospital
Rochester, New York

Gavin Hart, M.D., M.P.H.
Senior Medical Specialist
Information Services Division
South Australian Health Commission
South Australia

Jerome P. Kassirer, M.D., F.A.C.P.
Professor and Associate Chairman
Department of Medicine
Tufts University School of Medicine
     and
Associate Physician and Chief
New England Medical Center
Boston, Massachusetts

Anthony L. Komaroff, M.D.
Associate Professor of Medicine
Harvard Medical School
Boston, Massachusetts
     and
Chief
Division of General Medicine
Brigham and Women's Hospital
Boston, Massachusetts

Thomas H. Lee, M.D.
Assistant Professor of Medicine
Harvard Medical School
Boston, Massachusetts
     and
Associate Physician
Brigham and Women's Hospital
Boston, Massachusetts

Matthew H. Liang, M.D., M.P.H.
Associate Professor of Medicine
Harvard Medical School
Boston, Massachusetts
     and
Director
Robert B. Brigham Multi-Purpose Arthritis Center
Brigham and Women's Hospital
Boston, Massachusetts

Frederick A. Meier, M.D.
Assistant Professor of Pathology and Medicine
Medical College of Virginia
Richmond, Virginia

Alvin I. Mushlin, M.D., Sc.M., F.A.C.P.
Associate Professor of Medicine
Department of Medicine
University of Rochester School of Medicine and

Dentistry
Rochester, New York

Mark O'Konski, M.D.
Medical Resident
Department of Medicine
University of California, San Diego
La Jolla, California

Thomas A. Raffin, M.D.
Assistant Chief of Medicine
Associate Professor of Medicine
Department of Medicine
Stanford University School of Medicine
Stanford, California

Martin F. Shapiro, M.D., Ph.D.
Associate Professor of Medicine
Department of Medicine, UCLA
Center for the Health Sciences
Los Angeles, California

Harold C. Sox, Jr., M.D., F.A.C.P.
Professor of Medicine
Chief, Division of General Internal Medicine
Stanford University Medical Center
Stanford, California
        and
Veterans Administration Medical Center
Palo Alto, California

Anthony L. Suchman, M.D.
Assistant Professor of Medicine
Highland Hospital
Rochester, New York

Thomas G. Tape, M.D.
Assistant Professor of Medicine
University of Nebraska Medical Center
Section of General Internal Medicine
Omaha, Nebraska

A PROFESSION is defined in part by whether it commits itself to setting standards for the services society expects. The esteem society holds for a profession is determined largely by what standards it sets and how closely it meets them. One often professed standard in medicine is providing the best possible care at the lowest price.

The problems of excessive costs for medical care have to be attacked in various ways. One route is to eliminate the use of diagnostic tests when they do not contribute to the efficient practice of good medicine. Eliminating the use of even the low-cost tests that are frequently ordered can lead to substantial savings. The chapters in this manual represent efforts by standards-setters in American medicine to define the efficient use of commonly ordered tests.

This manual aims to help the physician decide when a diagnostic test is likely to make a desirable difference in care of a patient. Each chapter contains several recommendations for using a test, and each recommendation is based on critical review of published studies. When the published literature is silent on an issue, the authors have refrained from giving advice and have called for additional research. Thus the clinical investigator can use this manual to formulate an agenda for research.

The recommendations for test use are summarized in tabular form. Each recommendation has been closely scrutinized during three separate formal processes of review. Therefore the manual represents a remarkable degree of consensus about the use of these tests. Strongly held clinical opinion has been respected insofar as possible, without departing from the principle that the recommendations should have strong support from published clinical research. How consensus was reached may interest the reader.

This manual is the product of a long-standing working relationship between the American College of Physicians and the Blue Cross and Blue Shield Association. For the past decade, the Association has had a Medical Necessity

Project in which it develops guidelines for using medical procedures. In 1983 the Association asked the College for assistance in a review of common diagnostic tests ("little ticket technology"). The College's Clinical Efficacy Assessment Subcommittee approved the design of this project, which was at that time to be under the direction of J. Sanford Schwartz, M.D. With the additional assistance of Seymour Perry, M.D.; Paul Griner, M.D., Ph.D.; Howard Frazier, M.D.; and the Technology Assessment Committee of SREPCIM (the Society for Research and Education in Primary Care Internal Medicine), individuals were nominated to serve as consultants to the Blue Cross and Blue Shield Association and to prepare critical reviews from which the Blue Cross and Blue Shield Association would prepare medical necessity guidelines. These background papers became the chapters in this book. The papers were reviewed for the Blue Cross and Blue Shield Association by Jeremiah Barondess, M.D.; Charles Clayman, M.D.; David Eddy, M.D., Ph.D.; Paul Griner, M.D., Ph.D.; and Harold Sox, M.D. This phase of the project was coordinated by Ralph Schaffarzick, M.D., and David Tennenbaum. The guidelines for this series were written by Margaret Creditor of the Blue Cross and Blue Shield Association.

The papers were evaluated at the College by a process that included peer review by *Annals of Internal Medicine* and by several College committees. Because the papers were to appear in the Diagnostic Decision section of *Annals of Internal Medicine,* each paper was reviewed by the consulting editors for that section: John Eisenberg, M.D., and Sankey Williams, M.D. In addition, several manuscript consultants and the Associate Editors of *Annals* reviewed each paper.

The College's evaluation was equally thorough. First, its Clinical Efficacy Assessment Subcommittee reviewed the guidelines and the papers and modified the guidelines as necessary to achieve consensus. Members of the subcommittee included Earl Steinberg, M.D.; Paul Griner, M.D., Ph.D.; Lockhart McGuire, M.D.; John Davis, M.D.; Richard Hornick, M.D.; Harold Sox, M.D.; and Richard Farmer, M.D.; the review process was coordinated by Linda Johnson White. David B. Nash, M.D., and Diane McCabe provided editorial guidance for the project. Appropriate groups in a number of subspecialty societies also were given the opportunity to review the guidelines. The guidelines were then reviewed and approved by the College's Health and Public Policy Committee and by its Board of Regents. At each level of the review, the authors of the papers were asked to respond to criticisms, either by additional documentation or by modifying the paper or the recommendations. The guidelines have also been approved by the authors of the papers.

The reader will be the final judge of how well these chapters reflect our knowledge of these tests. If this manual proves to be as useful as we think it will, a second edition will have to be published. We shall welcome both criticisms of this edition and recommendations for the content of a new edition; the recommendations could be for additional content in present chapters and for chapters on other tests. Communications about this manual should be addressed to Edward J. Huth, M.D., Editor, *Annals of Internal Medicine,* 4200 Pine Street, Philadelphia, PA 19104, USA.

> Harold C. Sox Jr., M.D.
> Stanford University Medical Center
> Stanford, California
> and
> Veterans Administration Medical Center
> Palo Alto, California
>
> Edward J. Huth, M.D.
> *Annals of Internal Medicine*
> Philadelphia, Pennsylvania

Probability Theory in the Use of Diagnostic Tests

Application to Critical Study of the Literature

HAROLD C. SOX, Jr., M.D.

THE ARTICLE on serum carcinoembryonic antigen that appeared in January 1986 (1) was the first of a series of articles commissioned by the Blue Cross-Blue Shield Medical Necessity Project. In this series of articles, commonly used diagnostic tests are reevaluated critically. Their aim is to help the clinician identify the circumstances in which these tests are most likely to alter the care of the patient. This article reviews the terminology and analytic methods used by the authors in the series. These ideas are explained at greater length in standard references (2, 3). The approach to be taken in this series is based on two principles.

Principle I: Probability is a useful representation of diagnostic uncertainty.

Clinicians have always had to make decisions without definitive information. Consider a test whose *sensitivity* and *specificity* for a disease are both 0.90. According to the definition of these terms in Appendix 1, 90% of patients with the disease will have an abnormal test result (*true-positive result*) and 90% of patients who do not have the disease will have a normal test result (*true-negative result*). Conversely, 10% of patients with the disease will have a negative test result (*false-negative result*) and 10% of the patients who do not have the disease will have an abnormal result (*false-positive result*). When the test result for a patient is abnormal, the clinician cannot

▶ This chapter was originally published in *Annals of Internal Medicine.* 1986;**104**:60-6.

be certain that the patient has the disease, because abnormal results occur in patients both with the disease and without the disease. Thus, diagnostic tests often leave the physician still uncertain about the patient's true state.

Some clinicians express their uncertainty about the patient's true state by estimating the *probability* that the patient has a specified disease. By using probability (as defined in Appendix 1) rather than adjectives such as probably or possibly, the clinician expresses uncertainty quantitatively and unambiguously. Moreover, the effect of new information on the probability of disease may be calculated with *Bayes' theorem.* Bayes' theorem often provides insights that are not obtained by relying on intuition.

Principle II: Diagnostic tests should be obtained only when they can alter management in a case.

This principle does not take into account other possible reasons for obtaining tests, such as patient demand or fear of malpractice liability. Such reasons are not discussed here.

How does one decide if a test will alter management in a case? Often the answer to this question is self-evident: the clinician is committed to one course of action, and the test can have no bearing on management. When more than one management strategy is being considered, there are several ways to decide if a test can affect the choice.

Effect of a test result on the probability of disease: If the probability of disease after the test will be very similar to the probability of disease before the test, the test is unlikely to affect management. The authors in this series will use the probability of disease following a test (*post-test probability*) to identify situations in which a test may be useful. The post-test probability of disease can be predicted with Bayes' theorem, as discussed later in this article.

The threshold model of decision making: The threshold model is an extension of the idea that a test is judged by its effect on the probability of disease (4-6). The model postulates a *treatment threshold probability,* below which treatment is withheld and above which treatment is offered. If the *pretest probability* is below this threshold, treatment would not be offered unless the post-test probability equals or exceeds the treatment threshold. If the pretest probability is far from the treatment threshold probability or if the test is not specific for the disease, the test is unlikely to affect management. One must estimate the benefits and costs of treatment in order to set the treatment threshold probability.

Effect of test results on clinical outcomes: When a test result leads to a change in management that has no effect on clinical outcome, the test should not have been done. When the effect of a test result on longevity or functional status is known, the clinician can take into account the patient's attitudes towards changes in these outcomes. For example, investigators have calculated the average improvement in life expectancy from performing coronary arteriography in patients with stable angina pectoris (7). The decision to perform this procedure might well be affected by the patient's attitude toward its potential effect on longevity.

Marginal cost effectiveness of the test: This measure of test performance (as defined in Appendix 1) takes into account the increased costs from doing a test and the incremental benefit to the patient. A test result may lead to improved longevity, but the increase in cost per unit increase in longevity may be too large to warrant doing the test.

With the exception of a few studies, little is known about the effect of test results on clinical outcomes or the marginal cost effectiveness of tests. The authors in this series will use the effect of a test on the probability of disease as one guide to effective use of tests. Much can be learned from this approach, even though it is less conclusive than methods that take into account the cost and benefits of treatment. This introductory article describes the factors that determine the post-test probability of disease, the problems in measuring these factors, and potential problems in using Bayes' theorem. Information on cost-effectiveness analysis may be obtained from standard references (2, 8).

The Post-Test Probability of Disease

The probability of disease after the results of a diagnostic test are known (post-test probability of disease) depends on the pretest probability of disease and the sensitivity and specificity of the test. Several equivalent methods for calculating the post-test probability of dis-

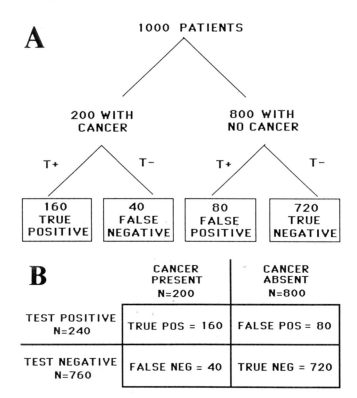

A

1000 PATIENTS

200 WITH CANCER

800 WITH NO CANCER

T+   T−   T+   T−

| 160 TRUE POSITIVE | 40 FALSE NEGATIVE | 80 FALSE POSITIVE | 720 TRUE NEGATIVE |

B

	CANCER PRESENT N=200	CANCER ABSENT N=800
TEST POSITIVE N=240	TRUE POS = 160	FALSE POS = 80
TEST NEGATIVE N=760	FALSE NEG = 40	TRUE NEG = 720

C PROBABILITY OF CANCER IF TEST IS POSITIVE

$$= \frac{\text{TRUE POS}}{\text{TRUE POS + FALSE POS}} = \frac{160}{160 + 80} = 0.67$$

PROBABILITY OF CANCER IF TEST IS NEGATIVE

$$= \frac{\text{FALSE NEG}}{\text{FALSE NEG + TRUE NEG}} = \frac{40}{40 + 720} = 0.05$$

Figure 1. Two methods for calculating the post-test probability of disease. Panels A and B show the effects of using a test with a sensitivity of 0.80 and a specificity of 0.90 in a population of 1000 patients in whom the prevalence of cancer is 0.20. Panel C shows that the probability of cancer is 0.67 if the test is positive (*T+*) and 0.05 if the test is negative (*T−*).

ease are shown in Figure 1 and Appendix 2. Figure 2A shows the post-test probability of disease after a "positive" result on a hypothetical test; a positive result is defined as a result that occurs more often in patients with a disease than in patients without the disease. Figure 2B shows the post-test probability after a "negative" test result, a result that occurs more often in patients without the disease than in patients with the disease. Several lessons can be learned from the relationship between the pretest probability of disease and the post-test probability of disease (Figure 2).

The interpretation of a test result depends on the pretest probability of disease: If a test is positive, the post-test probability increases as the pretest probability increases (Figure 2A). If a test is negative, the post-test probability decreases as the pretest probability decreases (Figure 2B).

The only exception to this relationship between pretest and post-test probability would be a perfect test. A test that is perfectly specific for one disease has no false-positive results; regardless of the pretest probability, the post-test probability if the test is positive is always 1.0. Conversely, when test sensitivity for a disease is 1.0, there are no false-negative results; regardless of the pretest probability, the probability of the disease if the test is negative is always 0. Few if any tests have these ideal characteristics.

The effect of a test result on the probability of a disease depends on the pretest probability: If the post-test probability is the same as the pretest probability, the post-test probability would lie on the 45-degree line in Figure 2. The vertical distance between the 45-degree line and the curve is the difference between the pretest and post-test probabilities:

When the pretest probability is *low,* a negative test has little effect, and a positive test has a large effect.

When the pretest probability is *high,* a negative test has a considerable effect, and a positive test has little effect.

Thus, when the clinician is already quite certain of the diagnosis, a confirmatory test result has little effect on the probability of disease. Tests have large effects when the probability of disease is intermediate or when the test result does not confirm the clinical impression.

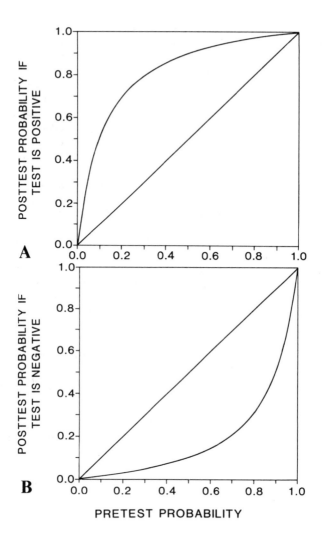

Figure 2. Relationship between pretest probability and post-test probability of disease. Sensitivity and specificity of the test were assumed to be 0.90 for the 3 examples. **Figure 2A.** The post-test probability of disease corresponding to a positive test result was calculated with Bayes' theorem for all values of pretest probability. **Figure 2B.** The post-test probability of disease corresponding to a negative test result was calculated with Bayes' theorem for all values of pretest probability. **Figure 2C.** The probability of a positive test result was calculated with the formula shown in Appendix 2. The probability of a negative test result is 1.0 minus the probability of a positive test.

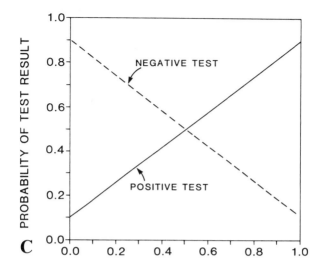

The pretest probability affects the probability that a test result will occur: Figure 2C shows that the higher the pretest probability, the more likely a positive test result is to occur. Conversely, a negative test result is less likely as the pretest probability increases.

The post-test probability depends on the sensitivity and specificity of the diagnostic test: As seen in the upper family of curves in Figure 3A, test *specificity* is an important factor in determining the post-test probability after a *positive* test result. Conversely, test specificity has relatively little effect on the post-test probability after a negative test result, as seen in the lower family of curves in Figure 3A. Thus, the importance of using a very specific test will depend on the pretest probability of disease and one's intent in testing. A test with high specificity is needed to verify the presence of a disease for which there is little clinical evidence or when the clinician must be virtually certain of a diagnosis.

Test *sensitivity* has relatively little effect on the post-test probability after a positive test, as seen in the upper family of curves in Figure 3B. Test *sensitivity* does affect the post-test probability after a *negative* test (lower family of curves in Figure 3B), particularly when the pretest probability is high. A test with high sensitivity is required to exclude a strongly suspected diagnosis or to confirm that a disease is not present when the clinician must be virtually certain.

The pretest probability of disease is an important factor in predicting the effect of a diagnostic test on management. Patients are particularly unlikely to benefit from testing when the pretest probability is very high or very low:

> If the pretest probability is very high, the physician is likely to treat the patient unless a negative test raises doubts about the diagnosis. The post-test probability of disease after a negative test result may be so high that treatment is still indicated. Thus, if the pretest probability is nearly 1.0, there is no point in testing unless the sensitivity of the test is very high (Figure 3B) and the clinician is willing to test even if the probability of a negative result is very low (Figure 2C).

> If the pretest probability is very low, as occurs in screening asymptomatic persons, the clinician is likely to do nothing unless a positive test raises concern. If, for example, the pretest probability is less than 0.001, the post-test probability may be less than 0.01. In this situation, a change in management is not indicated and the chance of a positive confirmatory test is very low (Figure 2C).

Patients are likely to benefit from tests when the pretest probability of disease is intermediate, which indicates considerable uncertainty about the patient's true state. As shown in Figure 3, the post-test probability may be close to 1.0 or 0 when the pretest probability is intermediate. Patients are also likely to benefit from testing when the pretest probability is close to a treatment threshold probability, because a small change in the probability of disease is sufficient to alter management.

To maximize the chance that a test will affect the management of a case, the clinician should choose a test whose sensitivity and specificity are appropriate to the pretest probability of disease. This series of articles will help to identify the circumstances in which commonly used tests are particularly useful. To read these articles critically, the clinician must understand the problems of estimating probability and measuring test sensitivity and specificity.

The Pretest Probability of Disease

Figure 2 shows the importance of the pretest probability in test-ordering decisions. When a physician classifies a patient as having a high, low, or intermediate probability of disease, the process is usually intuitive. The two principal influences on probability estimates are personal experience and the published literature.

PERSONAL EXPERIENCE

Personal experience with similar patients is the most important influence on probability estimates by clinicians. There are several cognitive principles, called *heuristics,* for using personal experience to estimate probability (9).

A clinician is using the *representativeness heuristic* when the probability that a patient has a disease is judged by the extent to which the patient's clinical findings resemble the essential features of the disease. Thus, if a patient has all the findings of Cushing's disease, the patient is judged highly likely to have Cushing's disease. This heuristic can be misleading if the disease is rare, if the patient's findings are poor predictors of disease or are redundant, or if the clinician's mental representation of the disease is based on a small, atypical experience.

Clinicians are using the *availability heuristic* when they judge the probability of an event by the ease with which similar events are remembered. This heuristic is often misleading. A physician who discovers porphyria in a patient with abdominal pain may overestimate the probability of porphyria in the next few patients with abdominal pain.

Clinicians often adjust from an initial probability estimate (the anchor) to take account of unusual features of a patient. The *anchoring and adjustment heuristic* is an important principle, but it is often used incorrectly. Many experiments have shown that clinicians do not adjust their initial estimate enough to take account of new information (9). Clinicians tend to be overconfident in their judgements and often overestimate the probability of disease (10).

PUBLISHED EXPERIENCE

The reported prevalence of a disease in a clinical population is a useful starting point for estimating the proba-

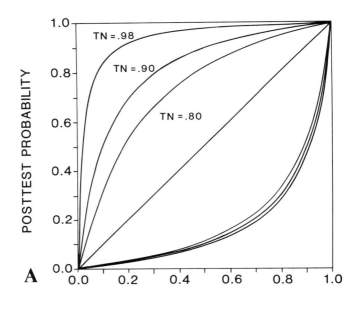

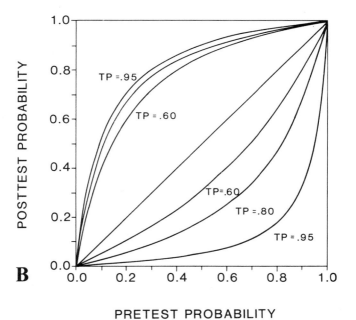

PRETEST PROBABILITY

bility of the disease. Applying the published literature to diagnostic judgements about individual patients may lead to error because many studies' conclusions are based on experience with patients who have been referred to subspecialists for care. This selection bias will lead to reported prevalences that are higher than prevalences in primary care patients.

Studies sometimes report the prevalence of clinical findings in patients with a disease, but this information is usually not useful for estimating probability because the prevalence of a finding in patients with a disease is not the same as the prevalence of disease in patients with a clinical finding. The most useful type of study also reports the prevalence of a finding in patients who were initially suspected of having the disease but were proved not to have it. The clinician can then calculate the *likelihood ratio* (Appendix 1), which is a measure of how well the finding predicts disease. Published studies seldom evaluate combinations of clinical findings. *Clinical prediction rules,* which are derived from systematic study of patients with a diagnostic problem, define how combinations of clinical findings may be used to estimate probability (11).

To take full advantage of the lessons in the Blue Cross-Blue Shield series of articles, clinicians will find it useful to do explicitly what they now do intuitively: estimate probability. Clinicians may improve their probability estimates by becoming aware of the types of errors that may occur.

Sensitivity and Specificity of Diagnostic Tests

As shown in Figure 3, the sensitivity and specificity of a test determine its effect on the probability of disease.

Figure 3. Effect of test sensitivity and specificity on post-test probability. Figures 3A and 3B are similar to Figures 2A and 2B except that the calculations have been repeated for several values of the sensitivity (*TP*, true-positive rate) and specificity (*TN*, true-negative rate) of the test. In Figure 3A, the sensitivity of the test was assumed to be 0.90, and the calculations were repeated for several values of test specificity. In Figure 3B, the specificity of the test was assumed to be 0.90, and the calculations were repeated for several values of the sensitivity of the test. In both panels, the top family of curves corresponds to positive test results, and the bottom family of curves correspond to negative test results.

Studies that measure the sensitivity and specificity of a test are important, but they are difficult to perform. Clinicians who take an interest in these matters will find that many studies are applicable only to a narrow spectrum of patients.

In the ideal study of a diagnostic test (or *index test*), all patients also undergo a definitive procedure (*"gold-standard" test*) to establish the true state of the patient. The "gold-standard" test is often costly, risky, or painful and is usually not done in patients with scant evidence for the disease. The sample population of a study may contain only a small fraction of patients who had the index test (12); consequently, the spectrum of patients in studies of a test often differs from the spectrum of patients in whom the test is typically used (13, 14). Therefore, published estimates of sensitivity and specificity may not be applicable to most patients.

Test performance may change as the test becomes more widely used (15). When a test is first introduced, the frequency of negative results in healthy volunteers is used to measure specificity. Unlike persons who are suspected of having the disease, healthy persons are unlikely to have other diseases that cause abnormal test results. Therefore, test specificity for a disease is apt to be overestimated in healthy persons. As the test becomes more widely used, an abnormal result on the index test becomes an indication to refer the patient for the definitive procedure. Patients with negative results on the index test are less likely to be referred and become enrolled in a study of test performance. Therefore, the frequency of true-negative results will be underestimated, and the reported test specificity will be lower than that in the population who had the index test. Referral bias is often unavoidable, but its effect may be minimized by performing the index test only after deciding to perform the "gold-standard" procedure (14).

Selection bias may also affect the measurement of test sensitivity. Early in the life of a test, study patients may be selected because they have extensive, easily detected disease. Later, an abnormal result on the index test becomes a criterion for referral. Patients with negative results on the index test, some of whom have disease, are less likely to be referred. Therefore, the frequency of false-negative results will be underestimated. Both types of selection bias result in overestimation of the sensitivity of the test.

Several other pitfalls can occur in measuring test performance. The "gold-standard" procedure may not be a perfect indicator of the disease. The interpretation of the index test may be influenced by the results of the "gold-standard" test (or vice versa). The association between the result of the "gold-standard" test and that of the index test will be artifactually strong, and test sensitivity and specificity will be overestimated.

Much information may be lost when studies of test performance define sensitivity and specificity in relation to a single cutoff value of a continuous variable. Many test results are expressed as a continuous variable, such as the serum concentration of creatine phosphokinase. A very high serum concentration of creatine phosphokinase is much more indicative of myocardial infarction than a serum concentration just above the upper limit of normal. When sensitivity and specificity are known for each point on a continuous scale, the post-test probability may be calculated for any test result.

Bayes' Theorem

One essential guidepost for interpreting test results and for deciding when a test is indicated is Bayes' theorem. This theorem is derived from first principles of probability theory. Errors in using Bayes' theorem occur because reported values for sensitivity and specificity are assumed to apply in all circumstances.

When Bayes' theorem is used, sensitivity and specificity are assumed to be constant, regardless of the pretest probability of disease. This assumption can be false. A test may be less sensitive in detecting a disease in an early stage, when the pretest probability is low, than it is in detecting disease in an advanced stage, when there are many signs and symptoms and the pretest probability is high (16). This error may be avoided by dividing the study population into subgroups that differ in the extent of clinical evidence for disease (14).

A second assumption is that the sensitivity and specificity of a test are independent of the results of other tests. This *independence assumption* is important when Bayes' theorem is used to calculate the probability of disease after a sequence of tests, in which the post-test probability after the first test in a sequence is used as the pretest probability for the second test. In the ideal study of this problem, both the index tests and a "gold-standard" procedure have been done in many patients. The sensitivity and specificity of the second test in the sequence should be calculated twice: in patients with a positive result on the first test and in patients with a negative result on the first test. If the sensitivity and specificity of the second test are the same regardless of the results of the first test, the independence assumption is valid. In practice, the independence assumption is seldom tested, and the clinician should be critical of recommendations for sequences of tests. The independence assumption is most likely to be correct when the tests measure different physiologic mechanisms of disease.

Appendix 1. Glossary of Terms

Anchoring and adjustment heuristic: a cognitive principle by which probability is estimated by starting from an initial value and adjusting to take account of additional information.

Availability heuristic: a cognitive principle by which the probability of an event is judged by the ease with which similar events can be remembered.

Bayes' theorem: an algebraic expression for calculating the post-test probability of disease if the pretest probability of disease [p(D)] and the sensitivity and specificity of a test are all known.

Clinical prediction rule: a rule, based on systematic clinical observations, for using the patient's findings to estimate the probability of a diagnosis or the outcome of an illness.

Cost-effectiveness analysis: comparison of clinical policies in terms of their cost per unit of outcome.

False-negative rate (FNR): the likelihood of a negative test in a patient with a disease.

False-negative result: a negative result in a patient with a disease.

False-positive rate (FPR): the likelihood of a positive test in a patient who does not have a disease.

False-positive result: a positive result in a person who does not have a disease.

"Gold-standard" test: the test or procedure that is used to define the true state of the patient (also definitive procedure).

Heuristic: serving to guide, discover, or reveal.

Independence assumption: the assumption that the sensitivity and specificity of a diagnostic test are independent of the results of prior tests.

Index test: the diagnostic test whose performance is being measured.

Likelihood ratio: a measure of discrimination by a test result. A test result with a likelihood ratio of greater than 1.0 raises the probability of disease and is often referred to as a "positive" test result. A test result with a likelihood ratio of less than 1.0 lowers the probability of disease and is often called a "negative" test result.

$$\text{Likelihood ratio} = \frac{\text{sensitivity}}{1 - \text{specificity}}$$

Marginal cost effectiveness: the increase in cost of a policy per unit increase in outcome.

Negative test-result: a test result that occurs more frequently in patients who do not have a disease than in patients who do have the disease.

Odds: the probability of an event.

$$\text{Odds} = \frac{\text{probability of event}}{1 - \text{probability of event}}$$

Positive test-result: a test result that occurs more frequently in patients with a disease than in patients without the disease.

Post-test probability: the probability of disease after the results of a test have been learned (also posterior probability or post-test risk).

Predictive value negative: probability of a disease being absent if a test result is negative.

Predictive value positive: probability of a disease if a test result is positive.

Pretest probability [p(D)]: the probability of disease before a test is done (also prior probability or pretest risk).

Probability: an expression of opinion, on a scale from 0 to 1.0, about the likelihood that an event will occur.

Representativeness heuristic: a cognitive principle by which the probability that an object belongs to a class of objects is judged by the degree to which the features of the object resemble the features of the class of objects.

Sensitivity: the likelihood of a positive test result in a person with a disease (also *true-positive rate,* TPR).

$$\text{Sensitivity} = \frac{\text{number of diseased patients with positive test}}{\text{number of diseased patients}}$$

Specificity: the likelihood of a negative test result in a patient without disease (also *true-negative rate,* TNR).

$$\text{Specificity} = \frac{\text{number of patients without disease with negative test}}{\text{number of patients without disease}}$$

Treatment threshold probability: the probability of disease at which the clinician is indifferent about withholding or giving treatment. Below the threshold probability, treatment is withheld; above the threshold, treatment is given.

True-negative result: a negative test result in a patient who does not have a disease.

True-positive result: a positive test result in a person with a disease.

Appendix 2. Bayes' Theorem for Calculating the Post-Test Probability of Disease

Probability of disease if test is positive =

$$\frac{p(D) \times TPR}{\{p(D) \times TPR\} + \{[1 - p(D)] \times FPR\}}$$

Probability of disease if test is negative =

$$\frac{p(D) \times FNR}{\{p(D) \times FNR\} + \{[1 - p(D)] \times TNR\}}$$

Probability of positive test result =
$$\{p(D) \times TPR\} + \{[1 - p(D)] \times FPR\}$$

Odds Ratio Form of Bayes' Theorem:

Post-test odds = pretest odds × likelihood ratio

Example: A clinician is planning to use a test with a sensitivity (TPR) of 0.8 and a false-positive rate (FPR) of 0.1. Suppose the pretest probability of disease [p(D)] is 0.20:

Probability of disease if test is positive =

$$\frac{p(D) \times TPR}{\{p(D) \times TPR\} + \{[1 - p(D)] \times FPR\}}$$

$$= \frac{0.20 \times 0.80}{\{0.20 \times 0.80\} + \{[0.80] \times 0.10\}} = \frac{0.16}{0.16 + 0.08} = 0.67$$

The pretest odds are 0.20/0.80 = 0.25 to 1. The likelihood ratio for the test is 0.80/0.10 = 8.0.

Post-test odds = pretest odds × likelihood ratio =
0.25 × 8.0 = 2.0 to 1

References

1. FLETCHER RJ. Carcinoembryonic antigen. *Ann Intern Med.* 1986;**104**:66-73.
2. WEINSTEIN MC, FINEBERG HV, ELSTEIN AS, et al. *Clinical Decision Analysis.* Philadelphia: W.B. Saunders Co.; 1980.
3. GRINER PF, MAYEWSKI RJ, MUSHLIN AI, GREENLAND P. Selection and interpretation of diagnostic tests and procedures: principles and applications. *Ann Intern Med.* 1981;**94**(4 pt 2):553-600.
4. PAUKER SG, KASSIRER JP. Therapeutic decision making: a cost-benefit analysis. *N Engl J Med.* 1975;**293**:229-34.
5. PAUKER SG, KASSIRER JP. The threshold approach to clinical decision making. *N Engl J Med.* 1980;**302**:1109-17.
6. DOUBILET P. A mathematical approach to interpretation and selection of diagnostic tests. *Med Decis Making.* 1983;**3**:177-95.
7. STASON WB, FINEBERG HV. Implications of alternative strategies to diagnose coronary artery disease. *Circulation.* 1982;**66**(5 pt 2):III80-6.
8. WEINSTEIN MC, STASON WB. Foundations of cost-effectiveness analysis for health and medical practices. *N Engl J Med.* 1977;**296**:716-21.
9. TVERSKY A, KAHNEMAN D. Judgment under uncertainty: heuristics and biases. *Science.* 1974;**185**:1124-31.
10. DESMET AA, FRYBACK DG, THORNBURY JR. A second look at the utility of radiographic skull examination for trauma. *AJR.* 1979;**132**:95-9.
11. WASSON JH, SOX HC, NEFF RK, GOLDMAN L. Clinical prediction rules: applications and methodological standards. *N Engl J Med.* 1985;**313**:793-9.
12. PHILBRICK JT, HORWITZ RI, FEINSTEIN AR, LANGOU RA, CHANDLER JP. The limited spectrum of patients studied in exercise test research: analyzing the tip of the iceberg. *JAMA.* 1982;**248**:2467-70.
13. RANSOHOFF DF, FEINSTEIN AR. Problems of spectrum and bias in evaluating the efficacy of diagnostic tests. *N Engl J Med.* 1978;**299**:926-30.
14. PHILBRICK JT, HORWITZ RI, FEINSTEIN AR. Methodologic problems of exercise testing for coronary artery disease: groups, analysis and bias. *Am J Cardiol.* 1980;**46**:807-12.
15. ROZANSKI A, DIAMOND GA, BERMAN D, FORRESTER JS, MORRIS D, SWAN HJC. The declining specificity of exercise radionuclide ventriculography. *N Engl J Med.* 1983;**309**:518-22.
16. WEINER DA, RYAN TJ, McCABE CH, et al. Exercise stress testing: correlations among history of angina, ST-segment response and prevalence of coronary-artery disease in the Coronary Artery Surgery Study (CASS). *N Engl J Med.* 1979;**301**:230-5.

Serum Enzyme Assays in the Diagnosis of Acute Myocardial Infarction

Recommendations Based on a Quantitative Analysis

THOMAS H. LEE, M.D.; and LEE GOLDMAN, M.D., M.P.H.

THE RECENT HISTORY of medicine has been characterized by the development of diagnostic tests of increasing sophistication. These tests have often enhanced our ability to detect diseases in subtle manifestations; in many instances, they have quickly become the "gold standard" by which even newer tests and physician judgments are measured.

In the last quarter century, serum enzyme assays have played such a role in the diagnosis of coronary artery disease. These tests have redefined the clinical entity that they are used to identify by revealing degrees of myocardial necrosis that previously could not be detected. Nevertheless, acute chest pain in a patient remains a difficult diagnostic problem (1-3), and autopsy results suggest that despite these technologic advances, physicians fail to diagnose myocardial infarctions with alarming frequency (4, 5), in part because serum enzyme levels are neither perfectly sensitive nor specific. This review recapitulates the basis of serum enzyme assays and discusses their limitations and indications in the patient with possible myocardial infarction as well as in other clinical settings.

Description

HISTORICAL BACKGROUND

In 1954, elevations of serum aspartate aminotransfer-

▶ This chapter was originally published in *Annals of Internal Medicine.* 1986;**105**:221-33.

ase (AST) levels were described in four of five patients with clinical diagnoses of myocardial infarction (6). Similar abnormal levels of lactate dehydrogenase (LDH) and its isoenzymes (7, 8) were reported in the next 3 years. Elevations of the third principal enzyme, creatine kinase (CK) (9), were found in patients with muscular dystrophy in 1959 (10) and, 1 year later, in patients with acute myocardial infarction (11). By 1962, the World Health Organization (12) had listed enzyme abnormalities among its diagnostic criteria for myocardial infarction. In 1966, CK isoenzymes were identified in different quantities in various tissues (13); subsequent studies in the early 1970s showed that CK-MB measurements added sensitivity and specificity to the diagnosis of myocardial infarction (14-17).

ENZYME CHARACTERISTICS

Creatine kinase is a dimeric enzyme that catalyzes the transfer of high-energy phosphate groups and is found predominantly in tissues that consume large amounts of energy. It has two subunits, each of which can be type M (for muscle) or B (for brain). In early fetal stages, only CK-BB is present; CK-MM and MB appear by the second trimester of gestation (18). The CK-MM isoenzyme is dominant in adult skeletal muscle, whereas CK-BB is found mostly in the central nervous system; myocardial CK is about 85% MM and 15% MB (16).

Only modest amounts of CK are found in other tissues (Table 1), but injury to these tissues can cause CK elevations. Creatine kinase-MB was initially thought to be found only in myocardial cells, but with the development of more sensitive assays, trace amounts have been found in several tissues including normal skeletal muscle (19, 20). Mild elevations have been found in athletes after vigorous exercise (21, 22); nevertheless, detectable rises in CK-MB levels from noncardiac sources are rare except when these organs are subjected to trauma or surgery (23). Abnormally high concentrations of CK-MB can be found in the skeletal muscle of marathon runners (24) and patients with muscular dystrophy (25), myositis (26), or rhabdomyolysis (27), reflecting abnormal enzyme differentiation or regeneration. Similarly, CK-MB and CK-BB have been reported in tumor homogenates from patients with lung cancer (28).

Lactate dehydrogenase is a ubiquitous tetrameric en-

Table 1. Characteristics of Enzymes Assayed in the Diagnosis of Myocardial Infarction

	Creatine Kinase	Creatine Kinase-MB
Molecular weight	86 000	86 000
Postinfarction characteristics		
Rises, *h*	4-8	4-8
Peaks, *h*	12-24	12-20
Returns to normal, *d*	3-4	2-3
Noncardiac sources	Muscle, liver, lung,* gastrointestinal tract,* brain, kidney, spleen	Muscle,* uterus,* diaphragm,* gastrointestinal tract,* thyroid,* prostate,* urethra*

	Lactate Dehydrogenase	Aspartate Aminotransferase
Molecular weight	135 000	47 000
Postinfarction characteristics		
Rises, *h*	8-12	8-12
Peaks, *h*	72-144	18-36
Returns to normal, *d*	8-14	3-4
Noncardiac sources	Most tissues	Muscle, liver, lung*

* Trace amounts. Data from references 19-32.

zyme that catalyzes the reversible reduction of pyruvate to lactate in the last step of glycolysis. Each of its subunits are type M (for muscle) or H (for heart), and the resulting five isoenzymes are named in the order of their rates of migration in an electrophoretic field. Most tissues contain all five isoenzymes, but LDH1 and, to a lesser extent, LDH2 predominate in the heart; skeletal muscle and the liver have mostly LDH5. Erythrocytes, kidneys, the brain, stomach, and pancreas are other important sources of LDH1 (29).

Serum AST is another widely distributed enzyme with high concentrations in the liver and skeletal muscles as well as the heart. Its major role is in the transfer of amine groups in amino acid synthesis.

RATES OF RELEASE

When myocardial cells are irreversibly damaged, their

cell membranes lose their integrity; enzymes diffuse into the interstitium and, from there, into the lymphatics and capillaries. Enzyme kinetics after infarction thus depend on several factors, including the size of the molecule, regional blood and lymphatic flow, and the rate of clearance of the enzyme (30). With conventional assays, the first detectable abnormalities after myocardial infarction are elevations of total CK and CK-MB levels (Table 1) (16). The level of CK-MB may return to normal slightly sooner than total CK levels, presumably because of faster clearance by the reticuloendothelial system (31).

Lactate dehydrogenase levels rise 8 to 12 hours after an infarction begins and remain elevated for 8 to 14 days (32). In contrast, AST activity rises within 8 to 12 hours of infarction and declines to normal levels within 3 to 4 days. Because either the CK or LDH level is abnormal during the periods when the AST level is elevated after myocardial infarction, the incremental benefit of an AST assay in diagnosis is small (33) and its routine use in evaluation of suspected myocardial infarction has been discouraged (32).

Peak levels of these enzymes are often higher and usually reached sooner after infarction in patients who have either spontaneous or iatrogenic thrombolysis leading to reperfusion of the area of infarction (34-40). For example, CK and CK-MB levels may peak at 8 to 14 hours in these patients. Moreover, the total amount of enzymes released into the blood may be greater when reperfusion occurs than when an infarction of the same size is not reperfused (40), presumably because of improved washout of released enzymes from the area of infarction. Similarly, some investigators have found that CK-MB appears in the serum sooner after small subendocardial myocardial infarctions than after major transmural infarctions, probably reflecting better perfusion of the area of cell necrosis (41).

ASSAYS

The performance of these tests depends not only on the assays themselves, but also on when and how the samples are collected. The level of CK-MM is stable for up to 48 hours at room temperature, but MB and BB isoenzymes may begin to dissociate within as little as 2 hours (31). With refrigeration, MB is stable for 24 hours, and fast-freezing can preserve isoenzymes for years. In contrast,

LDH is stable for days at room temperature, and the commonest problem in its collection is hemolysis, which causes high LDH1 levels.

Assays of CK (and most other enzymes) do not directly measure the level of the enzyme itself; instead, they estimate the CK concentration by assessing the enzyme's activity in standardized International Units per litre (42). Normal values vary depending on the assay used, but the upper limit of normal of CK for women is less than that of men by as much as one third (42). At very high concentrations, assays may underestimate total CK levels (43), but dilution of serum to a lower concentration allows accurate estimation of CK levels.

Creatine kinase isoenzyme levels can be measured in various ways. Qualitative assays use electrophoresis followed by fluorescence analysis of isoenzyme bands. These techniques take advantage of the negative charge on the B subunit at pH 8.0, which makes BB the most mobile isoenzyme in the electrophoretic field, whereas MM is neutral and MB is intermediate. Limiting the specificity of this approach is the occurrence of false-positive test results due to nonspecific fluorescing compounds such as tetracycline, aspirin, and chlorpromazine (31). As with total CK, very high concentrations of CK-MM can cause misleading results, because a broad MM band may carry over into the site of an expected MB band. Diluting the sample eliminates this problem (32).

In the early 1970s, quantitative assays were developed that used electrophoresis (44) or other techniques such as ion-exchange column chromatography (45) to separate the isoenzymes, which are then assayed for activity. Although the qualitative assays are considered to have a positive result if any MB band is found, the definition of the normal range with quantitative assays is less clear. Some laboratories use the actual CK-MB concentration to define the upper limit of normal, with thresholds ranging from 5 to 25 IU/L in different studies (31, 46). More commonly, the percentage of total CK concentration is calculated by dividing the CK-MB concentration by the total CK level. Again, there is little agreement on the threshold to be used to diagnose myocardial infarction; cutoffs ranging from 3% to 6% have been used in most studies.

Column chromatography assays have a high sensitivity (47), but specificity is limited by false-positive results, which, for example, can be caused by spillover of elevated MM isoenzyme into an apparent MB fraction (32). Another common problem is the occurrence of variant isoenzymes that migrate as a band between MM and MB on electrophoresis, but which can be interpreted as MB on quantitative assays (48-50). These variants occur in as much as 3% of the population (51) and are due, in at least some cases, to IgG complexed to CK-BB (52). An additional source may be mitochondrial CK, which differs from cytoplasmic CK in amino acid composition (53, 54). These variants can usually be identified by retesting the sample with a qualitative electrophoretic assay.

Instead of estimating enzyme activity, radioimmunoassays for CK-MB directly measure the isoenzyme level with antibodies to CK-BB that cross-react with MB (55) or, more recently, with antibodies to CK-MB itself (56, 57). In preliminary testing, these assays have been more sensitive than electrophoretic assays (57) and have detected increases in CK-MB levels within 2 to 4 hours of infarction (32). The radioimmunoassay and a glass-bead adsorption assay described by Herman and Roberts (58) can be done within a few minutes.

Assays for LDH also depend on measurement of the enzyme's activity. Isoenzymes of LDH are not readily quantitated, however. Therefore, most available assays separate isoenzymes by electrophoresis (59) and then estimate the ratio of LDH1 to LDH2, which is increased if there has been myocardial necrosis. The cutoff used to diagnose myocardial infarction is 1.0 in most series, but thresholds as low as 0.76 have been found useful (60). Because LDH1 specifically catalyzes the reduction of alpha-ketobutyrate to alpha-hydroxybutarate, this isoenzyme is also known as alpha-hydroxybutyrate dehydrogenase and can be assayed independently of the other isoenzymes (61). However, most clinical chemistry laboratories use assays that measure and compare the activities of all five isoenzymes.

OTHER ENZYMES

Concentrations of some enzymes, such as gamma-glutamyl transpeptidase, return to normal a month after myocardial infarction (62) and thus could theoretically be helpful for the late diagnosis of myocardial infarction. However, greater interest has focused on assays that might allow early detection of infarction, such as that for myoglobin, a small protein (molecular weight, 17 000) that appears in the serum as early as 90 minutes after the onset of chest pain (63) and is cleared rapidly by the kidneys (64). Unfortunately, many patients are hospitalized before myoglobin elevations are detectable or after the increases have resolved. Initial myoglobin levels were normal in 4 of 8 patients with acute myocardial infarction in one series (65), though all 21 patients in another series had elevations on their first sample (66). The specificity of myoglobin assays is compromised by the enzyme's wide distribution in skeletal muscle.

Recently, three subforms of CK-MM have been distinguished by variations in isoelectric points, and one of these "isoforms", $CK-MM_A$, is prevalent in myocardial tissue. Hashimoto and colleagues (67) have found that the relative proportions of CK-MM isoforms change as early as 1 hour after experimental coronary occlusion. However, the clinical role of assays for CK isoforms, myoglobin, and other enzymes has not yet been established.

CAUSES OF FALSE-POSITIVE AND FALSE-NEGATIVE VALUES

The lack of a definitive, alternate "gold-standard" test for diagnosis of myocardial infarction adds uncertainty to any description of the causes of false-positive or false-negative results for these enzyme assays. For example, in one series of patients admitted to a coronary care unit, 16% of patients with elevated MB levels had normal total CK levels, and within this group, only 17% had diagnostic QRS changes on electrocardiograms (as compared with 54% of patients with abnormal levels of both total CK and CK-MB) and only 28% had an LDH1/LDH2 ratio of greater than 1 (as compared with 79%) (68).

Although the diagnosis in such patients may remain unclear, clinical, electrocardiographic, and autopsy data suggest that the source of CK-MB elevations in patients with acute chest pain typical of myocardial ischemia is usually true infarction (68-71). Serial enzyme studies show that these patients often start with a low total CK level and have a typical rise and fall, all within the normal range—a so-called "intranormal bump." These "enzyme leaks" probably represent myocardial necrosis, not transient loss of cell membrane integrity due to ischemia, because histopathologic studies using microspheres to define areas of infarction in dogs have shown that viable cells have normal CK content (72, 73).

In patients with a low risk of myocardial infarction, however, the clinician should consider the laboratory artifacts that cause false-positive elevations of CK-MB levels and the nonischemic causes of true elevations of CK-MB levels (Table 2). The sources of CK-MB can be myocardial, peripheral, or both (18-28, 74-83). Alternatively, elevations can be caused by decreased clearance of

Table 2. Causes of Elevated Creatine Kinase (CK)-MB Levels

Cause (Reference)	Comment
False elevations	
Spillover of CK-MM (32)	Prevented by diluting samples
Isoenzyme variants (48-54)	Unmasked by electrophoresis
Nonspecific fluorescence (31)	Uncommon problem of qualitative electrophoretic assays
Myocardial damage	
Myocardial infarction (11)	. . .
Myocarditis (74)	Occasional finding
Pericarditis (75)	Rare reports
Myocardial puncture or trauma (76)	Including intracardiac injections
Systemic disease with cardiac involvement	
Muscular dystrophy (25)	Peripheral CK-MB also found
Hypothermia (77)	Probably reflects myocardial damage
Hyperthermia (78, 79)	Associated with anesthesia
Reye's syndrome (80)	Rare reports
Peripheral source of CK-MB	
Myositis (26)	May have cardiac involvement
Rhabdomyolysis (27)	Reflects abnormal regeneration
Athletic activity (21, 22)	Reflects abnormal regeneration
Prostate surgery (23)	Prostatic source
Cesarian section (23)	Uterine source
Gastrointestinal surgery (23)	Gastrointestinal source
Tumors (28)	Rare reports
Miscellaneous	
Renal failure (81, 82)	Source unknown
Subarachnoid hemorrhage (83)	May reflect myocardial damage
Hypothyroidism (84)	Decreased clearance

CK and CK-MB, as seen in patients with hypothyroidism (84). The clinical presentations of such processes can usually be distinguished from myocardial infarction, and the degree of CK-MB elevation is usually less (21, 82). Furthermore, these entities are unlikely to cause the acute rise and fall in total CK and CK-MB levels seen in myocardial infarction.

False-negative CK-MB results are usually due to inadequate sampling, such as once per 24 hours, or sampling too late after myocardial infarction when the CK-MB level has returned to normal. Otherwise, false-negative results are rare if assays are done properly on fresh or appropriately preserved samples.

False-positive elevations of total CK concentrations are much commoner than false-positive CK-MB results (29). In addition to the sources of CK-MB elevation described in Table 2, noncardiac causes of elevated total CK levels include skeletal muscle trauma, alcohol-related muscle damage, diabetes mellitus, seizures, and pulmonary embolism (29). False-negative total CK results in acute myocardial infarction usually reflect failure to sample frequently enough or soon enough or reflect small infarctions that cause only an intranormal bump (68-71).

False-positive elevations of the LDH1/LDH2 ratio can result from hemolyzed samples, pregnancy, or myopathies. Other tissues rich in LDH1 and LDH2 (kidney, pancreas, stomach, brain) tend to yield more LDH2 than LDH1 when injured (32). False-negative LDH isoenzyme assays are commoner if higher cutoffs (1.0 or more) are used or if samples are drawn more than a week after infarction (32, 60).

Clinical Applications

DIAGNOSIS OF MYOCARDIAL INFARCTION

Effect of Disease Detection on Outcome: The clinical suspicion of a myocardial infarction affects important short- and long-term management strategies, beginning with triage decisions. Although studies in Great Britain have raised questions about the impact of coronary care units on outcome after acute infarction (85, 86), those studies included an initial period of several hours during which patients were closely observed at home by a trained medical team, excluded potentially high-risk patients who would be more likely to benefit from intensive care, and involved too few patients to detect the expected degree of benefit from a coronary care unit (87, 88). In our ongoing investigation of patients presenting to the emergency room with acute chest pain, mortality among patients whose acute myocardial infarctions were not recognized and who were thus inappropriately sent home has been higher than the mortality among admitted patients, even though the discharged patients had less dramatic presentations than admitted patients (89). The high mortality among discharged patients presumably is due in part to the expected 4.5% rate of primary ventricular fibrillation that occurs with acute myocardial infarction (90) and perhaps to the difference between the conservative home care given to a patient with a recognized low-risk myocardial infarction and the higher complication rate to be expected in patients whose infarctions are not recognized. Thus, coronary care units remain the standard level of care in the United States for patients at moderate-to-high probability of myocardial infarction (91).

Even if admitted, patients who are diagnosed as having acute myocardial infarction have a higher short-term mortality than patients without infarction (92); thus, several management decisions made after admission are determined by whether or not a myocardial infarction is documented. First, rapid exclusion of this diagnosis with serial cardiac enzyme assays may permit early discharge of the patient from the coronary care unit (93), whereas patients who are diagnosed as having myocardial infarction commonly remain in the intensive care unit for a longer time (94). Second, patients with infarction do not require further tests to diagnose the presence of ischemic heart disease, whereas patients who do not meet diagnostic criteria for infarction may be studied with various invasive and noninvasive tests to establish the cause of their chest pain.

Because attempts to salvage threatened myocardium through reperfusion should be made within 4 hours after the onset of infarction (95), before CK or CK-MB elevations can be detected, these tests have not been used to identify patients with evolving infarction for whom such aggressive measures may be appropriate. It would be reasonable to hypothesize that patients who present with CK-MB elevations probably already have lost much of the jeopardized myocardium and therefore would be less likely to benefit from reperfusion, but no relevant data are available. Thus, the decision to attempt thrombolysis is currently based on information from the history and electrocardiogram.

After the initial period of management, long-term decisions are partly determined by whether infarction was documented. Follow-up studies indicate that the prognosis after hospitalization of a patient with a myocardial infarction may be no worse than that for patients with unstable angina (92). Nevertheless, randomized trials have indicated that therapy with a beta-adrenergic-blocking agent prolongs survival in patients in whom infarction is diagnosed even if angina is not present (96-98). The long-term consequences of such strategies make accurate diagnostic techniques critical to the care of these patients.

Studies of Test Performance: A major difficulty in determining the accuracy of these assays is the lack of a reliable alternative diagnostic standard for myocardial infarction. The limitations of other clinical data, including information from the history, physical examination, and electrocardiogram (17, 99-102), have forced investigations of the diagnostic performance of enzyme assays to define myocardial infarction by various criteria, none of which have proved satisfactory. In these studies, myocardial infarction has been diagnosed on the basis of clinical data, such as increased leukocyte count, body temperature, and erythrocyte sedimentation rate (14); the electrocardiogram (68-70); or combinations of clinical, electrocardiographic, and enzyme data (60, 99, 100, 103-106). This approach creates obvious possibilities for circular reasoning. For example, the diagnostic performance of LDH isoenzyme assays was measured using CK-MB elevations to define which patients had myocardial infarction (60), whereas the diagnostic performance of CK-MB assays has been studied using LDH isoenzymes to support the final diagnosis (17). One recent article has examined the diagnostic performance of total CK assays in a group of patients in whom myocardial infarction was diagnosed on the basis of CK-MB results (107). Unfortunately, these variables are not independent, and a small subendocardial myocardial infarction that does not present with a Q wave on the electrocardiogram may also be unlikely to yield clear enzyme abnormalities (46, 68-71).

To minimize the bias that these interrelationships invite, most studies have used diagnoses assigned by investigators who were blinded to the enzyme assay results under investigation. Some investigators also have reported data by patient subgroups with different combinations of criteria for myocardial infarction (17). In most studies, however, the number of patients who met various criteria for this multifactorial diagnosis has not been explicitly stated.

Test Performance of Serial Assays: Even the most rigorous investigative methods cannot remove uncertainty from the approximately 9% of cases in the coronary care unit in which enzyme and isoenzyme results fall into a "gray zone" where both diagnosis and prognosis are uncertain (46). In such cases, the diagnostic performance of these tests is unknown. However, in patients with Q-wave infarction, serial assays of each of these enzymes have proved highly sensitive (Table 3), despite wide variations among studies in assay techniques, definitions of abnormality, patient eligibility, sampling intervals, and criteria for myocardial infarction. The specificities are also high for CK and LDH isoenzyme assays, but less for the standard CK, LDH, and AST assays.

The "gold standard" that has emerged is the CK-MB test. Several series using different assays have confirmed that in patients who are evaluated within 24 hours of onset of chest pain, serial testing of CK-MB levels has a near-perfect sensitivity and high specificity (14, 16, 17, 51, 103-106, 109). Quantitative assays can detect CK-MB concentrations as low as 1 IU/L (46), but most studies using such assays have defined the upper limit of normal for CK-MB as 3% to 6% of the total CK. Whether different thresholds should be used if the total CK level is normal and whether higher cutoffs of 5% to 6% affect sensitivity and specificity have not been determined. Such issues do not arise with the qualitative electrophoretic assays, which can detect CK-MB concentrations of 5 IU/L (32, 100, 109). Despite being less sensitive than the quantitative assays, the electrophoretic assays have shown a sensitivity of over 95% in most studies (32, 103, 110).

Other enzyme assays also have high sensitivities but much lower specificities than those for CK-MB (Table 3). In patients seen early in the course of their infarction, the reported sensitivity of serial total CK measurements has been about 98% (17, 100, 106, 111), but false-positive rates have been 15% or more (17, 99, 100) due to the many causes of elevated CK levels. Similarly, the total LDH level has had a high sensitivity (98%) but a false-positive rate of about 30% (100).

Concentrations of LDH isoenzymes are considerably more specific than total LDH levels and are especially useful in patients presenting more than 24 hours after the onset of symptoms. In these patients, CK and CK-MB levels may already have returned to normal. Concentrations of LDH isoenzymes usually become abnormal within 14 hours of the onset of infarction and can remain diagnostic for as long as 2 weeks after the infarction. Studies of the diagnostic performance of this test have used serial samples (60, 105, 109), but whether assaying several specimens increases diagnostic yield over that of a single sample is not known. However, Irvin and coworkers (108) have shown that the LDH1/LDH2 ratio may revert to less than 1.0 within 2 to 3 days, and that the ratio often flips back and forth around 1.0 several times (109). Thus, some investigators recommend using a cutoff of 0.76, which in one study had a sensitivity and specificity over 90% (60). If the more commonly used definition of abnormal (LDH1/LDH2 > 1.0) is invoked, specificity remains high but sensitivity falls to 80% to 90% (17, 60).

To place these data in perspective, one can consider the performance of the alternative test for late detection of myocardial infarction, the technetium pyrophosphate scintiscan. These scans are much more expensive and show a regional defect in only about 37% of patients with non-Q-wave infarctions (112). Thus, technetium pyrophosphate scintigraphy contributes to changes in diagnosis and management only in a very selective group of patients (113).

Test Performance of a Single Assay: Although high sensitivities and specificities can be achieved through serial sampling, the diagnostic performance of a single value of any of these tests is not nearly as good (Table 3) (99). Furthermore, in populations with a low prevalence of myocardial infarction, such as patients in the emergency room or patients with atypical chest pain, false-positive results may be commoner than true-positive results; and the positive predictive value of an abnormal result will not be as high as that in the coronary care unit settings described in the literature (114).

Table 3. Diagnostic Accuracy of Cardiac Enzyme Assays in Patients in the Coronary Care Unit and Emergency Room

	Sensitivity	Specificity
	%	%
Serial studies in patients in the coronary care unit*		
Electrocardiogram	68	100
Creatine kinase-MB	100	98
Creatine kinase	98	67
Aspartate aminotransferase	97	86
Lactate dehydrogenase	98	72
LDH1:LDH2 > 1.0	81	94
LDH1:LDH2 > 0.76	92	94
Single test results in patients with chest pain in the emergency room†		
Creatine kinase-MB	34	88
Creatine kinase	38	80
Aspartate aminotransferase	53	82
Lactate dehydrogenase	60	66

* Data from Vasudevan and colleagues (60) and Grande and colleagues (100).
LDH = lactate dehydrogenase.
† Data from Lee and colleagues (99, 108).

Our data show that single values of CK-MB in patients with chest pain in the emergency room have a sensitivity of 34% and a specificity of 88% if the upper limit of normal for CK-MB levels is defined as 5% of an elevated total CK level (108), but we also found that the diagnostic performance of this test is influenced considerably by the degree of abnormality of the result and the time that has elapsed since the onset of symptoms. For example, a single CK-MB level drawn within 4 hours of the onset of symptoms may be nearly worthless; only 18% of patients in the emergency room with myocardial infarction in our series had elevated total CK and CK-MB levels of greater than 5% this soon after the onset of chest pain. However, with this same 5% threshold, single values of CK-MB had sensitivities of 50% and 57% if drawn 4 to 12 or more than 12 hours, respectively, after the onset of symptoms, whereas specificity remained constant at 88%. Higher CK-MB values were less sensitive but more specific; thus, a CK-MB threshold of greater than 9% had a sensitivity and specificity of 21% and 98%, respectively, compared with 34% and 88% for a threshold of greater than 5% in our 639 patients (108).

Pretest Probability: Although individual pieces of clinical data from the history and electrocardiogram cannot be used to diagnose or exclude myocardial infarction (99), this information can be used to calculate probabilities of myocardial infarction for individual patients. In prospective testing, multivariate statistical models have shown the potential to enhance the performance of physicians for diagnosing myocardial infarction (1) and other acute ischemic heart disease (2). Even without the assistance of computerized algorithms, rough estimates of the pretest probability of infarction can be made. For example, in our ongoing experience with patients with acute chest pain in the emergency room, a patient with 1-mm or greater ST elevation or Q waves in two or more leads that are not known to be old has approximately an 80% chance of having a myocardial infarction. In such a patient, a CK-MB result in the "gray zone" (46) would be more likely to reflect true myocardial necrosis than it would in a patient with a lower pretest probability of myocardial infarction (Table 4). Thus, one should interpret CK-MB and other laboratory tests only after assessing the pretest probability of myocardial infarction on the basis of clinical information with, if possible, the assistance of published data (1, 99, 115).

Table 4. Approximate Probability of Myocardial Infarction Among Certain Subsets of Patients with Acute Chest Pain in the Emergency Room

Finding	Approximate Probability of Myocardial Infarction*
	%
ST elevation or Q waves on ECG not known to be old	80
Ischemia or strain on ECG not known to be old	20-30
None of the preceding ECG changes but a prior history of angina or myocardial infarction	10
None of the preceding ECG changes and no prior history of angina or myocardial infarction	1-5

* These probabilities can be further refined by considering other clinical data; see, for example, references 1 and 99. ECG = electrocardiogram.

Post-Test Probability: In a Bayesian analysis, pretest probabilities of myocardial infarction can be modified by the results of enzyme assays (Table 5 and Figure 1A). Our calculation of post-test probabilities assumes that the sensitivity and specificity of serial sampling of CK-MB values in patients presenting within 24 hours of the onset of symptoms are about 95%, as suggested by a pessimistic interpretation of published data (14, 16, 17, 51, 103-106).

These figures should not be extended to interpretation of single test results of CK-MB. Calculations of post-test probabilities based on our overall data showing a sensitivity of 34% and a specificity of 88% for single CK-MB values using a greater than 5% threshold (108) are shown in Table 5 and Figure 1B. Not surprisingly, the effect of a single abnormal test result in the emergency room on pretest probabilities of myocardial infarction is less marked than the effect of abnormal results in serial testing. As noted previously, however, the interpretation of a single CK-MB level is also influenced by the degree

Table 5. Bayesian Analysis of the Effect of Creatine Kinase (CK)-MB Levels on the Probability of Myocardial Infarction in Patients Presenting Within 24 Hours of the Onset of Pain

Pretest Probability	Post-Test Probability	
	CK-MB Elevated	CK-MB Normal
Serial samples (sensitivity and specificity both = 95%)		
0.01	0.161	0.001
0.05	0.500	0.003
0.15	0.770	0.009
0.50	0.950	0.050
0.85	0.991	0.230
0.95	0.997	0.500
0.99	0.999	0.839
Single sample in patients in the emergency room		
(overall sensitivity = 34%; specificity = 88%*)		
0.01	0.028	0.008
0.05	0.130	0.038
0.15	0.333	0.117
0.50	0.739	0.429
0.85	0.941	0.810
0.95	0.982	0.934
0.99	0.996	0.987

* See text for discussion of how the sensitivity and specificity of a single CK-MB level also depend on the degree of abnormality of the CK-MB result and the time since the onset of the patient's symptoms.

Table 6. Charges for Cardiac Enzyme Assays at Brigham and Women's Hospital

Assay	Charge
	$
Creatine kinase	8
Creatine kinase and its isoenzymes	44
Lactate dehydrogenase	8
Lactate dehydrogenase and its isoenzymes	61
Aspartate aminotransferase	8
Battery of all five assays	129

of CK-MB elevation and the time that has elapsed since the onset of pain. Thus, a CK-MB elevation of greater than 9% in a patient seen more than 4 hours after the onset of symptoms would convert a 2% pretest probability of myocardial infarction into a 27% post-test probability, and a 5% pretest probability into a 48% post-test probability.

In all situations, it should be stressed that an abnormally elevated CK-MB level in a patient with a low clinical probability of myocardial infarction does not necessarily prove that ischemic damage has occurred. Conversely, the absence of detectable CK-MB elevation in a patient with high probability of myocardial infarction does not exclude the diagnosis, although it may lead to a reassessment of the time when infarction was likely to have occurred.

Recommendations: Deciding which tests to order and how often to order them involves weighing the potential benefits of accurate information against the cost of these assays (Table 6) and the implications of misleading results. From these considerations, reasonable recommendations for the use of cardiac enzyme assays to diagnose myocardial infarction can be proposed.

In the emergency room, total CK, AST, and LDH levels are often rapidly available, but the liabilities of these assays as indices of myocardial infarction have been shown (99, 108, 116). Their lack of specificity leads to high false-positive rates, and because many patients arrive early in the course of myocardial infarction, sensitivity is also poor. Rapidly available CK-MB levels may improve diagnostic specificity in the future (108), but false-negative results can be reduced only through serial

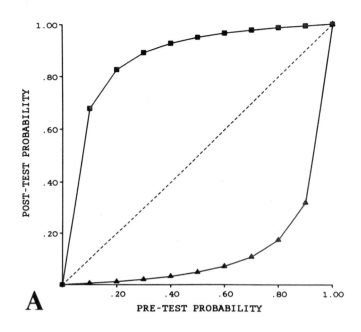

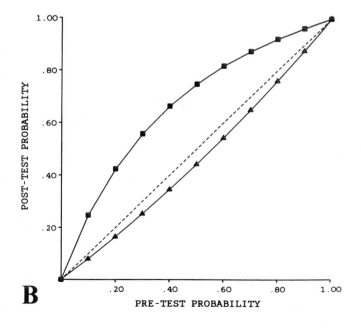

sampling. Because of the low sensitivity of a single assay, we do not recommend that these tests be used to exclude the diagnosis of myocardial infarction. Positive assays in the emergency room setting must be interpreted in light of the patient's clinical and electrocardiographic findings, though future research may identify situations in which an abnormal test result might appropriately convince the physician to admit or to continue to observe an otherwise low-risk patient. In some cases, an 8- to 12-hour observation period, sufficient for a second CK-MB level to be determined, may be an efficient and currently underused management strategy.

Once the patient has been admitted, serial enzyme levels will often be the key data in establishing or excluding myocardial infarction. There is no evidence that any combination of tests is more sensitive than the CK-MB assay alone if the patient has presented within 24 hours of infarction (100). Nevertheless, sampling the total CK level is also recommended (117), because total CK levels are needed to interpret quantitative CK-MB results.

Studies of the optimal sampling intervals have shown that virtually all early myocardial infarctions can be detected by measuring CK and CK-MB levels three times: on admission, 12 hours later, and 24 hours after admission (107, 118, 119). In one series of 581 patients with acute myocardial infarction, 98% had abnormal CK and CK-MB elevations within 24 hours of onset of symptoms

---

Figure 1A. Effect of serial creatine kinase (CK)-MB results on the probability of acute myocardial infarction. The pretest probabilities, as marked along the *x* axis, can be derived through use of computerized algorithms (1), personal experience, or analysis of published data (99, 115). Post-test probabilities are on the *y* axis. The curves correspond to post-test probabilities of infarction with normal (*triangles*) or elevated (*squares*) CK-MB results, assuming a 95% sensitivity and a 95% specificity for serial sampling of CK-MB levels (*see* text). **Figure 1B.** Effect of a single CK-MB value in the emergency room on the probability of acute myocardial infarction. As in Figure 1A, pretest probabilities are marked along the *x* axis; post-test probabilities are on the *y* axis; and the curves show the impact of a single normal (*triangles*) or a single abnormal (*squares*) CK-MB result. These curves are based on data showing an overall 34% sensitivity and 88% specificity for single CK-MB values obtained from patients with acute chest pain in the emergency room (108). See text for discussion of how the sensitivity and specificity of a single CK-MB level also depend on the degree of abnormality of the CK-MB result and the time since the onset of the patient's symptoms.

(119). In two other studies, CK-MB elevations were detectable in all 213 patients with acute infarction within 17 hours after admission (100, 109). Thus, further sampling is not needed after 24 hours of observation if ischemic pain has not recurred. However, insufficient data are available to compare a strategy in which enzyme levels are sampled at 0, 12, and 24 hours to a strategy in which enzymes are tested at shorter intervals, such as at 0, 8, and 16 hours.

If more than 24 hours have elapsed since the onset of pain and the total CK and CK-MB levels are not diagnostic, LDH isoenzyme assays may be useful. One study has shown that sensitivity and specificity for myocardial infarction are both about 90% if an LDH1/LDH2 ratio of 0.76 is used as the upper limit of normal (60). Because of the relative prices of a total LDH assay and an LDH isoenzyme determination (Table 6), it is recommended that LDH isoenzymes be assayed only when the total LDH level is elevated. No study has provided data showing that serial sampling of LDH isoenzyme levels increases diagnostic yield, but clinicians using a ratio of 1.0 as a cutoff should remember that the ratio in patients with myocardial infarction will sometimes flip back and forth just across this threshold (109).

After myocardial infarction has been diagnosed, CK and CK-MB levels may be useful for detecting extensions or reinfarctions, but routine daily samples in asymptomatic patients after an infarction have a low yield. In one series of 200 patients having daily enzyme assays, 35 had an early recurrence as confirmed by CK-MB assay (120), but these reinfarctions were usually associated with chest pain (94%) and electrocardiographic ST-T wave changes (91%). In patients who had reinfarction, inhospital mortality was high (20%); so if a patient has chest pain after infarction, electrocardiographic and enzyme evidence of recurrence should be sought. However, only 1% of these 200 patients had an asymptomatic extension. Therefore, routine daily assays of CK and CK-MB levels are not recommended.

ESTIMATION OF INFARCT SIZE AND PROGNOSIS

Effect of Test on Outcome: Enzyme assays can be used to make estimates of the size of a myocardial infarction (121, 122) that correlate with left ventricular ejection fraction (123), hemodynamics (124, 125), and arrhythmias (126, 127). The relation of enzyme values to morphologic data is stronger with CK-MB (128, 129) and total CK levels (130) than with LDH, though LDH isoenzymes can be used to estimate infarct size in patients presenting late after the onset of symptoms (131). Frequent sampling, such as every 4 hours, is more likely to detect the true enzyme peak, but major underestimation of CK peaks occurs rarely (3%) with 12-hour sampling intervals (118). Because enzyme peaks are also affected by other clinical events, such as spontaneous reperfusion and infarct extension (30, 39, 128-133), in routine clinical settings, CK and CK-MB levels allow only qualitative estimates of infarct size.

Peak enzyme levels have not been shown to have independent predictive value in multivariate analyses of mortality after myocardial infarction (134, 135). Long-term prognosis after myocardial infarction seems to be determined by how much myocardium has been lost in the past, remote as well as recent, and how much myocardium is in jeopardy (136). Thus, enzyme levels should not be used to predict mortality for individual patients (125).

Recommendations: Sampling CK-MB levels every 12 hours until the CK-MB level begins to decline allows a qualitative estimate of the size of a myocardial infarction, but these estimates should not be used to predict mortality or long-term prognosis. Therefore, frequent enzyme assays to estimate infarct size should not be a part of routine clinical care.

DIAGNOSIS OF PERIOPERATIVE MYOCARDIAL INFARCTION

Effect of Disease Detection on Outcome: As surgical techniques have become increasingly sophisticated, the percentage of perioperative morbidity and mortality attributable to cardiac complications rather than direct surgical problems has grown. To minimize cardiac risk in noncardiac surgery (137), the clinician must estimate preoperatively the risk of myocardial infarction and be able to detect perioperative infarctions and treat their often considerable complications. In some series, mortality for perioperative myocardial infarction is over 50% (138, 139).

One reason these rates are so high may be that the usual diagnostic criteria for myocardial infarction are so distorted in this setting that only large infarctions may be detected. Probably because of the effects of medications, half of perioperative patients do not note chest pain with their myocardial infarctions (140). Furthermore, metabolic abnormalities can mask electrocardiographic findings, and associated tissue damage often makes total CK and LDH levels uninterpretable. Thus, it is possible that only the most extensive myocardial infarctions were included in these series.

The difficulty of diagnosing myocardial infarction is even greater after cardiac surgery, because minor myocardial damage often leads to release of small amounts of CK-MB. However, when myocardial infarction is suggested by multiple tests, the prognosis is worse. In one recent series, 49% of patients having cardiac surgery who had perioperative infarctions had reinfarction or death within 2 years, as compared with 4% of patients who did not (141). Thus, the diagnosis of perioperative infarction has important prognostic implications for both cardiac and noncardiac surgery.

Studies of Test Performance: After surgery, the usual manifestations of myocardial infarction are distorted. Thus, pessimistic data on prognosis may reflect our lack of sensitivity for small infarctions. Fortunately, the percentage of CK-MB usually remains normal after noncardiac surgery, even when the total serum CK level is markedly elevated. As noted previously, tissue injury in this population can lead to false elevations of CK-MB levels due to spillover of MM into the MB band on either electrophoresis or column chromatography. Dilution of the sample will prevent misleading results.

The interpretation of CK-MB elevations after cardiac surgery is considerably more complex, and investigations of use of this assay have been hindered by the lack of an alternative "gold standard" for diagnosing myocardial infarction. In one series, CK-MB elevation was detected by electrophoresis in every patient (142). Peak CK-MB levels can be misleading but duration of elevation may be more useful, because elevations persisting longer than 12 to 18 hours correlate well with other evidence for myocardial infarction (142, 143). Other studies have suggested use of the total CK-MB released (144, 145) or a combination of clinical factors including CK-MB levels, electrocardiographic findings, and the results of technetium pyrophosphate scintiscans (146, 147).

Test Performance: Roberts and Sobel (148) have shown that in patients having noncardiac surgery, the CK-MB level is both a sensitive and a specific marker of myocardial infarction and can be used according to usual diagnostic strategies (148), with special emphasis on serial sampling to distinguish noncardiac from cardiac sources. Assays for LDH isoenzymes are less useful because hemolysis associated with surgical trauma can cause an isoenzyme profile similar to that of myocardial infarction.

Because of the lack of an alternative "gold standard," no sensitivities can be estimated for detection of myocardial infarction associated with cardiac surgery. The specificity of CK-MB levels, however, is known to be poor, though the false-positive rate can be decreased by requiring CK-MB elevations to last longer than 18 hours (142, 143).

Recommendations: Assays for CK-MB are useful for diagnosing myocardial infarction in patients having noncardiac surgery; diagnostic strategies should be similar to those used with patients not having surgery except that more care should be taken to exclude false-positive results (Table 2) through serial sampling. In the setting of cardiac surgery, several factors suggestive of myocardial infarction should be considered, including new Q waves on the electrocardiogram, a positive technetium pyrophosphate scintiscan, and prolonged CK-MB elevations. If any two of these factors are present, then the diagnosis of myocardial infarction is likely and the prognosis is worse (141).

OTHER SETTINGS

Studies have characterized CK isoenzyme profiles in several other settings. Roberts and colleagues (149) found that whereas total CK and other enzyme levels were usually elevated after cardiac catheterization, CK-MB levels remained normal unless there was other clinical evidence of myocardial infarction. In a recent series from the Mayo Clinic (150), CK-MB elevations were found in 20% of patients after successful percutaneous transluminal coronary angioplasty, and these patients were significantly more likely to have had chest pain or small-vessel occlusion during the procedure. Thus, eleva-

Table 7. Recommendations on the Use of Serum Enzyme Assays in the Diagnosis of Acute Myocardial Infarction

1. A single set of cardiac enzyme values in the emergency room is not sufficiently sensitive to exclude myocardial infarction. Although a single, markedly positive CK-MB value will greatly increase the probability of acute infarction, data are insufficient to support or reject a policy whereby low-risk patients, who otherwise would be sent home, would be observed until one or more CK-MB values are obtained.

2. If myocardial infarction is suspected, then samples of total CK and CK-MB levels should be measured on admission and about 12 and 24 hours later, although condensed versions of this strategy may ultimately prove to be equally efficacious and more cost effective. If myocardial infarction may have occurred more than 24 hours before admission, and if CK and CK-MB levels are not diagnostic, a total LDH level should be ordered. If the total LDH level is elevated, an assay of LDH isoenzymes should be obtained. If the first LDH1/LDH2 ratio is only slightly less than 1.0, a second assay is probably indicated.

3. If chest pain recurs after admission, CK and CK-MB assays should be done at 0, 12, and 24 hours. "Surveillance" enzyme assays are not recommended in asymptomatic patients without electrocardiographic changes.

4. Routine use of enzyme assays other than those for CK, CK-MB, and LDH isoenzymes is not recommended.

5. If more than 2 hours may pass before CK isoenzymes will be assayed, the serum sample should be preserved on ice.

6. Strategies including CK-MB assays can be used to diagnose myocardial infarction in the setting of noncardiac surgery and cardiac catheterization and after electrical countershock.

7. In the setting of cardiac surgery, myocardial infarction should be diagnosed if any two of the following are present: CK-MB elevation persisting more than 12 hours; new Q waves on an electrocardiogram; or regional defect on technetium pyrophosphate scintigraphy.

8. False-positive elevations of CK-MB can be minimized by diluting samples with marked elevations of total CK; detecting isoenzyme variants that masquerade as CK-MB on column chromatography assays by retesting the sample on an electrophoretic assay if the clinical presentation is atypical for myocardial infarction; or consideration of other sources of CK-MB (for example, myocarditis, renal failure, neuromuscular diseases, trauma) if a true elevation of CK-MB levels is found in the absence of a typical rise and fall of CK and CK-MB levels and other evidence for myocardial infarction.

tions of total CK levels probably reflected tissue injury, and increases in CK-MB levels after catheterization indicated myocardial damage during the procedure. However, some investigators have questioned whether morbidity and mortality with such procedure-induced CK-MB elevations have the same serious short-term consequences as other myocardial infarctions (150).

The cause of CK-MB elevations in patients with possible myocardial infarctions who undergo electrical countershock is sometimes questioned. Ehsani and colleagues (151) have shown that repetitive, intense countershocks in dogs could elevate CK-MB and produce myocardial necrosis but that CK-MB increases after countershock occurred in only 2 of 30 human patients. Thus, electrical countershock should rarely complicate the diagnosis of myocardial infarction.

Therefore, assays for CK-MB can be used to detect myocardial infarction after cardiac catheterization, percutaneous transluminal coronary angioplasty, or electrical countershock with the same diagnostic strategies as are recommended for patients with acute chest pain in the emergency room.

Conclusions

Based on this review of the characteristics of routinely used cardiac enzymes and data on their diagnostic performance and pitfalls, our recommendations are summarized in Table 7.

Appendix

Throughout this review, the following definitions are used to describe the diagnostic accuracy of tests:

Sensitivity = (all patients with myocardial infarction and with a positive test result)/(all patients with myocardial infarction).

Specificity = (all patients without myocardial infarction and with a negative test result)/(all patients without myocardial infarction).

Predictive value positive = (true-positive results)/(true-positive results + false-positive results).

Predictive value negative = (true-negative results)/(true-negative results + false-negative results).

ACKNOWLEDGMENTS: Grant support: in part by grant 83102-2H from the John A. Hartford Foundation. Dr. Lee is the recipient of a Public Health Service Clinical Investigator Award (HL01594-01) from the National Heart, Lung, and Blood Institute. Dr. Goldman is a Henry J. Kaiser Family Foundation Faculty Scholar in General Internal Medicine.

References

1. GOLDMAN L, WEINBERG M, WEISBERG M, et al. A computer-derived protocol to aid in the diagnosis of emergency room patients with acute chest pain. *N Engl J Med.* 1982;**307**:588-96.

2. POZEN MW, D'AGOSTINO RB, SELKER HP, SYTKOWSKI PA, HOOD WB JR. A predictive instrument to improve coronary-care-unit admission practices in acute ischemic heart disease: a prospective multicenter clinical trial. *N Engl J Med.* 1984;**310**:1273-8.

3. SOX HC JR, MARGULIES I, SOX CH. Psychologically mediated effects of diagnostic tests. *Ann Intern Med.* 1981;**95**:680-5.

4. ZARLING EJ, SEXTON H, MILNOR P JR. Failure to diagnose acute myocardial infarction: the clinicopathologic experience at a large community hospital. *JAMA.* 1983;**250**:1177-81.

5. GOLDMAN L, SAYSON R, ROBBINS S, COHN LH, BETTMANN M, WEISBERG M. The value of the autopsy in three medical eras. *N Engl J Med.* 1983;**308**:1000-5.

6. KARMEN A, WROBLEWSKI F, LADUE JS. Transaminase activity in human blood. *J Clin Invest.* 1954;**34**:126-33.

7. WROBLEWSKI F, LADUE JS. Lactic dehydrogenase activity in blood. *Proc Soc Exp Biol Med.* 1955;**90**:210-3.

8. VESSELL ES, BEARN AG. Localization of lactic acid dehydrogenase activity in serum fractions. *Proc Soc Exp Biol Med.* 1957;**94**:96-9.

9. LOHMANN K. Uber die enzymatische Aufspaltung der kreatin Phosphorsaure: zugleich ein Beitrag zum Chemismus der Muskelkontraktion. *Biochem Z.* 1934;**271**:264-77.

10. EBASHI A, TOYOKURA Y, MOMOI H, SUSITA H. High creatine phosphokinase activity of sera of progressive muscular dystrophy. *J Biochem.* 1959;**46**:103-4.

11. DREYFUS JC, SCHAPIRA G, RESNAIS J, SCEBAT L. Le creatine-kinase serique dans le diagnostic de l'infarctus myocardique. *Rev Fr Etud Clin Biol.* 1960;**5**:386-90.

12. Arterial hypertension and ischemic heart disease. *WHO Tech Rep Ser.* 1962;**231**:18.

13. VAN DER VEEN KJ, WILLEBRANDS AF. Isoenzymes of creatine phosphokinase in tissue extracts and in normal and pathological sera. *Clin Chim Acta.* 1966;**13**:312-6.

14. KONTTINEN A, SOMMER H. Determination of serum creatine kinase isoenzymes in myocardial infarction. *Am J Cardiol.* 1972;**29**:817-20.

15. ROE CR, LIMBIRD LE, WAGNER GS, NERENBERG ST. Combined isoenzyme analysis in the diagnosis of myocardial injury: application of electrophoretic methods for the detection and quantitation of the creatine phosphokinase MB isoenzyme. *J Lab Clin Med.* 1972;**80**:577-90.

16. ROBERTS R, GOWDA KS, LUDBROOK PA, SOBEL BE. Specificity of elevated serum MB creatine phosphokinase activity in the diagnosis of acute myocardial infarction. *Am J Cardiol.* 1975;**36**:433-7.

17. WAGNER GS, ROE CR, LIMBIRD LE, ROSATI RA, WALLACE AG. The importance of identification of the myocardial-specific isoenzyme of creatine phosphokinase (MB form) in the diagnosis of acute myocardial infarction. *Circulation.* 1973;**47**:263-9.

18. GOTO I, NAGAMINE M, KATSUKI S. Creatine phosphokinase isozymes in muscles: human fetus and patients. *Arch Neurol.* 1969;**20**:422-9.

19. JOCKERS-WRETOU E, PFLEIDERER G. Quantitation of creatine kinase isoenzymes in human tissues and sera by an immunological method. *Clin Chim Acta.* 1975;**58**:223-32.

20. NEUMEIER D. Tissue specific and subcellular distribution of creatine kinase isoenzymes: tissue specific distribution of creatine kinase isoenzymes. In: LANGE H, ed. *Creatine Kinase Isoenzymes: Pathophysiology and Clinical Application.* Berlin: Springer-Verlag; 1981:85-109.

21. JAFFE AS, GARFINKEL BT, RITTER CS, SOBEL BE. Plasma MB creatine kinase after vigorous exercise in professional athletes. *Am J Cardiol.* 1984;**53**:856-8.

22. SIEGEL AJ, SILVERMAN LM, HOLMAN L. Elevated creatine kinase MB isoenzyme levels in marathon runners: normal myocardial scintigrams suggest noncardiac source. *JAMA.* 1981;**246:**2049-51.

23. TSUNG SH. Several conditions causing elevation of serum CK-MB and CK-BB. *Am J Clin Pathol.* 1981;**75:**711-5.

24. SIEGEL AJ, SILVERMAN LM, EVANS WJ. Elevated skeletal muscle creatine kinase MB isoenzyme levels in marathon runners. *JAMA.* 1983;**250:**2835-7.

25. GOTO I. Creatine phosphokinase isozymes in neuromuscular disorders. *Arch Neurol.* 1974;**31:**116-9.

26. BROWNLOW K, ELEVITCH FR. Serum creatine phosphokinase isoenzyme (CPK2) in myositis: a report of six cases. *JAMA.* 1974;**230:**1141-4.

27. SIEGEL AJ, DAWSON DM. Peripheral source of MB band of creatine kinase in alcoholic rhabdomyolysis: nonspecificity of MB isoenzyme for myocardial injury in undiluted serum samples. *JAMA.* 1980;**244:**580-2.

28. LEE BI, BACH PM, HORTON JD, HICKEY TM. Elevated CK-MB and CK-BB in serum and tumor homogenate of a patient with lung cancer. *Clin Cardiol.* 1985;**8:**233-6.

29. SOBEL BE, SHELL WE. Serum enzyme determinations in the diagnosis and assessment of myocardial infarction. *Circulation.* 1972;**45:**471-82.

30. SOBEL BE, ROBERTS R, LARSON KB. Considerations in the use of biochemical markers of ischemic injury. *Circ Res.* 1976;**38**(5 suppl I):I-99-108.

31. ROBERTS R, SOBEL BE. Creatine kinase isoenzymes in the assessment of heart disease. *Am Heart J.* 1978;**95:**521-8.

32. ROBERTS R. Diagnostic assessment of myocardial infarction based on lactate dehydrogenase and creatine kinase isoenzymes. *Heart Lung.* 1981;**10:**486-506.

33. GOLDBERG DM, WINFIELD DA. Diagnostic accuracy of serum enzyme assays for myocardial infarction in a general hospital population. *Br Heart J.* 1972;**34:**597-604.

34. ONG L, REISER P, COROMILAS J, SCHERR L, MORRISON J. Left ventricular function and rapid release of creatine kinase MB in acute myocardial infarction: evidence for spontaneous reperfusion. *N Engl J Med.* 1983;**309:**1-6.

35. KHAJA F, WALTON JA JR, BRYMER JF, et al. Intracoronary fibrinolytic therapy in acute myocardial infarction: report of a prospective randomized trial. *N Engl J Med.* 1983;**308:**1305-11.

36. ANDERSON JL, MARSHALL HW, BRAY BE, et al. A randomized trial of intracoronary streptokinase in the treatment of acute myocardial infarction. *N Engl J Med.* 1983;**308:**1312-8.

37. KENNEDY JW, RITCHIE JL, DAVIS KB, FRITZ J. Western Washington randomized trial of intracoronary streptokinase in acute myocardial infarction. *N Engl J Med.* 1983;**309:**1477-82.

38. LEIBOFF RH, KATZ RJ, WASSERMAN AG, et al. A randomized, angiographically controlled trial of intracoronary streptokinase in acute myocardial infarction. *Am J Cardiol.* 1984;**53:**404-7.

39. TAMAKI S, MURAKAMI T, KADOTA K, et al. Effects of coronary artery reperfusion on relation between creatine kinase-MB release and infarct size estimated by myocardial emission tomography with thallium-201 in man. *J Am Coll Cardiol.* 1983;**2:**1031-8.

40. BLANKE H, VON HARDENBERG D, COHEN M, et al. Patterns of creatine kinase release during acute myocardial infarction after nonsurgical reperfusion: comparison with conventional treatment and correlation with infarct size. *J Am Coll Cardiol.* 1984;**3:**675-80.

41. SHELL WE, DEWOOD MA, KLIGERMAN M, GANZ W, SWAN HJC. Early appearance of MB-creatine kinase activity in nontransmural myocardial infarction detected by a sensitive assay for the isoenzyme. *Am J Med.* 1981;**71:**254-62.

42. ROSALKI SB. An improved procedure for serum creatine phosphokinase determination. *J Lab Clin Med*. 1967;**69**:696-705.

43. FARRINGTON C, CHALMERS AH. The effect of dilution on creatine kinase activity. *Clin Chim Acta*. 1976;**73**:217-9.

44. ROBERTS R, HENRY PD, WITTEEVEEN SAGJ, SOBEL BE. Quantification of serum creatine phosphokinase isoenzyme activity. *Am J Cardiol*. 1974;**33**:650-4.

45. MERCER DW. Separation of tissue and serum creatine kinase isoenzymes by ion-exchange column chromatography. *Clin Chem*. 1974;**20**:36-40.

46. WHITE RD, GRANDE P, CALIFF L, PALMERI ST, CALIFF RM, WAGNER GS. Diagnostic and prognostic signficance of minimally elevated creatine kinase-MB in suspected acute myocardial infarction. *Am J Cardiol*. 1985;**55**(13 pt 1):1478-84.

47. WONG PCP, SMITH AF. Comparison of 3 methods of analysis of the MB isoenzyme of creatine kinase in serum. *Clin Chim Acta*. 1975;**65**:99-107.

48. LJUNGDAHL L, GERHARDT W. Creatine kinase isoenzyme variants in human serum. *Clin Chem*.1978;**24**:832-4.

49. SAX SM, MOORE JJ, GIEGEL JL, WELSH M. Atypical increase in serum creatine kinase activity in hospital patients. *Clin Chem*. 1976;**22**:87-91.

50. FIOLET JWT, WILLEBRANDS AF, LIE KI, TER WELLE HF. Determination of creatine kinase isoenzyme MB (CK-MB): comparison of methods and clinical evaluation. *Clin Chim Acta*. 1977;**80**:23-35.

51. GERHARDT W, WALDENSTROM J, HORDER M, et al. Creatine kinase and creatine kinase B-subunit activity in serum in cases of suspected myocardial infarction. *Clin Chem*. 1982;**28**:277-83.

52. URDAL P, LANDAAS S. Macro creatine kinase BB in serum, and some data on its prevalence. *Clin Chem*. 1979;**25**:461-5.

53. ROBERTS R, GRACE AM. Purification of mitochondrial creatine kinase: biochemical and immunological characterization. *J Biol Chem*. 1980;**255**:2870-7.

54. STEIN W, BOHNER J, STEINHART R, EGGSTEIN M. Macro creatine kinase: determination and differentiation of two types by their activation energies. *Clin Chem*. 1982;**28**:19-24.

55. ROBERTS R, SOBEL BE, PARKER CW. Radioimmunosassay for creatine kinase isoenzymes. *Science*. 1976;**194**:855-7.

56. ROBERTS R, HERMAN C. An improved, rapid radioimmunoassay for individual human CK isoenzymes [Abstract]. *Am J Cardiol*. 1980;**45**:400.

57. AL-SHEIKH W, HEAL AV, PEFKAROS KC, et al. Evaluation of immunoradiometric assay specific for the CK-MB isoenzyme for detection of acute myocardial infarction. *Am J Cardiol*. 1984;**54**:269-73.

58. HERMAN CA, ROBERTS R. A sensitive, rapid and specific quantitative assay for plasma MB CK [Abstract]. *Circulation*. 1979;**59-60**(3 pt 2):II-13.

59. ROSALKI SB. Methods in the study of isoenzymes. *Histochem J*. 1974;**6**:361-8.

60. VASUDEVAN G, MERCER DW, VARAT MA. Lactic dehydrogenase isoenzyme determination in the diagnosis of acute myocardial infarction. *Circulation*. 1978;**57**:1055-7.

61. ORTEN JM, NEUHAUS OW. *Human Biochemistry*. 10th ed. St. Louis: C.V. Mosby Co.; 1982:86-96.

62. HEDWORTH-WHITTY RB, WHITFIELD JB, RICHARDSON RW. Serum gamma-glutamyl transpeptidase activity in myocardial ischaemia. *Br Heart J*. 1967;**29**:432-8.

63. GRENADIER E, KEIDAR S, KAHANA L, ALPAN G, MARMUR A, PALANT A. The roles of serum myoglobin, total CPK, and CK-MB isoenzyme in the acute phase of myocardial infarction. *Am Heart J*. 1983;**105**:408-16.

64. KLOCKE FJ, COPLEY DP, KRAWCZYK JA, REICHLIN M. Rapid renal clearance of immunoreactive canine plasma myoglobin. *Circulation.* 1982;**65:**1522-8.
65. TOMMASO CL, SALZEIDER K, ARIF M, KLUTZ W. Serial myoglobin vs. CPK analysis as an indicator of uncomplicated myocardial infarction size and its use in assessing early infarct extension. *Am Heart J.* 1980;**99:**149-54.
66. CAIRNS JA, MISSIRLIS E, WALKER WH. Usefulness of serial determinations of myoglobin and creatine kinase in serum compared for assessment of acute myocardial infarction. *Clin Chem.* 1983;**29:**469-73.
67. HASHIMOTO H, ABENDSCHEIN DR, STRAUSS AW, SOBEL BE. Early detection of myocardial infarction in conscious dogs by analysis of plasma MM creatine kinase isoforms. *Circulation.* 1985;**71:**363-9.
68. DILLON MC, CALBREATH DF, DIXON AM, et al. Diagnostic problem in acute myocardial infarction: CK-MB in the absence of abnormally elevated total creatine kinase levels. *Arch Intern Med.* 1982;**142:**33-8.
69. HELLER GV, BLAUSTEIN AS, WEI JY. Implications of increased myocardial isoenzyme level in the presence of normal serum creatine kinase activity. *Am J Cardiol.* 1983;**51:**24-7.
70. D'SOUZA JP, SINE HE, HORVITZ RA, KUBASIK NP, BRODY BB, BAROLD SS. The significance of the MB isoenzyme in patients with acute cardiovascular disease with a normal or borderline total CPK activity. *Clin Biochem.* 1978;**11:**204-9.
71. MCQUEEN MJ, STRICKLAND RD, MORI L. Detection of ischemic myocardial injury in patients with normal, or moderately elevated, serum CK and AST activities. *Clin Biochem.* 1982;**15:**138-40.
72. AHMED SA, WILLIAMSON JR, ROBERTS R, CLARK RE, SOBEL BE. The association of increased plasma MB CPK activity and irreversible ischemic myocardial injury in the dog. *Circulation.* 1976;**54:**187-93.
73. HIRZEL HO, SONNENBLICK EH, KIRK ES. Absence of a lateral border zone of intermediate creatine phosphokinase depletion surrounding a central infarct 24 hours after acute coronary occlusion in the dog. *Circ Res.* 1977;**41:**673-83.
74. JOHNSON RA, PALACIOS I. Dilated cardiomyopathies of the adult (second of two parts). *N Engl J Med.* 1982;**307:**1119-26.
75. TIEFENBRUNN AJ, ROBERTS R. Elevation of plasma MB creatine kinase and the development of new Q waves in association with pericarditis. *Chest.* 1980;**77:**438-40.
76. TONKIN AM, LESTER RM, GUTHROW CE, ROE CR, HACKEL DB, WAGNER GS. Persistence of MB isoenzyme of creatine phosphokinase in the serum after minor iatrogenic cardiac trauma: absence of postmortem evidence of myocardial infarction. *Circulation.* 1975;**51:**627-31.
77. CARLSON CJ, EMILSON B, RAPAPORT E. Creatine phosphokinase MB isoenzyme in hypothermia: case reports and experimental studies. *Am Heart J.* 1978;**95:**352-8.
78. ZSIGMOND EK. Isoenzymes in hyperpyrexia. *Anesth Analg.* 1971;**50:**1102.
79. ANIDO V, CONN RB, MENGOLI HF, ANIDO G. Diagnostic efficacy of myocardial creatine phosphokinase using polyacrylamide disk gel electrophoresis. *Am J Clin Pathol.* 1974;**61:**599-605.
80. ROCK RC, DRESKIN R, KICKLER T, WIMSATT T. Creatine kinase isoenzymes in serum of patients with Reye's syndrome. *Clin Chim Acta.* 1975;**62:**159-62.
81. MA KW, BROWN DC, STEELE BW, FROM AHL. Serum creatine kinase MB isoenzyme activity in long-term hemodialysis patients. *Arch Intern Med.* 1981;**141:**164-6.
82. JAFFE AS, RITTER C, MELTZER V, HARTER H, ROBERTS R. Unmasking artifactual increases in creatine kinase isoenzymes in patients with renal failure. *J Lab Clin Med.* 1984;**104:**193-202.

83. FABINYI G, HUNT D, MCKINLEY L. Myocardial creatine kinase isoenzyme in serum after subarachnoid haemorrhage. *J Neurol Neurosurg Psychiatry.* 1977;**40:**818-20.

84. GOLDMAN J, MATZ R, MORTIMER R, FREEMAN R. High elevations of creatine phosphokinase in hypothyroidism: an isoenzyme analysis. *JAMA.* 1977;**238:**325-6.

85. MATHER HG, MORGAN DC, PEARSON NG, et al. Myocardial infarction: a comparison between home and hospital care for patients. *Br Med J.* 1976;**1:**925-9.

86. HILL JD, HAMPTON JR, MITCHELL JRA. A randomised trial of home-versus-hospital management for patients with suspected myocardial infarction. *Lancet.* 1978;**1:**837-41.

87. GOLDMAN L. Coronary care units: a perspective on their epidemiologic impact. *Int J Cardiol.* 1982;**2:**284-7.

88. FREIMAN JA, CHALMERS TC, SMITH H JR, KUEBLER RR. The importance of beta, the type II error and sample size in the design and interpretation of the randomized control trial: survey of 71 "negative" trials. *N Engl J Med.* 1978;**299:**690-4.

89. LEE TH, BRAND D, WEISBERG M, et al. Patients sent home from emergency rooms with myocardial infarction—clinical characteristics and implications [Abstract]. *Clin Res.* 1985;**33:**257A.

90. GOLDMAN L, BATSFORD WP. Risk-benefit stratification as a guide to lidocaine prophylaxis of primary ventricular fibrillation in acute myocardial infarction: an analytic review. *Yale J Biol Med.* 1979;**52:**455-66.

91. FINEBERG HV, SCADDEN D, GOLDMAN L. Care of patients with a low probability of acute myocardial infarction: cost effectiveness of alternatives to coronary-care-unit admission. *N Engl J Med.* 1984;**310:**1301-7.

92. SCHROEDER JS, LAMB IH, HU M. Do patients in whom myocardial infarction has been ruled out have a better prognosis after hospitalization than those surviving infarction? *N Engl J Med.* 1980;**303:**1-5.

93. MULLEY AG, THIBAULT GE, HUGHES RA, BARNETT GO, REDER VA, SHERMAN EL. The course of patients with suspected myocardial infarction: the identification of low-risk patients for early transfer from intensive care. *N Engl J Med.* 1980;**302:**943-8.

94. THIBAULT GE, MULLEY AG, BARNETT GO, et al. Medical intensive care: indications, interventions, and outcomes. *N Engl J Med.* 1980;**302:**938-42.

95. BRAUNWALD E. The aggressive treatment of acute myocardial infarction. *Circulation.* 1985;**71:**1087-92.

96. BETA-BLOCKER HEART ATTACK TRIAL RESEARCH GROUP. A randomized trial of propranolol in patients with acute myocardial infarction: I. Mortality results. *JAMA.* 1982;**247:**1707-14.

97. NORWEGIAN MULTICENTER STUDY GROUP. Timolol-induced reduction in mortality and reinfarction in patients surviving acute myocardial infarction. *N Engl J Med.* 1981;**304:**801-7.

98. FRISHMAN WH, FURBERG CD, FRIEDEWALD WT. Beta-adrenergic blockade for survivors of acute myocardial infarction. *N Engl J Med.* 1984;**310:**830-7.

99. LEE TH, COOK EF, WEISBERG M, SARGENT RK, WILSON C, GOLDMAN L. Acute chest pain in the emergency room: identification and examination of low-risk patients. *Arch Intern Med.* 1985;**145:**65-9.

100. GRANDE P, CHRISTIANSEN C, PEDERSEN A, CHRISTENSEN MS. Optimal diagnosis in acute myocardial infarction: a cost-effectiveness study. *Circulation.* 1980;**61:**723-8.

101. KANNEL WB, ABBOTT RD. Incidence and prognosis of unrecognized myocardial infarction: an update on the Framingham Study. *N Engl J Med.* 1984;**311:**1144-7.

102. JOHNSON WJ, ACHOR RWP, BURCHELL HB, EDWARDS JE. Unrecognized myocardial infarction. *Arch Intern Med.* 1959;**103:**253-61.

103. ROARK SF, WAGNER GS, IZLAR HL JR, ROE CR. Diagnosis of acute myocardial infarction in a community hospital: significance of CPK-MB determination. *Circulation.* 1976;**53:**965-9.

104. VARAT MA, MERCER DW. Cardiac specific creatine phosphokinase isoenzyme in the diagnosis of acute myocardial infarction. *Circulation.* 1975;**51**:855-9.

105. GALEN RS, REIFFEL JA, GAMBINO R. Diagnosis of acute myocardial infarction: relative efficiency of serum enzyme and isoenzyme measurements. *JAMA.* 1975;**232**:145-7.

106. BLOMBERG DJ, KIMBER WD, BURKE MD. Creatine kinase isoenzymes: predictive value in the early diagnosis of acute myocardial infarction. *Am J Med.* 1975;**59**:464-9.

107. TURI ZG, RUTHERFORD JD, ROBERTS R, et al. Electrocardiographic, enzymatic and scintigraphic criteria of acute myocardial infarction as determined from study of 726 patients (A MILIS study). *Am J Cardiol.* 1985;**55**(13 pt 1):1463-8.

108. LEE TH, WEISBERG M, COOK EF, DALEY K, BRAND DA, GOLDMAN L. Clinical impact of creatine kinase and creatine kinase-MB for diagnosis of myocardial infarction in the emergency room. *Arch Intern Med.* 1986. (In press).

109. IRVIN RG, COBB FR, ROE CR. Acute myocardial infarction and MB creatine phosphokinase: relationship between onset of symptoms of infarction and appearance and disappearance of enzyme. *Arch Intern Med.* 1980;**140**:329-34.

110. OGUNRO EA, HEARSE DJ, SHILLINGFORD JP. Creatine kinase isoenzymes: their separation and quantitation. *Cardiovasc Res.* 1977;**11**:94-102.

111. SMITH AF. Diagnostic value of serum-creatine-kinase in a coronary-care unit. *Lancet.* 1967;**2**:178-82.

112. OLSON HG, LYONS KP, BUTMAN S, PITERS KM. Validation of technetium-99m stannous pyrophosphate myocardial scintigraphy for diagnosing acute myocardial infarction more than 48 hours old when serum creatine kinase-MB has returned to normal. *Am J Cardiol.* 1983;**52**:245-51.

113. GOLDMAN L, FEINSTEIN AR, BATSFORD WP, COHEN LS, GOTTSCHALK A, ZARET BL. Ordering patterns and clinical impact of cardiovascular nuclear medicine procedures. *Circulation.* 1980;**62**:680-7.

114. RANSOHOFF DF, FEINSTEIN AR. Problems of spectrum and bias in evaluating the efficacy of diagnostic tests. *N Engl J Med.* 1978;**299**:926-30.

115. RUDE RE, POOLE WK, MULLER JE, et al. Electrocardiographic and clinical criteria for recognition of acute myocardial infarction based on analysis of 3,697 patients. *Am J Cardiol.* 1983;**52**:936-42.

116. EISENBERG JM, HOROWITZ LN, BUSCH R, ARVAN D, RAWNSLEY H. Diagnosis of acute myocardial infarction in the emergency room: a prospective assessment of clinical decision making and the usefulness of immediate cardiac enzyme determination. *J Community Health.* 1979;**4**:190-8.

117. ALPERT JS. Serum enzyme determination in patients with suspected myocardial infarction [Editorial]. *Arch Intern Med.* 1983;**143**:1522-3.

118. FISHER ML, CARLINER NH, BECKER LC, PETERS RW, PLOTNICK GD. Serum creatine kinase in the diagnosis of acute myocardial infarction: optimal sampling frequency. *JAMA.* 1983;**249**:393-5.

119. HERLITZ J, HJALMARSON A, WALDENSTROM J. Time lapse from estimated onset of acute myocardial infarction to peak serum enzyme activity. *Clin Cardiol.* 1984;**7**:433-40.

120. MARMOR A, SOBEL BE, ROBERTS R. Factors presaging early recurrent myocardial infarction ("extension"). *Am J Cardiol.* 1981;**48**:603-10.

121. SHELL WE, KJEKSHUS JK, SOBEL BE. Quantitative assessment of the extent of myocardial infarction in the conscious dog by means of analysis of serial changes in serum creatine phosphokinase activity. *J Clin Invest.* 1971;**50**:2614-25.

122. SOBEL BE, BRESNAHAN GF, SHELL WE, YODER RD. Estimation of

infarct size in man and its relation to prognosis. *Circulation.* 1972;**46**:640-8.

123. HORI M, INOUE M, FUKUI S, et al. Correlation of ejection fraction and infarct size estimated from the total CK released in patients with acute myocardial infarction. *Br Heart J.* 1979;**41**:433-40.

124. KAHN JC, GUERET P, MENIER R, GIRAUDET P, FARHAT MB, BOURDARIAS JP. Prognostic value of enzymatic (CPK) estimation of infarct size. *J Mol Med.* 1977;**2**:223-31.

125. BLEIFELD W, MATHEY D, HANRATH P, DUSS H, EFFERT S. Infarct size estimated from serial serum creatine phosphokinase in relation to left ventricular hemodynàmics. *Circulation.* 1977;**55**:303-11.

126. ROBERTS R, HUSAIN A, AMBOS HD, OLIVER GC, COX JR JR, SOBEL BE. Relation between infarct size and ventricular arrhythmia. *Br Heart J.* 1975;**37**:1169-75.

127. GELTMAN EM, EHSANI AA, CAMPBELL MK, SCHECHTMAN K, ROBERTS R, SOBEL BE. The influence of location and extent of myocardial infarction on long-term ventricular dysrhythmia and mortality. *Circulation.* 1979;**60**:805-14.

128. GRANDE P, CHRISTIANSEN C, ALSTRUP K. Comparison of ASAT, CK, CK-MB, and LD for the estimation of acute myocardial infarct size in man. *Clin Chim Acta.* 1983;**128**:329-35.

129. GRANDE P, HANSEN BF, CHRISTIANSEN C, NAESTOFT J. Estimation of acute myocardial infarct size in man by serum CK-MB measurements. *Circulation.* 1982;**65**:756-64.

130. RYAN W, KARLINER JS, GILPIN EA, COVELL JW, DELUCA M, ROSS J JR. The creatine kinase curve area and peak creatine kinase after acute myocardial infarction: usefulness and limitations. *Am Heart J.* 1981;**101**:162-8.

131. SHIBATA T, HASHIMOTO H, ITO T, OGAWA K, SATAKE T, SASSA H. Late estimation of myocardial infarct size by total creatine kinase nomogram. *Am Heart J.* 1985;**109**:1238-43.

132. BLEIFELD WH, HANRATH P, MATHEY D. Serial CPK determinations for evaluation of size and development of acute myocardial infarction. *Circulation.* 1976;**53**(3 pt 1):I-108-11.

133. SMITH JL, AMBOS HD, GOLD HK, et al. Enzymatic estimation of myocardial infarct size when early creatine kinase values are not available. *Am J Cardiol.* 1983;**51**:1294-300.

134. MADSEN EB, GILPIN E, HENNING H, et al. Prediction of late mortality after myocardial infarction from variables measured at different times during hospitalization. *Am J Cardiol.* 1984;**53**:47-54.

135. MADSEN EB, GILPIN E, HENNING H. Short-term prognosis in acute myocardial infarction: evaluation of different prediction methods. *Am Heart J.* 1984;**107**:1241-51.

136. PITT B. Prognosis after acute myocardial infarction [Editorial]. *N Engl J Med.* 1981;**305**:1147-8.

137. GOLDMAN L. Cardiac risks and complications of noncardiac surgery. *Ann Intern Med.* 1983;**98**:504-13.

138. TARHAN S, MOFFITT EA, TAYLOR WF, GIULIANI ER. Myocardial infarction after general anesthesia. *JAMA.* 1972;**220**:1451-4.

139. MAUNEY FM JR, EBERT PA, SABISTON DC JR. Postoperative myocardial infarction: a study of predisposing factors, diagnosis and mortality in a high risk group of surgical patients. *Ann Surg.* 1970;**172**:497-503.

140. GOLDMAN L, CALDERA DL, SOUTHWICK FS, et al. Cardiac risk factors and complications in non-cardiac surgery. *Medicine (Baltimore).* 1978;**57**:357-70.

141. GUITERAS VAL P, PELLETIER LC, HERNANDEZ MG, et al. Diagnostic criteria and prognosis of perioperative myocardial infarction following coronary bypass. *J Thorac Cardiovasc Surg.* 1983;**86**:878-86.

142. DELVA E, MAILLE JG, SOLYMOSS BC, CHABOT M, GRONDIN CM, BOURASSA MG. Evaluation of myocardial damage during coronary

artery grafting with serial determinations of serum CPK MB isoenzyme. *J Thorac Cardiovasc Surg.* 1978;**75:**467-75.

143. WARREN SG, WAGNER GS, BETHEA CF, ROE CR, OLDHAM HN, KONG Y. Diagnostic and prognostic significance of electrocardiographic and CPK isoenzyme changes following coronary bypass surgery: correlation with findings at one year. *Am Heart J.* 1977;**93:**189-96.

144. DU CAILAR C, MAILLE JG, JONES W, et al. MB creatine kinase and the evaluation of myocardial injury following aortocoronary bypass operation. *Ann Thorac Surg.* 1980;**29:**8-14.

145. BAUR HR, STEELE BW, PREIMESBERGER KF, GOBEL FL. Serum myocardial creatine kinase (CK-MB) after coronary arterial bypass surgery. *Am J Cardiol.* 1979;**44:**679-86.

146. BALDERMAN SC, BHAYANA JN, STEINBACH JJ, MASUD ARZ, MICHALEK S. Perioperative myocardial infarction: a diagnostic dilemma. *Ann Thorac Surg.* 1980;**30:**370-7.

147. RAABE DS JR, MORISE A, SBARBARO JA, GUNDEL WD. Diagnostic criteria for acute myocardial infarction in patients undergoing coronary artery bypass surgery. *Circulation.* 1980;**62:**869-78.

148. ROBERTS R, SOBEL BE. Elevated plasma MB creatine phosphokinase activity: a specific marker for myocardial infarction in perioperative patients. *Arch Intern Med.* 1976;**136:**421-4.

149. ROBERTS R, LUDBROOK PA, WEISS ES, SOBEL BE. Serum CPK isoenzymes after cardiac catheterization. *Br Heart J.* 1975;**37:**1144-9.

150. OH JK, SHUB C, ILSTRUP DM, REEDER GS. Creatine kinase release after successful percutaneous transluminal coronary angioplasty. *Am Heart J.* 1985;**109:**1225-31.

151. EHSANI A, EWY GA, SOBEL BE. Effects of electrical countershock on serum creatine phosphokinase (CPK) isoenzyme activity. *Am J Cardiol.* 1976;**37:**12-8.

Utility of the Routine Electrocardiogram Before Surgery and on General Hospital Admission

Critical Review and New Guidelines

ARY L. GOLDBERGER, M.D.; and MARK O'KONSKI, M.D.

A 12-LEAD ELECTROCARDIOGRAM (ECG) has been recommended for adult patients before various operations involving general or regional anesthesia (1-3) as well as in adult patients on general hospital admission (4). However, opinion differs widely on specific guidelines for ordering this test in such patients (1-13). The key issue centers on whether the ECG should be ordered routinely or reserved for selected groups of patients.

This problem may have important implications for the cost and quality of health care. Whereas the ECG is non-invasive and relatively inexpensive, it is not without possible "adverse" effects. If, for example, tens of thousands of tests are being done unnecessarily, a change in ordering practices could result in substantial cumulative savings. Another consideration is that obtaining an ECG on patients with an extremely low prevalence of important organic heart disease is likely to yield a relatively high percentage of false-positive results. Such apparent ECG abnormalities may, in turn, engender additional, expensive, time-consuming, and invasive procedures in the search for nonexistent or insignificant cardiac disease. On the other hand, the ECG may provide the first clue to life-threatening metabolic disturbances such as hyperkalemia and hypokalemia. In some patients, the routine preoperative or admission ECG also could be the first and sole indication of major underlying heart disease

▶ This chapter was originally published in *Annals of Internal Medicine.* 1986;**105**:552-7.

and, perhaps most important, of a recent unrecognized myocardial infarction.

The detection of such previously unrecognized diagnoses is a measure of the marginal benefit of the ECG— that is, of how often the test uncovers abnormalities not apparent through pertinent clinical evaluation using history, physical examination, and laboratory testing. Aside from its use as a screening test, the routine ECG has also been recommended as a potentially valuable source of baseline information (3).

This review critically reassesses the indications for the routine use of the ECG preoperatively and on general hospital admission. Unfortunately, there are important gaps and weaknesses in the data needed to resolve definitively many of the major questions. Particular emphasis therefore is given to the limitations of relevant studies. After focusing on the use of the ECG preoperatively and on general hospital admissions, we present new guidelines for ordering the test based on available data and suggest directions for future clinical research.

Preoperative Electrocardiograms

PREVALENCE OF ABNORMALITIES

Several studies on the yield of the routine preoperative ECG have indicated that abnormalities are relatively common and that a major determinant of their prevalence is patient age (1, 2, 5-13). A plot of the mean frequency of abnormal ECG results against age derived from data in four studies (2, 9, 12, 13) reveals an exponential relationship ($r = 0.99$; Figure 1). According to this regression, a 10% prevalence of abnormal preoperative ECG results is predicted by about age 35 and a 25% prevalence by about age 57. It should be noted that these estimates are based on pooled data combining a variety of ECG findings in both sexes.

The relatively high frequency of ECG abnormalities in patients scheduled for noncardiac surgery focuses attention on the potential positive or negative effects of these findings. Positive effect refers to the capacity of any ECG finding to aid independently in assessing the risk of cardiac complications or to alter patient management so as to reduce risk. Negative effect refers to the capacity of any ECG finding to cause unnecessary further evaluation or postponement of needed surgery.

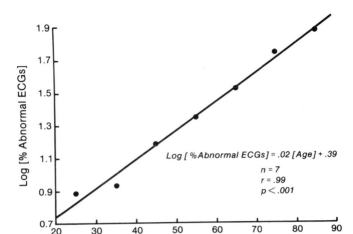

Figure 1. Prevalence of electrocardiographic (*ECG*) abnormalities increases exponentially with age. The mean frequency of abnormal ECG findings in seven age groups, weighted by the total number of patients in each population in four studies (2, 9, 12, 13), is plotted.

POSITIVE EFFECTS

Diagnosis of Myocardial Infarction: Several studies (14-19) on large numbers of patients having various elective and urgent operative procedures involving regional or general anesthesia have indicated that recent myocardial infarction, particularly within the preceding 6 months, is a major risk factor for life-threatening cardiac complications. Preoperative recognition of recent myocardial infarction is also important because careful intraoperative and postoperative management may reduce the complication rate in high-risk patients (20). Furthermore, certain patients may derive long-term benefits from treatment with beta-blocking drugs (21). Finally, postponement of elective surgery in patients with recent infarction may lessen operative risk.

A key question therefore is, how often will a routine preoperative ECG provide the major, or even sole, evidence of previously unrecognized infarction? In an update of the Framingham study, Kannel and Abbott (22) have reported that about 28% of infarcts were discovered only through the appearance of new ECG changes

(Q-waves or loss of R-waves) observed on a routine biennial study. These infarctions had been previously unrecognized by the patient and attending physician. The estimated semiannual incidence of unrecognized myocardial infarctions based on these ECG criteria increases with advancing age (Table 1), exceeding 0.25 to 0.5/1000 in men aged 40 to 45 years or more and women aged 55 years or more. These findings are consistent with those of other studies (23, 24) which also show a clinically important incidence of unrecognized infarctions increasing with age. Hypertension has been significantly correlated with the risk of unrecognized infarction (24, 25), but the common clinical impression (25) that diabetes mellitus is associated with unrecognized infarction has not been proved (24). Although not reported in any of the pertinent studies, the risk of unrecognized myocardial infarction in patients in younger age groups may also be enhanced by other conditions associated with premature coronary disease, including atherosclerotic peripheral vascular disease (26) and renal hemodialysis (27).

These studies (23-25) may underestimate the incidence of unrecognized Q-wave myocardial infarctions because the ECG characteristics may normalize or become nondiagnostic within a few months after Q-wave infarction (28, 29). On the other hand, overestimation of the incidence of unrecognized Q-wave infarcts may have occurred to the extent that false-positive (pseudo-infarct) ECG patterns were not recognized. Data regarding the incidence of unrecognized non-Q-wave infarction are not

Table 1. Estimated Semiannual Incidence of Q-Wave Myocardial Infarction in Men and Women by Age Groups*

Age	Men		Women	
	Unrecognized Infarctions	All Infarctions	Unrecognized Infarctions	All Infarctions
yrs	←―――――――――	*n/1000*	―――――――――→	
30-34	0.13	0.64	0.0	0.11
35-44	0.32	1.91	0.13	0.26
45-54	0.83	3.61	0.14	0.65
55-64	1.41	5.40	0.90	2.35
65-74	2.69	7.05	1.06	2.78
75-84	3.01	5.64	1.70	6.42

* These estimates assume a constant 10-year incidence. Data derived from 2282 men and 2845 women at risk reported by Kannel and Abbott (22).

available. According to two large autopsy series (30, 31) suggesting that the sensitivity of standard Q-wave criteria for all infarctions is in the range of 33% to 62%, the actual incidence of unrecognized (Q-wave and non-Q-wave) infarction could be twice as high as that shown in Table 1.

Although the ECG may provide the major and perhaps sole clue to the diagnosis of a previously unrecognized infarction, the presence of such abnormalities usually does not indicate the timing of the event. Without historical data, ancillary laboratory tests (for example, cardiac enzyme levels with acute infarction), a previous ECG for comparison, or serial tracings showing evolving ischemic changes, Q-waves, ST-deviations, or T-wave inversions per se will not distinguish between recent and remote infarction. Because operative risk is highest within 6 months after myocardial infarction, ECG evidence of an unsuspected infarct will be of limited value in precisely assessing cardiac risk. No study has addressed the prognosis of patients discovered by routine preoperative ECG screening to have an unrecognized myocardial infarction of indeterminate age.

In conclusion, the major positive effect of a preoperative ECG is related to the detection of previously unrecognized myocardial infarction, the risk of which increases with advancing age. However, even in the highest risk group (men 75 years old or more), the estimated incidence of unrecognized Q-wave infarction within the preceding 6 months is relatively small (< 0.5%). Furthermore, the presence of Q waves (or ischemic ST-T changes associated with non-Q-wave infarction) does not necessarily indicate that the infarct occurred within the preceding 6 months. The absence of Q-wave or ischemic ST-T changes is strong, but not absolute, evidence against a recent unrecognized infarction.

Other Electrocardiographic Findings: Aside from the diagnosis of unrecognized myocardial infarction, do any other ECG findings affect surgical morbidity or mortality? Using multivariate analysis techniques, Goldman and colleagues (16) retrospectively identified two ECG findings that contributed independently to the risk of postoperative myocardial infarction, pulmonary edema, or ventricular tachycardia. One was a rhythm on the last preoperative ECG other than sinus or premature atrial contractions, including atrial fibrillation, atrial flutter, junctional rhythm, junctional tachycardia, wandering atrial pacemaker, multifocal atrial tachycardia, paroxysmal atrial tachycardia, or electrically paced rhythm. The other important arrhythmia was ventricular ectopy with five or more premature ventricular beats per minute documented at any time before surgery. Ventricular and serious supraventricular arrhythmias probably correlate with increased cardiac risk because of their association with advanced coronary artery disease or myocardial dysfunction. Whereas such arrhythmias may be markers of increased cardiac risk, there is no evidence that specific antiarrhythmic therapy will reduce this risk. In this regard, Goldman and colleagues observed that the patients in their study with frequent premature ventricular contractions who died usually did not have a primary fatal ventricular tachyarrhythmia.

A related question is, how much information does a routine ECG add to physical examination in the diagnosis of arrhythmias? Although palpation of peripheral pulses and cardiac auscultation are likely to be helpful in screening for arrhythmias, physical examination has important limitations. For example, distinction between supraventricular and ventricular ectopy may be difficult, and certain rhythm disturbances such as nonparoxysmal junctional tachycardia, wandering atrial pacemaker, or atrial flutter with 3:1 or 4:1 conduction are easily overlooked on examination and may not be associated with symptoms. The prevalence of such "silent" arrhythmias is not known, but the yield of the ECG would be predicted to be greatest in asymptomatic older patients (2, 9, 12, 13) and in patients in all age groups with other cardiac complaints or physical findings.

Other ECG abnormalities related to QRS-axis deviation, PR-interval prolongation, QRS voltage, QRS duration, P-waves, R-wave progression, or ST-T changes not associated with infarction in the preceding 6 months were not identified as independent risk factors for preoperative cardiac morbidity or mortality by Goldman and colleagues (16). However, two potential limitations of their analysis in assessing the prognostic value of ECG variables should be considered. First, the power of a "negative" study was reduced by the relatively small number of endpoints (patient complications) and the small number of patients with any particular ECG abnormality. Second, the study included data only on patients who actually had surgery. Patients whose surgery was cancelled or postponed because of ECG abnormalities would not have been enrolled. Therefore, the significance of preoperative ECG abnormalities would have been undervalued by this analysis if certain undisclosed, presurgical ECG findings lessened morbidity or mortality by leading to cancellation or deferral of procedures.

The risk of surgery in patients with chronic bundle branch block appears to be related to the underlying myocardial, valvular, or coronary disease commonly present in this setting (32, 33). However, bundle branch block per se has not been identified as an independent risk factor for cardiac complications (16). Furthermore, asymptomatic chronic bifascicular block (as evidenced by complete left bundle branch block or by complete right bundle branch block with left anterior or left posterior fascicular block) does not require prophylactic placement of a temporary pacemaker in patients having surgery under general anesthesia (33, 34).

In conclusion, the ECG may be of small marginal benefit in detecting certain arrhythmias associated with increased perioperative risk that are not always apparent on routine physical examination. The yield should be greatest in patients with the highest risk of arrhythmias, including those with a positive cardiovascular history or physical findings and asymptomatic older patients.

NEGATIVE EFFECTS

Routine application of a test with limited specificity for a disease will lead to the generation of abnormal (false-positive) results in patients who do not have the disease. Problems in the diagnosis of myocardial infarction, for example, arise because Q-waves and prominent ST- and T-wave changes are sometimes seen either in normal persons or in patients with noncoronary heart disease (35). The specificity of Minnesota Code Q-wave criteria for the diagnosis of recent or old infarction has been reported by Uusitupa and colleagues (31) on the basis of findings at autopsy in a university hospital in Finland. Specificity values ranging from 88% to 98% were obtained in a group of 1194 men and women aged 30 years or older who had an ECG recorded "shortly" before death. These estimates are similar to the 89% specificity for Q-wave criteria reported by Horan and colleagues (30) in an earlier postmortem series. Specificity data for various ST-T abnormalities in the diagnosis of infarction are not available.

The likelihood that an abnormal ECG finding represents a false-positive result depends in part on the prevalence of the particular disease in the population being tested as well as on the specificity of the test (36). The prevalence of unrecognized infarction increases progressively with advancing age in both sexes but is higher for men in all age groups (Table 1). Thus, Q-waves or ST-T abnormalities are less likely to indicate ischemic heart disease in young adult men or women compared with older persons. As a corollary, the vigorous diagnostic investigation of borderline ECG abnormalities noted at the time of routine or "baseline" preoperative evaluation in low-risk subsets may lead to costly and time-consuming cardiac evaluations. However, data are not available for estimating the cost of such false-positive diagnoses in various subsets of patients who have routine ECG testing done preoperatively.

BASELINE PREOPERATIVE ELECTROCARDIOGRAMS

Distinct from the utility of the ECG as a screening test is the question of obtaining a routine ECG as a baseline test in all adults preoperatively. The rationale, as explained by the 1977 Task Force of the Tenth Bethesda Conference on Optimal Electrocardiography (3), would be to "provide a recent baseline record to help manage surgical complications (for example, cardiac or pulmonary complications, electrolyte imbalance)." In other patients, the surgical procedure itself (for example, neurosurgery [37]) might induce ECG changes that could be a source of diagnostic confusion without a baseline tracing. However, the utility of such baseline data obtained as part of routine preoperative assessment has not been studied, and the cost effectiveness requires prospective evaluation. For example, obtaining baseline ECG data may be justified only in selected subsets of patients such as those having intrathoracic, intraperitoneal, or aortic procedures or emergency surgery, because these types of surgery independently correlate with increased cardiac risk (16).

SUMMARY

1. There is no consensus on the indications for an ECG in adult patients before surgery with general or regional anesthesia.

2. Abnormalities in an ECG are common in patients having surgery, and the prevalence of these abnormalities increases exponentially with age (Figure 1).

3. The most important role for the ECG may be to detect a recent unrecognized myocardial infarct, because an infarction within the preceding 6 months is a risk factor for perioperative morbidity and mortality. The estimated semiannual incidence of unrecognized Q-wave infarction increases progressively with age and exceeds 0.25 to 0.5/1000 in men aged 40 to 45 years or more and women aged 55 years or more. However, even in the highest risk group (men 75 years or older), the estimated incidence of unrecognized Q-wave myocardial infarction within the preceding 6 months is quite low (< 0.5%).

4. Standard ECG criteria for Q-wave myocardial infarction are relatively specific but do not distinguish recent from remote events. Furthermore, false-positive findings may lead to costly evaluations in the search for insignificant or nonexistent heart disease. The predictive value of prominent Q-waves (or ST-T abnormalities) for recent unrecognized myocardial infarction will be lowest in subsets with the lowest prevalence of this condition, including asymptomatic men less than 40 to 45 years of age and women less than 55 years old who do not have important risk factors for coronary disease.

5. Two preoperative arrhythmias are independent risk factors for perioperative cardiac morbidity or mortality. In particular, increased risk is associated with the presence of a rhythm other than sinus or premature atrial contractions on the last preoperative ECG. The other important arrhythmia is ventricular ectopy (more than five premature ventricular beats per minute) documented at any time before surgery.

6. There is no evidence that supports the utility of obtaining a routine ECG in all patients preoperatively solely as a baseline for comparison. Whether a baseline ECG is useful in selected subsets of patients preoperatively who do not have evidence of cardiac disease remains to be determined.

Electrocardiograms on General Hospital Admissions

Although an ECG has been recommended (4) for patients without apparent heart disease when they are admitted to the hospital, there is little evidence to support this practice. In the only study that addresses the utility of the routine admission ECG, Moorman and colleagues (38) prospectively surveyed 1410 patients admitted to a general medical service. They excluded patients admitted to intensive care units and those transferred from other services (Table 2). In the 635 patients with cardiac findings on history or physical examination, the admission ECG in 44 (6.9%) added new information. In contrast, in the 775 patients with no evidence of cardiac abnormalities, the admission ECG added new information in only 8 (1.0%). Furthermore, for patients without cardiac abnormality shown by history or physical examination, the yield was primarily noted in patients 45 years or older (Table 2). Only 2 of the 775 patients (a 49-year-old man and a 72-year-old woman) appeared to receive lasting benefit from information added by a screening ECG.

Although this well-designed study (38) casts doubt on the utility of the routine screening admission ECG in patients less than 45 years of age without apparent cardiac abnormalities, the findings must be interpreted cautiously. Because no clinical importance was assigned to ECG abnormalities that were either previously known or readily predicted from clinical data, the practical value of the ECG in the initial assessment of patients with previously recognized cardiac disease may have been underestimated. Furthermore, the quantitative assessment of the cost effectiveness of the ECG performed in this study was

Table 2. Yield of Admission Electrocardiogram According to Age and Diagnosis*

	n/n(%)
Without cardiac abnormality	
≥ 45 years old	7/500 (1.4)
< 45 years old	1/275 (0.4)
With cardiac abnormality	
≥ 45 years old	40/472 (8.5)
< 45 years old	4/163 (2.5)

* Data adapted from those of Moorman and colleagues (38). Yield was defined as positive if the electrocardiogram provided information not obtained by the admission history or physical examination.

based on only two patients, and therefore further studies are needed.

This study also was not designed to investigate the value of the admission ECG as a baseline for future evaluation. The authors did note that in no case was the admission ECG "indispensable" to the care of patients who developed symptoms after admission. This observation complements Rubenstein and Greenfield's (39) finding that a baseline ECG was infrequently essential in the emergency room evaluation of patients with chest pain. However, in both studies the assessment of the utility of the baseline ECG was made exclusively by retrospective analysis.

Finally, the study of Moorman and colleagues does not have sufficient power to evaluate the utility of a baseline or screening ECG in selected subsets of patients without overt cardiac disease, such as those with systemic conditions (for example, certain malignancies, collagen vascular diseases, or infectious diseases) that may be associated with cardiac involvement, patients at risk for major electrolyte disorders, and patients using or about to receive noncardiac medications that are associated with potential cardiac toxicity or important ECG alterations (phenothiazines, tricyclic antidepressants, doxorubicin and its congeners, and so on).

Recommendations and Future Directions

The recommendations given in Table 3 are based on the present review. In light of the deficiencies of existing data, the tentative nature of the guidelines must be emphasized. At the same time, this critical review highlights the need for further clinical research. Some key questions remain unanswered: What are the consequences of a false-positive ECG in surgical patients? How often does an abnormal preoperative ECG provide the first clue to a previously unrecognized infarction in a patient? What is the outcome of surgery in patients with ECG evidence of previously unrecognized myocardial infarction of indeterminate age? How often does the routine preoperative ECG lead to the detection of clinically important, unsuspected arrhythmias?

In addition, better data on the sensitivity and specificity of ST-T criteria for infarction in the preceding 6 months would be helpful. Generally speaking, under-

Table 3. Guidelines for Ordering an Electrocardiogram in Adult Patients Before Surgery and on General Hospital Admission*

An ECG is not routinely indicated before noncardiac surgery.

An ECG is not routinely indicated solely because of general hospital admission.

Clinical judgment should guide the ordering of an ECG preoperatively and on general hospital admission. Subsets of patients in whom an ECG may be helpful include, but are not limited to, the following:

Patients with a history or physical findings suggesting clinically important heart disease, including arrhythmias.

Men aged 40 to 45 years or more and women aged 55 years or more.

Patients with systemic diseases or other conditions that may be associated with clinically important but previously *unrecognized* cardiac abnormalities. Such conditions include, but are not limited to, hypertension, atherosclerotic peripheral vascular disease, or diabetes mellitus, which may be associated with unrecognized coronary atherosclerosis. Others include certain malignancies, collagen vascular diseases, or infectious diseases, which may be associated with unrecognized cardiac involvement.

Patients concurrently using or about to be prescribed noncardiac medications that can cause potentially serious cardiac toxicity or that may be associated with important ECG alterations (for example, phenothiazines, tricyclic antidepressants, doxorubicin and related drugs).

Patients at risk for major electrolyte abnormalities.

Additional preoperative considerations. Patients having elective intrathoracic, intraperitoneal, or aortic surgery or emergency operations under general or regional anesthesia are at increased risk for cardiac complications. In addition, major neurosurgical operations may be associated with ECG changes. The value of a preoperative ECG in these settings, however, has not been ascertained. Clinical judgment therefore should be applied in individual patients with respect to conditions not already included in the previous categories.

---

* For purposes of this discussion, an electrocardiogram (ECG) consists of 12 conventional leads and is taken at rest. The preoperative category includes patients scheduled to have surgery under general anesthesia or regional anesthesia with sedation. General admission includes other patients admitted to medical and nonmedical services but excludes those admitted to intensive care units.

standing of the diagnostic accuracy of the ECG is based on the detection not of recent infarcts, but of all infarcts. Future prospective studies will also be useful in defining the utility of the routine admission ECG in selected groups of patients without overt cardiac disease (for example, men aged 40 to 45 years or older and women aged 55 years and older, or patients with systemic diseases that may be associated with unrecognized cardiac abnormalities— *see* Table 3). Finally, prospective evaluation of the utility of the ECG as a baseline for future comparison in different subsets of medical and surgical patients would be helpful.

The age criteria suggested in Table 3 are necessarily arbitrary and arguments could be made to adjust the age cutoffs at higher or lower levels or to have different age-related criteria for medical and surgical patients. Moorman and colleagues (38) were appropriately cautious in interpreting the results of their study, and they did not make any explicit recommendations regarding the routine admission ECG in patients without cardiac signs or symptoms. These guidelines also are not intended to cover all contingencies. Should an obese 39-year-old man who smokes cigarettes and has hypercholesterolemia have a routine preoperative ECG? Clinical judgment rather than arbitrary rules obviously must guide physicians in making such decisions. It should be emphasized that a careful history and physical examination are essential in the evaluation of all hospitalized patients.

References

1. HOWLAND WS, SCHMEITZER O, LADUE JS. Evaluation of routine postoperative electrocardiography. *NY State J Med.* 1962;**62**:1941-5.
2. FERRER MI. The value of obligatory preoperative electrocardiograms: a survey of 1260 patients. *J Am Med Wom Assoc.* 1978;**33**:459-64.
3. RESNEKOV L, FOX S, SELZER A, et al. The quest for optimal electrocardiography: task force IV: use of electrocardiograms in practice. *Am J Cardiol.* 1978;**41**:170-5.
4. KRUPP MA, TIERNEY LM, JAWETZ E, et al. *Physician's Handbook.* 21st ed. Los Altos, California: Lange Medical Publications;1985:29.
5. RABKIN SW, HORNE JM. Preoperative electrocardiography: its cost-effectiveness in detecting abnormalities when a previous tracing exists. *Can Med Assoc J.* 1979;**121**:301-6.
6. ROBBINS JA, MUSHLIN AI. Preoperative evaluation of the healthy patient. *Med Clin North Am.* 1979;**63**:1145-56.
7. BLERY C, CHASTANG C, GAUDY J. Critical assessment of routine preoperative investigations. *Eff Health Care.* 1983;**1**:111-4.

8. Diagnostic and therapeutic technology assessment: mandatory ECG before elective surgery. *JAMA*. 1983;**250**:540.

9. PATERSON KR, CASKIE JP, GALLOWAY DJ, MCARTHUR K, MCWHINNIE DL. The pre-operative electrocardiogram: an assessment. *Scott Med J*. 1983;**28**:116-8.

10. RABKIN SW, HORNE JM. Preoperative electrocardiography effect of new abnormalities on clinical decisions. *Can Med Assoc J*. 1983;**128**:146-7.

11. SEYMOUR DG, PRINGLE R, MACLENNAN WJ. The role of the routine pre-operative electrocardiogram in the elderly surgical patient. *Age Ageing*. 1983;**12**:97-104.

12. ELSTON RA, TAYLOR DJ. The preoperative electrocardiogram [Letter]. *Lancet*. 1984;**1**:349.

13. JAKOBSSON A, WHITE T. Routine preoperative electrocardiograms [Letter]. *Lancet*. 1984;**1**:972.

14. MAUNEY FM JR, EBERT PA, SABISTON DC JR. Postoperative myocardial infarction: a study of predisposing factors, diagnosis and mortality in a high risk group of surgical patients. *Ann Surg*. 1970;**172**:497-503.

15. TARHAN S, MOFFITT EA, TAYLOR WF, GIULIANI ER. Myocardial infarction after general anesthesia. *JAMA*. 1972;**220**:1451-4.

16. GOLDMAN L, CALDERA DL, NUSSBAUM SR, et al. Multifactorial index of cardiac risk in noncardiac surgical procedures. *N Engl J Med*. 1977;**297**:845-50.

17. COOPERMAN M, PFLUG B, MARTIN EW JR, EVANS WE. Cardiovascular risk factors in patients with peripheral vascular disease. *Surgery*. 1978;**84**:505-9.

18. STEEN PA, TINKER JH, TARHAN S. Myocardial reinfarction after anesthesia and surgery. *JAMA*. 1978;**239**:2566-70.

19. VON KNORRING J. Postoperative myocardial infarction: a prospective study in a risk group of surgical patients. *Surgery*. 1981;**90**:55-60.

20. RAO TLK, JACOBS KH, EL-ETR AA. Reinfarction following anesthesia in patients with myocardial infarction. *Anesthesiology*. 1983;**59**:499-505.

21. BETA-BLOCKER HEART ATTACK TRIAL RESEARCH GROUP. A randomized trial of propranolol in patients with acute myocardial infarction: I. Mortality results. *JAMA*. 1982;**247**:1707-14.

22. KANNEL WB, ABBOTT RD. Incidence and prognosis of unrecognized myocardial infarction: an update on the Framingham study. *N Engl J Med*. 1984;**311**:1144-7.

23. ROSENMAN RG, FRIEDMAN M, JENKINS CD, STRAUS R, WURM M, KOSITCHEK R. Clinically unrecognized myocardial infarction in the Western Collaborative Group study. *Am J Cardiol*. 1967;**19**:776-82.

24. MEDALIE JH, GOLDBOURT U. Unrecognized myocardial infarction: five-year incidence, mortality, and risk factors. *Ann Intern Med*. 1976;**84**:526-31.

25. KANNEL WB, DANNENBERG AL, ABBOTT RD. Unrecognized myocardial infarction and hypertension: the Framingham Study. *Am Heart J*. 1976;**109**(3 pt 1):581-5.

26. KANNEL WB, SHURTLEFF D. The natural history of arteriosclerosis obliterans. *Cardiovasc Clin*. 1971;**3**:37-52.

27. LINDNER A, CHARRA B, SHERRARD DJ, SCRIBNER BH. Accelerated atherosclerosis in prolonged maintenance hemodialysis. *N Engl J Med*. 1974;**290**:697-701.

28. KAPLAN BH, BERKSON DM. Serial electrocardiograms after myocardial infarction. *Ann Intern Med*. 1964;**60**:430-5.

29. KALBFLEISCH JM, SHADAKSHARAPPA KS, CONRAD LL, SARKAR NK. Disappearance of the Q-deflection following myocardial infarction. *Am Heart J*. 1968;**76**:193-8.

30. HORAN LG, FLOWERS NC, JOHNSON JC. Significance of the diagnostic Q wave of myocardial infarction. *Circulation*. 1971;**43**:428-36.

31. UUSITUPA M, PYÖRÄLÄ K, RAUNIO H, RISSANEN V, LAMPAINEN E. Sensitivity and specificity of Minnesota Code Q-QS abnormalities in the diagnosis of myocardial infarction verified at autopsy. *Am Heart J.* 1983;**106**(4 pt 1):753-7.
32. SMITH S, HAYES WL. The prognosis of complete left bundle branch block. *Am Heart J.* 1965;**70**:157-9.
33. BELLOCCI F, SANTARELLI P, DI GENNARO M, ANSALONE G, FENICI R. The risk of cardiac complications in surgical patients with bifascicular block: a clinical and electrophysiologic study in 98 patients. *Chest.* 1980;**77**:343-8.
34. PASTORE JO, YURCHAK PM, JANIS KM, MURPHY JD, ZIR LM. The risk of advanced heart block in surgical patients with right bundle branch block and left axis deviation. *Circulation.* 1978;**57**:677-80.
35. GOLDBERGER AL. *Myocardial Infarction: Electrocardiographic Differential Diagnosis.* 3rd ed. St. Louis: C.V. Mosby Co.; 1984.
36. GRINER PF, MAYEWSKI RJ, MUSHLIN AL, GREENLAND P. Selection and interpretation of diagnostic tests and procedures: principles and applications. *Ann Intern Med.* 1981;**94**(4 pt 2):557-92.
37. FINKLESTEIN D, NIGAGLIONI A. Electrocardiographic alterations after neurosurgical procedures. *Am Heart J.* 1961;**62**:772-84.
38. MOORMAN JR, HLATKY MA, EDDY DM, WAGNER GS. The yield of the routine admission electrocardiogram: a study in a general medical service. *Ann Intern Med.* 1985;**103**:590-5.
39. RUBENSTEIN LZ, GREENFIELD S. The baseline ECG in the evaluation of acute cardiac complaints. *JAMA.* 1980;**244**:2536-9.

The Utility of Routine Chest Radiographs

THOMAS G. TAPE, M.D.; and ALVIN I. MUSHLIN, M.D., Sc.M.

Chest radiographs account for a major portion of diagnostic medical expenditures. The World Health Organization (1) has estimated that 50% of all radiologic procedures worldwide are chest radiographs. Many of these are done routinely on hospital admission and preoperatively; it has been estimated that over 30 million such films were taken in hospitals in the United States in 1980 with an associated $1.5 billion in charges to consumers (2).

Historically, the major reason for obtaining routine chest radiographs on all hospital admissions and before surgery was to identify patients with clinically silent pulmonary tuberculosis. The declining prevalence of this disease and the development of better screening tests led to the abandonment of mass screening programs. Although some hospitals continue to mandate routine chest radiographs for newly admitted patients and patients having surgery, it is difficult to find specific justification for such a practice. Screening can probably be explained in part by the ready availability of equipment to do chest radiographs and by the widely held belief that radiography is a more sensitive means of detecting occult chest disease than the clinical examination. Indeed, many clinicians consider chest radiography an extension of the routine clinical examination (3). Other reasons for obtaining routine chest films preoperatively include the establishment of a baseline against which to assess future (postoperative) changes as well as medicolegal reasons (4-6).

Recently, enthusiasm for the use of routine chest radiography has been waning, and several letters and edito-

▶ This chapter was originally published in *Annals of Internal Medicine.* 1986;**104**:663-70.

rials have questioned the practice (7-12). Studies of patients in psychiatric wards and pregnant women have shown a lack of utility of routine radiographs (13-16). Several specialty societies (17-19) as well as ad hoc committees of the Food and Drug Administration (20) and the World Health Organization (1) have issued opinions supporting the abandonment of routine chest radiography.

This article critically examines the literature pertaining to admission and preoperative chest radiography and presents evidence that such routine radiography is not indicated in either instance. First, we discuss the technique, limitations, and accuracy of chest radiography. We then focus on studies of the diagnostic yield of routine chest radiography and the impact of its findings on patient management; possible adverse effects are also considered. Finally, we suggest strategies for identifying subgroups of patients in whom screening chest films might be beneficial.

Technique and Accuracy

For routine or screening purposes, chest radiographs are usually taken as posteroanterior and lateral projections with the patient standing. If the patient is too ill to stand, anteroposterior upright or supine projections are alternative but less satisfactory views. The charge for a standard two-view examination at our institution is $62. The radiation exposure is relatively low compared with that from other natural and artificial sources of radiation (6); the average skin exposure is 63 mrem and the average bone marrow exposure is 4.3 mrem. The risk of malignancy at these levels is exceedingly small (21).

As with any diagnostic test, there are inherent limitations to its accuracy. False-positive and false-negative results may arise for several reasons. Suboptimal technique, poor exposure, poor patient positioning, patient motion, and lack of cooperation may lead to artifacts and may obscure significant findings on the film. Even with perfect technique, lesions may be hidden by overlying shadows; also, overlapping shadows of normal structures may be incorrectly interpreted as pathologic findings.

The accuracy of the chest film has not been studied adequately, perhaps because of the major methodologic problems in evaluating a test that can have many abnor-

Table 1. Studies of the Accuracy of Chest Radiography

Study Population	Methodologic Biases	"Gold-Standard" Test	Sensitivity	Specificity
			%	%
Yerushalmy (22)				
14 000 college students	Incorporation bias*	Bacteriologic or radiographic evidence of active tuberculosis	75	98
Nicklaus et al. (26)				
VA autopsy series, 73 patients	Selection bias†	Pathologic criteria for severe COPD	91	96
Baumstark et al. (27)				
50 patients having cardiac catheterization without past chest surgery or COPD	Selection bias‡	Pulmonary wedge pressure	74	88

* Incorporation bias occurred because the radiographic result was used in the determination of the "gold-standard" diagnosis, resulting in the overestimation of specificity.

† Selection bias occurred because only patients who had macrosections of the lungs prepared at autopsy were studied. Accuracy for detecting chronic obstructive pulmonary disease (COPD) in hospitalized patients is probably much lower.

‡ Selection bias occurred because only patients with chronic heart conditions having catheterization were studied, thus selecting for patients with severer cardiac disease. Accuracy for detecting less severe disease may be lower.

mal findings and that can detect many diseases for which there is no suitable "gold-standard" test. Probably the major cause of inaccurate results is interpreter (perceptive) variability. In several studies reviewed by Yerushalmy (22, 23), a single reader missed 32% of the "true-positive" cases of tuberculosis, which were agreed on by a group of radiologists. Herman and colleagues (24) reported data from 100 admission chest radiographs independently reviewed by five staff radiologists. Forty-one percent of the individual reports contained potentially significant errors of interpretation. In another study, Herman and Hessel (25) randomly selected 100 chest radiographs and had them independently interpreted by ten readers. For each radiograph, a "gold-standard" report was prepared by a consensus panel using both clinical and radiologic data. Twenty-one percent of the 2224 total statements made by the readers were incorrect: 15% of the errors were false-positive and 85% were false-negative. The sensitivity and specificity of the procedure could not be calculated from the reported findings.

A few studies of the accuracy of chest radiography for specific diseases have been done (Table 1) but have serious methodologic biases in patient selection and the definition of "gold standard" (22, 26, 27). The nature of the biases is such that the values for both sensitivity and specificity are likely to be significantly overestimated. Although not yielding a useful measure of the accuracy of chest radiography, these studies show that the procedure may be less accurate than is commonly assumed by practicing clinicians.

Clinical Applications

The major reasons for admission and preoperative chest radiographs are to screen for silent disease, evaluate suspected chest disease, and establish a baseline for future comparison. We first discuss the characteristics of the ideal study assessing the usefulness of routine chest films. Then, after a brief discussion of baseline radiographs, we focus on screening radiographs done preoperatively and on admission, and show that they are rarely helpful in patient care. Finally, we discuss circumstances in which chest radiography is indicated, including the evaluation of suspected chest disease.

THE IDEAL STUDY OF ROUTINE CHEST RADIOGRAPHY

To be ideal, a study would show improved health outcome in a randomized trial allocating patients without clinical indications for chest radiography to receive or not receive the procedure. Lower rates of perioperative complications and mortality would be sought in the screened group. The major problem with this approach is the large number of patients required when the frequency of adverse outcomes is low in the control group. For example, if the mortality of a procedure is 2% and a chest radiograph can reduce this rate by one fourth, then more than 20 000 patients would be needed to have an 80% chance of showing the difference (28).

Most studies of routine chest radiography are not randomized and lack a control group. However, such studies may still be valid if they show that unexpected findings on routine chest films do not result in changes in patient management. If no management changes occur in the screened group, a control group is unnecessary. Also, when no management changes occur, it can be inferred that no change in health outcome will occur. Whether such a study is valid depends on its use of an adequate sample size and controls for methodologic biases.

To ensure a clinically significant result, we believe that at least 1000 patients should be studied. Four other criteria must be met to control for bias: The study sample should be representative of the general population of hospitalized patients, including patients with a broad spectrum of diseases and severity of illness. Patients should be followed up completely during the hospitalization. Criteria for defining a change in management due to findings on routine chest radiographs should be objective and reproducible. Ideally, physicians should prospectively record their treatment plans before the radiograph is done and then revise their plan if warranted by the results. In a retrospective study, cancellation of surgery and documented changes in the treatment plan are objective outcomes, but there may be other, undocumented changes in patient management that cannot be measured by such a study. Finally, only unexpected radiographic findings should be considered significant, so that the independent contribution of the radiograph to patient care can be assessed. The investigator should carefully define the criteria used to label a finding "unexpected" to avoid bias. A summary of designs used in studies of chest radiography is presented in the Appendix. Few studies meet our criteria.

BASELINE CHEST RADIOGRAPHS

One frequent argument for obtaining chest films is to establish a baseline for comparison should chest problems arise. We are aware of only one study of adequate sample size that has addressed this issue directly. Thomsen and colleagues (29) identified 198 patients who had a postoperative chest radiograph from among 1823 surgical patients. Although 88 patients had abnormal findings on the postoperative radiographs, the authors stated that "comparing a postoperative x-ray with a preoperative x-ray did not have therapeutic consequence in any case." This statement must be interpreted cautiously, because no explicit criteria were provided for deciding whether postoperative films were helpful. Other studies of the value of baseline chest radiographs have been too limited in scope (30, 31) or have reported insufficient data (18) to draw valid conclusions.

A second argument against obtaining routine baseline films relates to logistics: many ill patients needing chest radiographs can tolerate only portable or anteroposterior supine studies. Under these circumstances, baseline posteroanterior and lateral films may not be useful for comparison. Although this issue deserves further study, the current evidence does not justify the practice of routinely obtaining baseline chest films.

SCREENING CHEST RADIOGRAPHS

An effective screening test must be able to detect efficiently a disease before symptoms arise and thereby lead to improved health outcome. (In a technical sense, admission and preoperative films are casefinding rather than screening, because they are applied to patients rather than the general population. However, we use the term screening to encompass both uses of routine radiographs.) In the perioperative period, the outcomes of importance are operative mortality and morbidity. A change in the decision to operate or in perioperative management is an important intermediate outcome that may result in reduced morbidity and mortality.

Diagnostic Yield of Routine Radiographs: Several conditions detectable with chest radiography may not be apparent on clinical evaluation of the patient. Some of these conditions, which may influence operative or anesthetic decisions, include tracheal deviation, mediastinal masses, pulmonary nodules, solitary lung masses, aortic aneurysm, pulmonary edema, pneumonia, atelectasis, dextrocardia, cardiomegaly, and new fractures of the vertebrae, ribs, and clavicles (5). Some retrospective series have shown the frequency of such abnormalities on preoperative chest radiographs to be 1% to 8% in pediatric patients (30-32), 6% to 39% in adults (33-39), and 43% in geriatric patients (40). In assessing the utility of the preoperative chest film, however, these data are of little use because the presence of an abnormality does not always imply a negative outcome or the need for a change in patient management. Simply finding an abnormality on a chest film does not necessarily justify the examination.

Impact of Routine Preoperative Chest Radiographs on Patient Care: Fifteen studies, listed in the Appendix, have attempted to address the contribution of preoperative or admission chest radiographs to patient care. Five are not helpful in determining the value of routine chest radiographs because they lack any consideration of the impact of abnormal radiographic findings. Two studies that have assessed intermediate outcomes are not discussed here because of their incomplete outcome assessment (36) and inadequate sample size (41). We assess the study designs and results of the remaining eight studies.

The largest study was done by the Royal College of Radiologists (18) and is a multicenter study of preoperative chest radiography in 10 619 patients. A fivefold variation in utilization rates occurred among the eight centers involved. Most of the variation was explained by differences among individual centers and not by differences in severity of illness or case mix, suggesting wide variation in ordering habits for chest radiographs. This result is also the major weakness of the study: because physicians decided who would receive radiography, many examinations were undoubtedly nonroutine, a serious selection bias but one that would tend to overestimate the value of routine films. Outcome was assessed by whether the patient had surgery as planned and by what type of anesthesia was used. (It was implied that the radiographic result might influence the choice of anesthetic.) Of patients with significant abnormalities found on chest films, 92.0% had surgery, compared with 96.2% of patients with normal findings. In addition, 26% of patients had surgery before the radiographic report was available, despite the fact that a quarter of these patients ultimately had a significant abnormality reported. Inhalation anesthesia was used in the same proportion of patients (about 96%), regardless of whether the preoperative radiograph was ordered because of a specific clinical finding, was done routinely, or was not done at all. Similarly, the results of the chest radiograph did not change the rate of use of inhalation anesthesia.

The importance of this study is its large number of patients and their broad spectrum of diseases. However, because of the limitations in study design, we cannot conclude from it that routine preoperative chest radiographs are unjustified. We can say that there is great variability in test-ordering behavior among physicians that is not accounted for by differences in case mix, and that the decision to operate and type of anesthesia used are rarely influenced by an abnormal radiographic report.

Three studies have examined the effect of routine chest radiographs done before surgery in adult patients (Table 2). Haubek and Cold (34) retrospectively reviewed 400 consecutive patients admitted for surgery and classified them into three groups: patients with cardiopulmonary disease or other clinical indications for radiography, patients having upper abdominal laparotomy, and patients without clinical indications for radiography. One hundred seventy-four patients had routine chest films done solely because of age over 40. Six radiographs showed pathologic findings (chronic obstructive pulmonary disease on four, cardiomegaly on one, and intrathoracic goiter on one), but none had any consequences for perioperative management. Management changes sought were postponed surgery, changed form of anesthesia, added or changed treatment, or medical consultation. Thirty patients had routine radiographs solely because of upper abdominal surgery; no abnormalities were detected. The 75 patients under 41 years old who did not have chest radiography had no postoperative cardiopulmonary complications.

Table 2. Studies Showing Changes in Patient Therapy Due to Abnormal Findings on Routine Chest Radiographs

	Patients Screened	Abnormalities Detected	Changes in Surgical Plan
	n	*n*	*n(%)*
Haubek and Cold (34)	204*	6	0
Thomsen et al. (29)	1227*	75	2(0.2)
Rucker et al. (33)	368†	1	0
Hubbell et al. (2)	294‡	106	12(4)
Wood and Hockelman (30)	749§	35	3(0.4)
Farnsworth et al. (31)	350§	31	0
Sane et al. (32)	1500§	111	45(3)

* Patients are over 40 years old; includes only routine radiographs.
† Patients are under 60 years old; includes only routine radiographs.
‡ Patients were admitted to a medical service from the emergency room; includes only routine radiographs.
§ Patients are from the pediatrics service; includes both routine and clinically indicated radiographs.

Thomsen and colleagues (29) reviewed the cases of all patients over age 40 who were admitted to surgical services (excluding thoracic, otologic, and ophthalmologic services) and searched for clinical evidence of chest disease, the chest radiographic interpretation and any resulting changes in patient care (not explicitly defined), and postoperative complications. Unexpected findings were defined as those that provided new information about the patient. Patients were labeled retrospectively as either healthy or not healthy from a cardiopulmonary standpoint on the basis of history and physical examination alone. Among the healthy patients, 1089 had normal radiographic findings, 42 had cardiomegaly, 10 had previously expected abnormalities, 23 had unexpected abnormalities (11 with infiltrates, 6 with fibrosis, 3 with pleural effusions, 2 with emphysema, and 1 with thyroid adenoma), and 63 did not have chest radiographs done. Five patients with unexpected abnormalities had further testing. Two patients had treatment changes related to the radiographic findings: a malignant hydrothorax was found in a patient with a suspected gynecologic malignancy, and a pulmonary nodule, later found to be a hamartoma, was detected in an apparently healthy patient.

Rucker and associates (33) postulated that certain clinical features could be used to classify patients as being at low or high risk of having a serious abnormality on preoperative chest radiographs. These "risk factors" included age over 60; history of cardiac or pulmonary disease, malignancy, or stroke; signs and symptoms of chest disease; and recent thoracic surgery. The study population consisted of 905 consecutive patients admitted for surgery (excluding thoracic surgery) of whom 368 had no risk factors. Only 1 patient with no risk factors had a significant abnormality (an elevated hemidiaphragm) on chest radiography. No perioperative complications occurred in the low-risk group.

These three studies provide evidence that routine chest radiographs do not enhance patient care. All identified a cohort of patients without apparent chest disease and showed a very low yield (2 of 1718) of unexpected radiographic abnormalities with implications for patient care. However, their retrospective study designs raise some potential problems. All of the studies were prone to investigator bias, because explicit criteria were not developed for attributing management changes to results of chest films. In addition, incomplete documentation of the physicians' decision-making process in the chart may have resulted in undervaluing the contribution of the chest radiograph. Incomplete documentation may also have led to patients with significant chest disease being misclassified as healthy. However, the possible inclusion of some patients with chest disease in the group labeled as healthy should strengthen the conclusion of a study finding no benefit from routine radiography.

Another problem is that the clinical features used to define high and low risk may have been chosen after the data were examined. Using these criteria to select patients likely to have an abnormality on chest films should be validated in a prospective study. Although not explicitly stated, all studies implied that these predictors were chosen on the basis of prior hypotheses, which lessens the need for validation. Only one investigation (33) adequately described the study population, which was typical of those of university teaching hospitals. All three studies were probably subject to expectation bias in which prior knowledge of the patients' clinical status may have influenced the radiologic interpretation. In studies with negative conclusions, such a bias strengthens the conclusions, because interpretation of radiographs with knowledge of clinical information should improve test sensitivity and make a negative conclusion less likely. In summary, although the yield of screening is probably low, the problems associated with retrospectively measuring the effect of routine chest radiographs suggest that the test's value may have been underestimated by these studies. However, even if all the unexpected chest film abnormalities led to improved patient outcome, only 30 of 1718 (<2%) patients would have benefited from routine radiographs.

Effect of Routine Admission Chest Radiographs on Patient Care: The usefulness of routine chest films for all hospital admissions has not been as well studied as the usefulness of preoperative radiography (2, 41-44). Most studies have been retrospective and do not consider the implications of abnormal findings on chest radiographs. One good study identified prospectively those films that were done routinely and then examined their impact on patient care (2) (Table 2). The study population consisted of medical patients (all of whom had chest radiographs) admitted from the emergency department of a Veterans Administration hospital. There were 106 abnormalities detected among the 294 routine films, but only 20 findings were new or worse. In only 12 patients was a change in therapy indicated (according to the opinions of three independent reviewers), 8 of whom had signs or symptoms of chest disease noted on the chart. Thus, only 4 patients had truly occult chest disease identified by routine chest films (2 with pneumonia, 1 with congestive heart failure, and 1 with a pulmonary nodule). According to the authors, "It is likely that historical or physical evidence of their disease would have been found during hospitalization . . ."(2). The patient with a pulmonary nodule died despite early detection of cancer. Therefore, like preoperative screening, the routine chest radiograph on admission does identify unexpected abnormalities in a substantial proportion of patients (20 of 294), but its potential for affecting patient management is very small.

The three remaining studies measuring the effect of routine admission radiographs on patient care were limited to children (Table 2). Two studies (30, 31) reported results similar to those of the preoperative studies. The other study (32) reported a higher rate of changes in patient care resulting from radiographic findings and deserves further comment. Sane and colleagues (32) studied 1500 consecutive chest radiographs done preoperatively at the Minneapolis Children's Health Center and reported that 71 (4.7%) of the children were considered to have significant radiographic abnormalities that were not expected by the primary physician. Surgery was postponed in 11 patients because of unsuspected pneumonic consolidations. The authors also reported 34 minor changes in anesthetic technique. However, "There was no record of unexpected roentgenographic findings altering surgical technique or leading to postoperative complications" (32). The higher rate of significant abnormalities could be explained by the inclusion in the study of patients having thoracic surgery (although the primary chest disease was not counted as an abnormality). In addition, the finding of 38 (2.5%) patients with cardiac abnormalities, including 8 with dextrocardia or dextroversion, suggests a higher than average prevalence of chest disease. The preoperative clinical evaluation of these 1500 patients may have been inadequate because 11 had unsuspected pneumonia (45). Thus, the results of this study may not be generalizable to the typical patient having surgery.

Conclusions: In summary, the studies of the diagnostic yield of routine chest radiographs and their impact on patient management show that screening preoperative films seldom enhance patient care. Estimates of disease prevalence from other sources support these conclusions. Robbins and Mushlin (46), using data from population surveys in England and the United States, have estimated that in asymptomatic populations, the prevalence of tuberculosis is 0.045%, that of chronic interstitial lung disease is 0.01%, and that of chronic obstructive lung disease is 1.9%. Because the prevalence of occult disease is so small, the aggregate benefit of screening chest radiographs is at best slight. However, the decision of whether to use the routine chest film preoperatively depends also on the possible negative consequences related to false-positive and false-negative results. Because no studies have directly addressed these consequences, in the next section we first consider these issues qualitatively and then present examples using hypothetical data to show when routine chest radiographs would and would not be useful.

POTENTIALLY HARMFUL EFFECTS OF SCREENING
CHEST RADIOGRAPHY

Significant abnormal findings on chest films in patients without chest disease (false-positive results) may lead to an undesirable change in patient therapy, delay of surgery, prolonged hospitalization, and additional diagnostic tests to prove the radiographic finding false. Secondary negative effects include possible deterioration of the primary disease while definitive therapy is delayed, as well as the cost and potential complications of those additional diagnostic tests. Patients having unsuspected chest disease not identified by chest radiography (false-negative results) are also subject to harmful effects. Not only will appropriate changes in patient care not be made, but the clinician may be less vigilant in seeking evidence of chest disease and may monitor the patient less intensively because of the false reassurance of the normal chest radiograph.

Whether there is more potential for good or harm from routine chest radiographs can be determined by comparing the consequences of accurate and inaccurate results weighted by their respective likelihoods of occurrence. The likelihood of a particular radiographic result being correct can be determined from the prevalence (or estimated likelihood) of occult chest disease in the group of patients being considered combined with the sensitivity and specificity of chest radiography.

Example 1: Because of the lack of reliable data on the prevalence of occult disease or the accuracy of chest radiography, we must use estimates. In the previously reviewed studies (29-34), the prevalence of clinically important findings on chest radiographs in asymptomatic patients was generally less than 0.5%; this rate will be used as an estimate of the prevalence of occult disease. We will assume that the accuracy of chest radiography is very high—sensitivity of 90% and specificity of 95%— similar to the rates described in published studies (Table 1), which overestimate sensitivity and specificity.

The likelihood that a radiograph with positive findings is a true-positive is calculated as follows: Given a hypothetical group of 10 000 patients with a 0.5% prevalence of occult chest disease, 50 will have the disease. A chest film will identify 45 (90% of 50) of them as having true-positives but will also misclassify 498 ([100% − 95%] of 9950) as having false-positives. The likelihood of a positive radiograph being a true-positive is then 45/(45 + 498), or 0.08. In this example, only 1 of 12 positive chest radiographs (8%) represents a truly significant finding; the remainder are false-positives with potentially harmful effects. Unless the benefit from a true-positive result is many times greater than the potential for harm from a false-positive result, the net effect in this example is that routine radiographs cause more harm than good. Even if the benefit does outweigh the harm, the cost may be prohibitive because of the large number of negative studies done to find the few significant abnormalities as well as the cost of evaluating the many associated false-positive tests.

Example 2: For chest radiography to be useful, the prevalence of chest disease would have to be much higher than 0.5%. Consider a patient with a 10% likelihood of chest disease. If we assume the same sensitivity and specificity as in Example 1, the likelihood of a positive finding on a radiograph being a true-positive is 0.67. Now, unless the potential harm from a false-positive result is very high, radiographs in such patients will do more good than harm. Chest radiography targeted at patients likely to have chest disease will probably be beneficial.

These examples were partly simplified for clarity. A full decision analysis would include the costs and consequences stemming from all possible results of chest radiographs. We omitted consideration of false-negative results because they occur with negligible frequency when disease prevalence is low. Adequate consideration of the different consequences from various radiographic results is not possible with the data presently available.

CHEST RADIOGRAPHY TO EVALUATE SUSPECTED CHEST DISEASE

The preceding discussion of screening is limited to patients in whom there is no clinical suspicion of active chest disease after a history and physical examination have been done. The situation in patients with signs and symptoms of chest disease is quite different, as in Example 2. These patients have symptoms, physical findings, or other disease states associated with chest disease, and chest radiography should be helpful in their assessment. The literature supports this view. Thomsen and colleagues (29) found significant abnormalities on preoperative chest films in 24% of 695 patients with cardiopulmonary problems, although only 2 patients had changes in therapy. Haubek and Cold (34) identified 64 patients with suspected cardiopulmonary disease; 24 of these patients had abnormal findings on chest radiographs, 11 of whom had changes in preoperative planning.

In contrast to suspected active chest disease, a history of cardiac or pulmonary disease has not been associated with the need for a repeat chest radiograph. In the series reported by Hubbell and coworkers (2), 86 of 106 abnormal "routine" chest radiographs simply confirmed previously known findings. In only three patients (with lung carcinoma) was there worsening of disease in the absence of clinical clues.

VALUE OF THE HISTORY AND PHYSICAL EXAMINATION

Some have justified doing routine chest radiographs by arguing that the cursory history and physical examination sometimes done on hospital admission may not be sensitive enough to replace the chest radiograph as a screening test. They argue that rather than spending money on a more thorough clinical evaluation, perhaps we should instead do a screening chest radiograph. This issue has been partially addressed by the studies of the impact of routine chest radiographs on patient management (discussed earlier). Four of the seven studies have relied on retrospective study designs (29-31, 33) in which the clinical evaluations consisted of routine presurgical evaluations. The extremely low yield of unknown or unsuspected abnormalities on radiographs indicates that these routine examinations did not miss many significant diseases. Apparently, the current standard of preoperative clinical assessment is adequate for screening purposes. Furthermore, a good preoperative clinical evaluation has the added benefits of searching for multiple problems other than chest disease, allowing assessment of risk factors, establishing a clinical baseline, reassuring the patient through physician-patient contact, and reducing medicolegal risk. Indeed, the basic history and physical examination make up the one diagnostic maneuver that cannot be eliminated.

SITE OF OPERATION

Although not explicitly studied, it seems clear that patients having procedures involving the chest cavity should have routine chest radiographs to define the anatomy of that area. It may also be prudent to obtain routine films on patients having operations in sites close to the chest (for example, upper abdomen) or procedures with a high risk of postoperative chest complications. However, these issues remain unstudied.

Unresolved Issues

Although many studies present evidence that routine preoperative chest radiographs do not enhance patient care, a carefully designed, large prospective study, as discussed earlier, is needed to eliminate the possibility that investigator bias has resulted in underestimating the benefits of this procedure. In addition, by including a group of patients with clinical evidence of chest disease, such a study could also attempt to relate clinical factors to chest radiographic findings that result in improved patient outcomes. This study would enable physicians to be selective in the use of radiography for symptomatic patients. Better data are also needed on the operating characteristics (sensitivity and specificity) of the chest radiograph in identifying clinically important chest conditions in the selected population of patients without apparent chest disease. This information, combined with accurate prevalence data, might identify certain target populations in whom the effectiveness of screening chest radiography could be shown. Lacking these data, we recommend that physicians use clinical judgment in selecting patients who are at high risk for chest disease.

Although several studies (2, 3, 33, 40, 43, 44) have shown an increasing prevalence of chest radiographic abnormalities with advancing patient age (Table 3), the presence of these abnormalities does not necessarily justify the procedure. Well-designed studies of routine radio-

Table 3. Chest Radiographic Abnormalities in Patients Stratified by Age

	Patient Age					
	< 30	31-40	41-50	51-60	61-70	> 70
	n/n					
Hubbell et al. (2)	0/12	5/22	5/28	32/87	34/94	30/51
Rees et al. (3)	2/108	12/93	23/119	48/121	58/134	58/92
Rucker et al. (33)	26/392	6/148	14/114	38/114	41/104*	...
Tornebrandt and Fletcher (40)	...	...	...	...	...	43/91
Fink et al. (43)	1/3	1/6	3/10	20/38	12/22	15/24
Sagel et al. (44)	9/1415	22/942	66/928	179/833	290/997	347/832
Total	38/1930 (2.0%)	46/1211 (3.8%)	111/1199 (9.3%)	317/1193 (27%)	394/1247 (32%)	493/1090 (45%)

* Includes patients greater than age 60; data not pooled in totals.

Table 4. Recommendations on the Routine Use of Chest Radiographs*

A chest radiograph is not routinely indicated solely because of hospital admission.

A chest radiograph is not routinely indicated as part of a preoperative evaluation, before administration of anesthesia, or for a baseline assessment.

Patients in whom an admission or preoperative chest radiograph is indicated should be identified on the basis of a clinical suspicion of active chest disease identified during a history and physical examination.

A chest radiograph is not indicated solely because of advanced age. However, because of the high prevalence of symptoms and signs of chest disease in this age group, many elderly patients will require a chest film for their evaluation.

A routine preoperative chest radiograph is generally indicated for patients scheduled for intrathoracic surgery.

---

* These guidelines are intended to assist physicians in assessing the need for a chest radiograph. The history and physical examination and the clinical judgment of the physician will determine the need for the procedure.

graphs in the elderly are lacking. Nevertheless, patients with clinically significant chest conditions in any age group should have signs or symptoms that will identify the problem or lead the physician to pursue further evaluation including chest radiography.

A history of smoking is another area that deserves study. We are not aware of any studies demonstrating that smokers should have routine preoperative or admission chest radiographs. Significant smoking-related chest disease should be apparent on the history and physical examination. Clinically silent disease related to smoking, such as early carcinoma, would be unlikely to affect short-term patient outcomes adversely and is not currently recommended as a target for screening chest radiography (47).

Summary

Routine screening chest radiographs done at the time of hospital admission or before surgery will identify various abnormalities. However, most of these abnormal findings will not have a significant impact on patient management or outcome. The likelihood of finding clinically occult but significant disease is probably extremely small. If routine chest radiographs are done, a large number of false-positive results will occur with possible adverse consequences for these patients. A history and physical examination can be used to select a group of patients who are suspected of having chest disease and in whom chest radiography is indicated to evaluate the suspected disease further. Table 4 lists our proposed indications for ordering chest radiographs.

Appendix: Methodologic Criteria for Evaluating Studies of Routine Chest Radiography

Population Studied and Selection Criteria	Expectation Bias*	Independent Contribution from Film Assessed†	Outcome Assessed‡
Preoperative radiographs			
Rees et al. (3)			
Large hospital in Wales; 667 consecutive patients admitted for elective surgery	Probable	Yes	No
Royal College of Radiologists (18)			
8 hospitals; 10 619 patients with a wide spectrum of diseases; consecutive admissions for elective surgery§	Probable	No	Yes
Thomsen et al. (29)			
Amt Hospital, Copenhagen; 1823 consecutive surgical patients	Probable	Yes	Yes
Wood and Hoekelman (30)			
2 university teaching hospitals; 1924 consecutive patients admitted for elective surgery, age < 19§	Probable	Yes	Yes
Farnsworth et al. (31)			
County hospital; 350 patients admitted for elective surgery; multiple exclusions	No	Yes	Yes
Sane et al. (32)			
Children's hospital; 1500 consecutive patients, age < 20	Probable	Yes	Yes
Rucker et al. (33)			
University hospital; 905 consecutive surgical patients	Probable	Yes	Yes

Appendix: (Continued)

Population Studied and Selection Criteria	Expectation Bias*	Independent Contribution from Film Assessed†	Outcome Assessed‡
Haubek and Cold (34)			
Hvidovre Hospital, Copenhagen; 400 consecutive patients admitted for elective surgery	Probable	Yes	Yes
Loder (35)			
District general hospital; 1000 consecutive patients; routine preoperative films	Probable	No	No
Maigaard et al. (36)			
1256 consecutive patients from surgery and obstetrics/gynecology department	?	Yes	Yes
Tornebrandt and Fletcher (40)			
University hospital, Sweden; 100 consecutive patients admitted for elective surgery, age > 70	Probable	Yes	Yes, but inadequate
Radiographs other than preoperative			
Hubbell et al. (2)			
Veterans Administration Hospital; 742 consecutive patients admitted to medicine service from emergency room	Probable	Yes	Yes
Sewell et al. (41)			
50 elderly patients (mean age, 81); selection criteria not specified	Probable	Yes	Yes
Fink et al. (43)			
Veterans Administration Hospital; 113 patients; all medical admissions	Probable ‖	No	No
Sagel et al. (44)			
University hospital; 10 597 patients from all services; selection criteria not specified	Probable	Yes	No

* Expectation bias occurs when the clinical diagnosis is known to the interpreter of the radiograph. *Probable* indicates that the radiographic reports were the basis of the diagnosis; in most settings, radiographs are read with knowledge of the clinical diagnosis.

† The independent contribution of the chest radiograph is diagnostic information that was not suspected from a prior clinical evaluation.

‡ Relevant outcomes are perioperative complications or changes in surgical, anesthetic, or medical management.

§ Fewer than 50% of patients in these series had chest radiographs.

‖ Radiographs were interpreted by both medical residents and radiologists.

References

1. WHO SCIENTIFIC GROUP ON THE INDICATIONS FOR AND LIMITATIONS OF MAJOR X-RAY DIAGNOSTIC INVESTIGATIONS. *A Rational Approach to Radiodiagnostic Investigations.* Geneva, Switzerland: World Health Organization; 1983:7-28. (*WHO Technical Report Series* No. 689).
2. HUBBELL FA, GREENFIELD S, TYLER JL, CHETTY K, WYLE FA. The impact of routine admission chest x-ray films on patient care. *N Engl J Med.* 1985;**312:**209-13.
3. REES AM, ROBERTS CJ, BLIGH AS, EVANS KT. Routine preoperative chest radiography in non-cardiopulmonary surgery. *Br Med J.* 1976;**1:**1333-5.
4. KERR IH. The preoperative chest x-ray. *Br J Anaesth.* 1974;**46:**558-63.
5. ROIZEN MF. Routine preoperative evaluation. In: MILLER RD, ed. *Anesthesia.* New York: Churchill Livingstone; 1981:3-19.
6. MILNE ENC. Chest radiology in the surgical patient. *Surg Clin North Am.* 1980;**60:**1503-18.
7. MANUEL FR. Hospital admission chest x-rays [Letter]. *Can Med Assoc J.* 1974:**110:**889-90.
8. POLLARD B. Routine investigations in elective surgical patients [Letter]. *Med J Aust.* 1979;**2:**370.
9. AINLEY-WALKER JC. Routine preoperative chest x-rays [Letter]. *Anaesthesia.* 1979;**34:**686.
10. JACOBS JC. Chest x-ray screening for tuberculosis [Letter]. *JAMA.* 1974;**228:**24-5.
11. The preoperative chest x-ray [Editorial]. *NZ Med J.* 1980;**91:**18.
12. Preoperative chest x-rays [Editorial]. *Lancet.* 1979;**1:**141.
13. LISTON EH, GERNER RH, ROBERTSON AG, FORD CV. Routine thoracic radiography for psychiatric inpatients. *Hosp Community Psychiatry.* 1979;**30:**474-6.
14. HUGHES J, BARRACLOUGH BM. Value of routine chest radiography of psychiatric patients. *Br Med J.* 1980;**281:**1461-2.
15. HADLOCK FP, PARK SK, WALLACE RJ. Routine radiographic screening of the chest in pregnant women: is it indicated? *Obstet Gynecol.* 1979;**54:**433-6.
16. BONEBRAKE CR, NOLLER KL, LOEHNEN CP, MUHM JR, FISH CR. Routine chest roentgenography in pregnancy. *JAMA.* 1978;**240:**2747-8.
17. AMERICAN ACADEMY OF PEDIATRICS COMMITTEE ON HOSPITAL CARE. Preoperative chest radiographs. *Pediatrics.* 1983;**71:**858.
18. ROYAL COLLEGE OF RADIOLOGISTS WORKING PARTY ON THE EFFECTIVE USE OF DIAGNOSTIC RADIOLOGY. Preoperative chest radiology: national study by the Royal College of Radiologists. *Lancet.* 1979;**2:**83-6.
19. AMERICAN COLLEGE OF RADIOLOGY. *Referral Criteria for Chest X-ray Examinations.* [Policy Statement]. Chicago: American College of Radiology; 1982.
20. NATIONAL CENTER FOR DEVICES AND RADIOLOGICAL HEALTH. *The Selection of Patients for X-ray Examinations: Chest X-ray Screening Examinations.* Rockville, Maryland: Food and Drug Administration; 1983. HHS publication no. (FDA) 83-8204.
21. GREENE R. Screening chest radiography: its role in modern medicine. *Australas Radiol.* 1982;**26:**10-6.
22. YERUSHALMY J. The statistical assessment of the variability in observer perception and description of roentgenographic pulmonary shadows. *Radiol Clin North Am.* 1969;**7:**381-92.
23. YERUSHALMY J. Reliability of chest radiography in the diagnosis of pulmonary lesions. *Am J Surg.* 1955;**89:**231-40.
24. HERMAN PG, GERSON DE, HESSEL SJ, et al. Disagreements in chest roentgen interpretation. *Chest.* 1975;**68:**278-82.

25. HERMAN PG, HESSEL SJ. Accuracy and its relationship to experience in the interpretation of chest radiographs. *Invest Radiol.* 1975;**10**:62-7.
26. NICKLAUS TM, STOWELL DW, CHRISTIANSEN WR, RENZETTI AD JR. The accuracy of the roentgenologic diagnosis of chronic pulmonary emphysema. *Am Rev Respir Dis.* 1966;**93**:889-99.
27. BAUMSTARK A, SWENSSON RG, HESSEL SJ, et al. Evaluating the radiographic assessment of pulmonary venous hypertension in chronic heart disease. *AJR.* 1984;**142**:877-84.
28. YOUNG MJ, BRESNITZ EA, STROM BL. Sample size nomograms for interpreting negative clinical studies. *Ann Intern Med.* 1983;**99**:248-51.
29. THOMSEN HS, GOTTLIEB J, MADSEN JK, et al. [Routine radiographic examination of the thorax prior to surgical intervention under general anaesthesia]. *Ugeskr Laeger.* 1978;**140**:765-8.
30. WOOD RA, HOEKELMAN RA. Value of the chest x-ray as a screening test for elective surgery in children. *Pediatrics.* 1981;**67**:447-52.
31. FARNSWORTH PB, STEINER E, KLEIN RM, SANFILIPPO JA. The value of routine preoperative chest roentgenograms in infants and children. *JAMA.* 1980;**244**:582-3.
32. SANE SM, WORSING RA, WIENS CW, SHARMA RK. Value of preoperative chest x-ray examinations in children. *Pediatrics.* 1977;**60**:669-72.
33. RUCKER L, FRYE EB, STATEN MA. Usefulness of screening chest roentgenograms in preoperative patients. *JAMA.* 1983;**250**:3209-11.
34. HAUBEK A, COLD G. [The indications and consequences of preoperative radiography of the thorax]. *Ugeskr Laeger.* 1978;**140**:772-3.
35. LODER RE. Routine pre-operative chest radiography: 1977 compared with 1955 at Peterborough District General Hospital. *Anaesthesia.* 1978;**33**:972-4.
36. MAIGAARD S, ELKJAER P, STEFANSSON T. [Value of routine preoperative radiographic examination of the thorax and ECG]. *Ugeskr Laeger.* 1978;**140**:769-71.
37. CATCHLOVE BR, WILSON RM, SPRING S, HALL J. Routine investigations in elective surgical patients: their use and cost effectiveness in a teaching hospital. *Med J Aust.* 1979;**2**:107-10.
38. DELAHUNT B, TURNBULL PRG. How cost effective are routine preoperative investigations? *NZ Med J.* 1980;**92**:431-2.
39. ROBERTS CJ, FOWKES FGR, ENNIS WP, MITCHELL M. Possible impact of audit on chest x-ray requests from surgical wards. *Lancet.* 1983;**2**:446-8.
40. TORNEBRANDT K, FLETCHER R. Pre-operative chest x-rays in elderly patients. *Anaesthesia.* 1982;**37**:901-2.
41. SEWELL JMA, SPOONER LLR, DIXON AK, RUBENSTEIN D. Screening investigations in the elderly. *Age Ageing.* 1981;**10**:165-8.
42. FEINGOLD AO. Routine chest roentgenograms on hospital admission do not discover tuberculosis. *South Med J.* 1977;**70**:579-80.
43. FINK DJ, FANG M, WYLE FA. Routine chest x-ray films in a Veterans Hospital. *JAMA.* 1981;**245**:1056-7.
44. SAGEL SS, EVENS RG, FORREST JV, BRAMSON RT. Efficacy of routine screening and lateral chest radiographs in a hospital-based population. *N Engl J Med.* 1974;**291**:1001-4.
45. NEUHAUSER D. Cost effective clinical decision making: are routine pediatric preoperative chest x-rays worth it? *Ann Radiol (Paris).* 1978;**21**:80-3.
46. ROBBINS JA, MUSHLIN AI. Preoperative evaluation of the healthy patient. *Med Clin North Am.* 1979;**63**:1145-56.
47. EDDY E. ACS report on the cancer-related health checkup. *CA.* 1980;**30**:193-240.

Indications for Arterial Blood Gas Analysis

THOMAS A. RAFFIN, M.D.

ARTERIAL BLOOD GAS analysis is done to evaluate oxygen and carbon dioxide gas exchange and acid-base status. In assessing the current state of arterial blood gas analysis for pH, Pco_2, Po_2, and calculated bicarbonate, I have reviewed techniques for measuring arterial blood gases, quality control, normal values, and indications in clinical practice, as well as the role of newer noninvasive techniques. In conclusion, I offer recommendations for appropriate use of arterial blood gas analysis. Other tests less commonly done on arterial blood samples, including oxyhemoglobin saturation, determination of oxygen content, carboxyhemoglobin, methemoglobin, and P_{50}, are not discussed.

In the 1950s significant advances were achieved in the development of efficient electrodes that could accurately measure pH, Pco_2, and Po_2 (1, 2). Presently, automated blood gas analyzers are available that can measure pH, PCo_2, Po_2 and calculated bicarbonate in arterial blood samples within 1 minute (3). The stimuli for this development are a result of the remarkable growth of intensive care units and life-support equipment (including sophisticated ventilators and pulmonary function and exercise testing) and the practice of open-heart surgery.

Currently, general indications for arterial blood gas analysis are remarkably broad and little clinical investigation has been done to show validity or generalizability. One recent study of 227 laboratories doing arterial blood gas analysis reported the number of analyses done in a 24-hour period (4). By taking their most conservative data, one can compute that approximately 6.7 million analyses were done in these 227 laboratories in 1 year.

▶ This chapter was originally published in *Annals of Internal Medicine*. 1986;105:390-8.

Charges per analysis usually average from $60 to $80. Thus, these 227 laboratories accounted for at least $402 million in charges. Given that there are over 6000 acute care hospitals and 50 000 beds in critical care wards in this country, the cost for all analyses is probably far greater than this figure.

During the enormous growth in the number of arterial blood gas analyses performed, concurrent technologic development has produced devices with the potential for noninvasively analyzing blood gases. Ear and finger oximeters, mass spectrometry for evaluating inspired and expired gas concentrations, and transcutaneous electrodes are all in different stages of clinical study and use. Thoughtful and scientific quality control for arterial blood gas analysis only began in the early 1980s (5). It is hoped that current noninvasive technology development will fall under more stringent quality control before there is widespread clinical application.

Obtaining the Sample

An arterial blood gas sample can be obtained either by an arterial puncture with a needle and syringe or by withdrawing a sample from an indwelling arterial line (6). Contamination of the arterial blood sample with room air or excess heparin must be minimized (7). Clean, sterile, closely fitting glass syringes should be used to minimize leakage or diffusion of gases from the sample. Plastic syringes may allow loss of gas or contamination (8). Special preheparinized plastic syringes have been developed, but their efficacy has not yet been established.

The optimal site for sampling is the radial artery (9). An Allen test should be done to assess adequacy of collateral circulation (10). The second choice for an arterial puncture is the brachial artery; if necessary the femoral artery can be used. In infants, the temporal artery is an effective site for obtaining blood gases. Very small diameter needles (25 gauge) minimize trauma and pain, although larger needles (20 to 23 gauge) are easier to use (11). The sample should be transferred in ice and evaluated using a blood gas analyzer as soon as possible because delay, especially when leukocyte counts are high, can markedly decrease the Po_2 due to metabolism (12).

Intra-arterial catheters are usually placed in the radial artery and sometimes in the femoral, axillary, or brachial arteries (6). Femoral artery placement is not preferred because the catheter may be dislodged and the risk of infection is relatively high. A continuous flushing system with a low dose of heparin is used to maintain the patency of the line. Intra-arterial catheters facilitate the drawing of blood, especially when blood gas analyses are done at frequent intervals (greater than five per day); when the exact timing of the sample is important as in an exercise study; and when arterial punctures might interfere with a test, as during a sleep study (13). Complications of arterial puncture or cannulation are infrequent but include hematoma, bleeding, arterial thrombosis, arterial occlusion, local infection, and sepsis (14).

Analyzing the Sample

The most widely used analyzers are equipped with electrodes for measuring pH, P_{CO_2}, and P_{O_2} (3). The amount of bicarbonate is either obtained from a nomogram or calculated by a computer program. Oxyhemoglobin saturation is measured only by a co-oximeter, not by routine arterial blood gas analyzers. If a value for oxyhemoglobin saturation is read from a nomogram and reported, it can be misleading because the true oxyhemoglobin saturation might be significantly different. Manual blood gas analyzers have been widely replaced by automated machines capable of rapid analysis of blood samples as small as 0.15 mL (6).

Measurement Errors

Errors can occur during sampling, transport to the blood gas analyzer, or during analysis of the blood sample. Excessive amounts of heparin in the syringe should be avoided and small air bubbles should be removed. The temperature of the electrodes and the calibration gases must be 37 °C. It is important to know the temperature of the patient, because there are significant temperature corrections used in determining pH, P_{CO_2}, and P_{O_2} (15). Protein contamination of the blood gas analyzer will also cause errors. Contamination can be avoided by ensuring heparinization of samples and by following recommended cleaning procedures.

Range of Normal Values

The normal values for pH, P_{CO_2}, and P_{O_2} are based on a limited number of studies of arterial blood gas results in normal persons (9). The accepted range of two standard deviations for a normal pH is 7.35 to 7.45 (16). Only healthy, nonsmoking subjects were studied to measure this range (17). The accepted range of two standard deviations for a normal PCO_2 is 35 to 45 mm Hg (18). Of the several studies attempting to identify the normal range for PCO_2, Minty and Nunn (19) determined the 95% confidence limit for normal persons to be 30 to 45.8 mm Hg from a review of seven published studies. Filley and associates (20) studied 19 normal men and found a mean PCO_2 of 38.8 ± 3.16 mm Hg (one standard deviation).

Hypoxemia can be defined as a PO_2 less than 80 mm Hg (9). However, a number of investigators have analyzed PO_2 values in normal persons and have developed regression equations. Mellemgaard (21) studied 80 patients and calculated a predictive regression equation of $PO_2 = 104.2 - 0.27 \times$ age (in years). Sorbini and associates (22) studied 152 normal persons and calculated a predictive equation of arterial $PO_2 = 109 - 0.43 \times$ age (in years). Sorbini and associates had a greater age regression but it is important to note that they excluded smokers and subjects who were supine during sampling.

Reproducibility of arterial blood gas values has not been well studied. Estimates of the range of repeated measurements are: pH ± 0.02, PCO_2 ± 3.0 mm Hg, and PO_2 ± 3.0 mm Hg (17).

Quality Control

Uniform blood gas quality control is vital if data are to be accurate, reproducible, and comparable among different institutions (5). In 1982 blood gas quality control and proficiency testing materials were evaluated by tonometry in two geographically separate laboratories (5). Using three models of semi-automated blood gas machines, PO_2 and PCO_2 concentrations in fresh blood, plasma, and several commercial quality-control materials were systematically evaluated by tonometry, sampled, and measured. No significant difference was discovered between materials or machines for PCO_2 between 25 to 72 mm Hg. For PO_2 values of approximately 25 to 100 mm Hg, however, there were significant differences when using quality-control materials with hemoglobin, fluorocarbons, or low-oxygen-capacity materials. It was determined that significant contamination of blood gas machines with fluids other than the samples was occurring. This contamination resulted in quality-control materials of low oxygen capacity being inadequate for proficiency testing when the Po_2 was below 100 mm Hg. Thus, this study identified a need for better quality control and standardization of proficiency testing materials.

As a result of this study, the American Thoracic Society began a blood gas survey in an attempt to standardize quality control and identify uniform proficiency testing materials. In 1984, results of a monthly interlaboratory pH and blood gas survey were reported (23). Data were collected from 131 laboratories. Average errors were characterized on a percentile ranking basis that enabled participating laboratories to assess their performance as compared with that of peer laboratory results. When samples had normal Pco_2 levels, 95% of reported laboratory results had an error of 4.5 mm Hg or less. When samples had normal Po_2 levels, 95% of reported results had an error of 13 mm Hg or less and 95% of the pH results had an error of 0.05 pH units or less. This type of interlaboratory pH and blood gas survey is essential to quality control.

A recent survey of 227 acute care and blood gas laboratories was done through the memberships of the Society of Critical Care Medicine and the National Association of Medical Directors of Respiratory Care (4). Key findings included uneven quality control in terms of types and frequencies of procedures and variable education of laboratory personnel. Certification of laboratory personnel was mainly through the National Board for Respiratory Care, but 36% of the personnel had no certification or registration. Thus, uniform quality control and utilization of established proficiency testing materials has not yet been achieved in analyzing arterial blood gas.

General Indications

Although the general indications for arterial blood gas sampling and analysis proposed in medical and pulmonary textbooks are extremely broad, few of these indications have been shown to be clinically valid or applicable to the broad patient population. Fundamentally, if the physician suspects that the patient has a significant aberration in oxygen or carbon dioxide gas exchange or acid-base balance, then arterial blood gas analysis is recom-

Table 1. Common Reasons for Doing Arterial Blood Gas Analysis

Gas exchange abnormalities (P_{O_2}, P_{CO_2})
  Acute and chronic pulmonary disease
    Obstructive (bronchitis, emphysema, chronic obstructive
      pulmonary disease, asthma)
    Restrictive (pneumonia, atelectasis, pulmonary edema,
      acute or chronic infiltrative lung disease)
    Pulmonary vascular (pulmonary embolism, vasculitis)
    Ventilatory control (sleep apnea syndromes,
      hyperventilation syndrome, central nervous system
      disease)
  Acute respiratory failure
    Any obstructive disease (bronchitis, emphysema, chronic
      obstructive disease, asthma)
    Adult respiratory distress syndrome
    Trauma
    Drugs and toxins
  Cardiovascular diseases
    Congestive heart failure
    Shock (with pulmonary shunt)
  Rest and exercise pulmonary function tests
  Monitoring acute and chronic oxygen therapy
  Sleep disorder studies
Acid-base disturbances
  Metabolic acidosis
    Lactic acidosis
    Renal failure
    Ketoacidosis
    Poisons (carbon monoxide, methanol, ethylene glycol)
  Metabolic alkalosis
    Hypochloremia, hypokalemia
    Gastric suctioning or vomiting
    Sodium bicarbonate administration

mended (9, 24-26). Most reviews point out that the entire therapeutic approach to patients with pulmonary disease and especially patients with respiratory failure is based on the presence and extent of blood gas and pH abnormalities. Some authors refer to lists of diseases and pathophysiologic processes that often will require arterial blood gas analysis. For example, in one textbook (9) devoted to the clinical application of blood gases, at least 31 common clinical diseases were discussed with reference to arterial blood gas results.

Critically ill patients in intensive care units are evaluated by serial arterial blood gas analyses, and there are very few studies of how many samples are actually necessary in the management of these patients. The same is true of postoperative patients and patients with chronic respiratory failure who are not critically ill. A complete list of clinical situations involving significantly ill patients where an analysis of arterial blood gas might be indicated would consist of most of the table of contents of a general medical or pulmonary textbook. Table 1 shows an abbreviated list of indications. However, criteria for performing this analysis are largely lacking, and only a few indications have been studied specifically.

Specific Indications

The role of arterial blood gas analysis in patient care has been studied in several clinical situations. In these studies the clinical rationale for the application of this analysis is presented. Validity can be determined by ascertaining whether arterial blood gas analysis identifies patients at an increased risk for a bad outcome or whether the result can reveal an effective intervention. Finally, if the clinical premise is valid then it must be shown to apply to other patient populations.

PATIENTS WITH ACUTE ASTHMA IN THE EMERGENCY ROOM

Arterial blood gas analysis is recommended for acutely ill asthmatic patients presenting to emergency rooms (27, 28). However, arterial blood gas tensions are poorly correlated with the severity of asthma as measured by pulmonary function testing (29, 30).

Peak expiratory flow rates (PEFR) and forced expiratory volume in 1 second (FEV_1) can identify asthmatic patients at risk for hypercarbia, hospitalization, and respiratory failure. Therefore, measurement of PEFR or FEV_1 might help to avoid the use of this analysis in patients not at risk. In one study (31), data resulting from 89 emergency visits by 51 asthmatic patients showed a small but statistically significant correlation between arterial blood gas parameters and PEFR ($p < 0.05$). No patient who had a PEFR greater than 25% of predicted had a Pco_2 greater than 45 mm Hg or pH less than 7.35. These authors (31) proposed that only patients with a PEFR less than 25% predicted are at risk for significant hypercarbia or acidosis and should have routine arterial blood gas analysis done. The authors estimated that if PEFR is used as a simple screening tool, it may be possible to safely eliminate at least 40% of these analyses in acute asthmatic patients.

A more recent study prospectively evaluated pre- and post-treatment arterial blood gas and pulmonary function testing measurements in order to compare their ability to assess asthma severity and to predict outcome in patients with acute asthma attacks initially seen in an emergency room (32). This analysis (pH, Pco_2, Po_2) could not be used to separate patients requiring admission from those that could be confidently discharged. However, FEV_1 and PEFR before and after treatment were sufficient to do so. In this study, patients with hypercarbia (Pco_2 greater than 42 mm Hg) or severe hypoxemia (Po_2 less than 60 mm Hg) had a PEFR below 200 L/min or an FEV_1 below 1.0 L. The authors (32) concluded that restrictive use of this analysis by means of PEFR should substantially decrease both diagnostic cost and patient discomfort without jeopardizing health care. However, the authors did not check the accuracy of their rule by evaluating a new set of patients. In other words, the generalizability of their rule has not been assessed. Also, it should be emphasized that these findings were in asthmatic patients and should not be applied to patients with chronic obstructive pulmonary disease.

Therefore, a significant percentage of analyses might be avoided if acute asthmatic patients are evaluated by simple pulmonary function testing. Furthermore, pulmonary function predicts the need for admission whereas arterial blood gas analysis is often not helpful. However, it is not yet clear if the cost effectiveness of routine pulmonary function testing (PEFR or FEV_1) in acute asthmatic patients is superior to more frequent blood gas analyses.

AFTER CORONARY ARTERY BYPASS GRAFT SURGERY

Coronary artery bypass graft surgery is one of the commonest surgical procedures. Patients often remain intubated until the first morning after surgery. The mean time on the ventilator is approximately 16 hours (33), and approximately 11 analyses are done during this time. If patients could be extubated earlier after coronary artery bypass graft surgery, fewer analyses would be required because patients normally require at the most one analysis to assess oxygen therapy after extubation.

In 1972, Klineberg and associates (34) reported that 62% of 72 patients receiving narcotic anesthesia were able to be safely extubated within 5 hours after cardiac surgery. Quasha and coworkers (35) compared 18 patients extubated early with 20 patients extubated later after coronary artery bypass graft surgery. The 38 patients were randomly assigned and all received inhalational anesthesia. The late extubation group had more than twice the number of "morbid events." Lichtenthal and colleagues (36) reported in 1983 that 40 of 100 patients undergoing cardiac surgery met criteria for extubation 90 minutes after surgery and were extubated without any problems. The authors stated that the use of inhalational anesthesia was the major factor that minimized the time on postoperative mechanical ventilation. Most cardiac surgery is done with high-dose narcotic anesthesia, which is thought to be safer but requires a longer time on the ventilator after surgery.

In 1984 Foster and associates (33) did a prospective study of ventilator management and weaning after coronary artery bypass graft surgery using narcotic anesthesia. Twenty-seven of sixty-three patients in the study were managed by a standard weaning protocol, and 36 were managed by a newly developed (and more efficient) ventilation and weaning protocol. By applying this new protocol the mean time to extubation was decreased by 41% (from 16 to 11 hours) and arterial blood gas sampling was reduced 42%. There were no deaths in either group. Of significant interest was the fact that respiratory therapists were able to carry out this protocol without close physician supervision.

Thus, several studies show that decreasing the time of intubation after coronary artery bypass graft surgery can safely reduce the number of arterial blood gas analyses. This result has been shown in patients receiving narcotic anesthesia and inhalational anesthesia. Even though inhalational anesthesia requires a shorter period of postoperative mechanical ventilation, there is still controversy over which anesthetic technique is superior.

PULMONARY EMBOLISM

In the past, it was thought that a low Po_2 was consistent with a diagnosis of pulmonary embolism and a normal Po_2 essentially ruled out this diagnosis (37, 38). However, in 1973 the published results from the National Heart and Lung Institute's Urokinase Pulmonary Embolism Trial (38) revealed that 11.5% of patients with significant pulmonary embolism had an arterial oxygen tension above 80 mm Hg. Thus, although a normal Po_2 reduced the probability of pulmonary embolism, the finding could no longer be said to exclude the diagnosis.

Respiratory alkalosis is also commonly seen in patients with acute pulmonary embolism. However, patients with previous cardiopulmonary disease sometimes do not develop hypocarbia with acute pulmonary embolism and thus there is no predictive value in the extent of arterial hypocarbia (39, 40). Furthermore, hypercarbia is common in acute respiratory disease.

Thus, at the present time arterial blood gas analysis cannot definitely rule out the diagnosis of pulmonary embolism, and a finding of significant hypoxemia is nonspecific. Of interest, Dantzker and Bower (39) have collected blood gas samples from 54 patients involved in three separate studies who had pulmonary embolism shown by angiography, and 13% of these patients had an arterial Po_2 of 80 mm Hg or more. However, in those patients where an alveolar-arterial oxygen difference could be calculated, when the arterial Po_2 was 80 mm Hg or greater, the alveolar-arterial Do_2 was always abnormally widened. Therefore, data are accumulating to suggest that, although significant pulmonary embolism can have occurred when there is a normal arterial Po_2, the alveolar-arterial Do_2 will usually be abnormally widened.

STABLE PATIENTS IN INTENSIVE CARE UNITS

Frequent measurement of arterial blood gases is a routine component of intensive care management. Serial arterial blood gases are evaluated to monitor a patient's progress; to adjust oxygen and other medication regimens; and to make management decisions concerning assisted ventilation, positive end-expiratory pressure, and weaning from ventilatory support. Clinicians occasionally make management decisions based on small isolated changes in arterial blood gas values, but little information was available concerning spontaneous fluctuations in arterial blood gases in seriously ill patients until the study of Thorson and associates (41). These authors measured the degree of variation in arterial blood gas values when there were no apparent changes in the patient's clinical condition. The lowest and highest Po_2 and Pco_2 ranged from 1 to 45 mm Hg (16.2 ± 10.9 mm Hg) and 1 to 8 mm Hg (3 ± 1.9 mm Hg), respectively. The pH varied within 0.03 ± 0.02 units. The average change in PO_2 between sequential intrapatient samples was $5.3 \pm 2.8\%$ and $7.1 \pm 7.9\%$ over 10- and 50-minute intervals, respectively. Thus, considerable spontaneous variation occurs, even in stable patients. The authors recommended that clinicians take care not to base therapeutic decisions on small changes in PO_2 that were unrelated to changes in clinical status.

This study (41) is important because it gives insight into the sampling variation expected to occur between sequential blood gas values over a brief time in clinically stable but critically ill patients. Clinicians should be careful when interpreting PO_2 changes in such patients. Also, clinical research that evaluates changes in PO_2 should take into account the variability of arterial blood gas values in stable patients in intensive care units.

INDICATIONS AND MONITORING OF OXYGEN THERAPY

In 1984 the American College of Chest Physicians and the National Heart, Lung and Blood Institute sponsored a National Conference on Oxygen Therapy (13). It was recognized that there were few studies that identified indications for arterial blood gas analysis or guidelines for monitoring oxygen therapy. Thus, the conference attempted to establish criteria in large part on the basis of clinical practice. The subcommittee reporting on indications for oxygen therapy recognized that the cost of an arterial blood gas analysis approximates that of 24 to 48 hours of in-hospital oxygen therapy. Thus, the subcommittee concluded it is not always cost effective to document hypoxemia when it is suspected on a clinical basis. Furthermore, they stated that stopping oxygen therapy when the clinical condition of the patient is improved does not necessarily require documentation by arterial blood gas analysis.

The conference (13) supported the position that arterial blood gas analysis is seldom indicated in patients with acute uncomplicated myocardial infarction. These patients are routinely placed on moderate-flow supplemental oxygen. In the only prospective, controlled, double-blind clinical trial on the use of oxygen in patients with myocardial infarction, there was no significant difference between the oxygen-treated and control groups in mortality, incidence of arrhythmias, use of analgesics, or systolic time intervals (42, 43).

The report (13) from the national conference also presented guidelines for institution of long-term supplemental oxygen therapy. It was emphasized that long-term oxygen therapy should only be considered for patients who have been on an optimal medical regimen for 30 days or more before evaluating arterial blood gases. If patients have an arterial Po_2 of 55 mm Hg or less, as measured at rest in the nonrecumbent position, long-term oxygen therapy is recommended. Clearly, in this patient subpopulation, arterial blood gas analysis would be necessary to identify patients meeting the guidelines.

In the conference subgroup on monitoring oxygen therapy, although attention was paid in a broad sense to the consideration of cost and benefit when performing arterial blood gas analysis, no effort was made to identify general or specific indications for this analysis.

ARTERIAL OXYGEN TENSION AT DIFFERENT
CONCENTRATIONS OF INSPIRED OXYGEN

Many formulas have been proposed to calculate the expected response of arterial oxygen tension to different fractions of inspired oxygen being delivered to patients (44, 45). These equations cannot be used when patients receive fluctuating fractions of inspired oxygen, as occurs when oxygen is delivered by nasal cannula or mask. However, such formulas could be of value in patients who are on assisted ventilation because the fraction of inspired oxygen (Fio_2) remains relatively constant and the ability to predict arterial oxygen tensions accurately at different concentrations of inspired oxygen may enable physicians to decrease the number of serial arterial blood gases drawn in the intensive care unit. However, difficult and time-consuming calculations would certainly impede the acceptance of such formulas.

In 1981, Gross and Israel (46) developed a nomogram that would allow rapid and simple prediction of arterial oxygen tensions at different concentrations of inspired oxygen in mechanically ventilated patients. They assumed that the ratio of arterial to alveolar oxygen tension provides an index of respiratory impairment that remains relatively unchanged over the range of Fio_2 from 0.21 to

1.0. They prospectively studied nine patients and used their nomogram to evaluate 16 changes in FIO_2 that were all judged desirable by the attending physicians. When Gross and Israel compared the predicted PO_2 with that actually obtained by arterial blood gas analysis, there was a mean difference of only 4.6%, or 2.6 mm Hg. Thus, in patients who do not have rapidly changing pulmonary function, a predictive nomogram could possibly decrease the number of serial arterial blood gases taken over a circumscribed period of time. If the patient's pulmonary status changes—for example if atelectasis, increased lung water, or infection develops—the relationship between the PO_2 and the alveolar oxygen tension would change and the nomogram would no longer be accurate.

VENOUS BLOOD GAS ANALYSIS

Since 1959 there has been interest in venous blood gas analysis (47-50). Because venous blood is easier to draw, it was hoped that its accuracy would be similar to arterial blood gas analysis. Early work suggested that peripheral venous acid-base status was closely correlated to arterial acid-base status (47, 48). However, there were few patients with abnormal blood gas results.

More recent studies generally agree that although gross abnormalities of gas exchange can be found in blood gas analysis of samples from a central venous line (not a pulmonary artery catheter), that procedure is at best recommended only for screening because of its inaccuracy (49, 50). Periodically, peripheral venous sampling has been proposed for critically ill patients when rapid acid-base analysis would be of importance. However, on theoretical grounds peripheral venous sampling is significantly less reliable in defining acid-base status than central venous sampling (50). Thus, although there continues to be interest in both central venous and peripheral venous blood gas analysis for estimation of acid-base status in critically ill patients, the literature and present standard of practice do not support such procedures.

DIRECT POSTOPERATIVE MEASUREMENT OF WOUND AND TISSUE OXYGEN TENSIONS

Adequate tissue perfusion after surgery is important for wound healing (51, 52). Chang and associates (53) in 1983 studied oxygen tension in the wounds of 33 post-operative patients using an implanted catheter. They discovered that wound hypoxia was common, and that hypovolemia was a common cause of postoperative tissue hypoxia. The authors stated that measurements of tissue oxygen tension, coupled with a single arterial oxygen determination, constitute a clinically useful means of monitoring tissue perfusion. This study (53) sheds light on tissue oxygenation in postoperative patients. However, studies of this nature should not be translated into clinical practice until controlled, prospective trials that show the cost effectiveness of the proposed laboratory test are done.

Alternatives to Analyzing Arterial Blood Samples

Over the past two decades, noninvasive means of assessing oxygen and carbon dioxide gas exchange have been investigated. Although little progress has been made in noninvasive pH measurement, there have been four important areas of technologic development: oximetry; transcutaneous gas measurement; inspired-expired gas measurements; and indwelling intravascular electrodes or fiberoptic systems.

OXIMETRY

An oximeter is a spectrophotometer that measures the absorbency of light due to oxyhemoglobin and can be used to determine the concentration of oxyhemoglobin in blood. A co-oximeter is found in many arterial blood gas laboratories and can simultaneously analyze arterial blood samples and report the amount of reduced hemoglobin, oxyhemoglobin, carboxyhemoglobin, and methemoglobin (54). Oximetry only identifies oxyhemoglobin saturation and gives no insight into PCO_2 or pH. Furthermore, marked changes in PO_2 can occur with small corresponding changes in saturation if the pH is above 90%.

Ear oximetry is a noninvasive method for evaluating arterial oxygenation (55). Ear oximeters are commonly used in both sleep studies and exercise laboratories (56). Ear oximeters are accurate in selected patients although caution must be used in the presence of jaundice, carboxyhemoglobin levels above 3%, or reduced blood flow (57).

The National Conference on Oxygen Therapy pointed

out that ear oximetry can be valuable in various clinical settings when intermittent arterial blood gas sampling is likely to miss important variations (13). Examples included using ear oximetry during bronchoscopy in patients at risk for desaturation, and to assess oxygen requirements in hypoxemic patients.

Recently, simplified ear oximeters have been marketed and are claimed to be as accurate as and have equivalent response characteristics to the older, more elaborate oximeters (56). Also, finger pulse oximeters have recently been developed and are presently being used in operating rooms to detect sudden arterial desaturation (57, 58). A finger pulse oximeter is similar to a classical oximeter in that discrete wave lengths of light are used to measure the optical density due to hemoglobin. However, the unique feature of the finger pulse oximeter is that it distinguishes arterial blood from venous blood and tissue.

However, there have been no prospective, controlled studies of oximeters involving patients with acute or chronic respiratory failure or patients in intensive care units. The effects of significant alterations in blood pressure, tissue perfusion, temperature, or the relative concentrations of hemoglobin on the oximeter reading must be studied. More importantly, do oximeters improve patient care by reducing the need for arterial blood gas measurements, reduce hospitalization, and prolong life?

TRANSCUTANEOUS OXYGEN AND CARBON DIOXIDE MEASUREMENTS

The Clark and Severinghaus electrodes can be adapted to measure the gas tension of oxygen and carbon dioxide through the skin (59, 60). Transcutaneous oxygen electrodes require high blood flow in the skin. Currently available transcutaneous electrodes heat the skin under the sensor to 43 to 45 °C to increase local blood flow. Because of the elevation in skin temperature there is often local erythema under the electrodes and a potential for significant burns unless the electrode is periodically moved to different sites.

Transcutaneous oxygen electrode measurements correlate well with arterial oxygen tensions as long as there is adequate tissue perfusion (61, 62). However, some anesthetic agents have caused incorrect transcutaneous oxygen electrode data (63). A recent study showed that transcutaneous Po_2 measurements correlate poorly with arterial Po_2 in adults during general anesthesia (64). Other factors that can cause inaccurate measurements include increased oxygen consumption at the skin site; a shift in the oxyhemoglobin dissociation curve; variability in skin permeability; and insufficient skin perfusion.

Noninvasive monitoring of blood gases using skin electrodes has been studied best in critically ill neonates (57, 65, 66). Transcutaneous carbon dioxide electrode measurements correlate well with arterial Pco_2 measurements when perfusion is adequate. A recent retrospective study compared transcutaneous Po_2 and Pco_2 values to simultaneously drawn arterial blood gas values in 500 neonates. Transcutaneous Pco_2 measurements are a reliable substitute for arterial or capillary Pco_2. Transcutaneous Po_2, on the other hand, was not the same as arterial or capillary Po_2, although the direction of changes in transcutaneous Po_2 measurements reflected trends in arterial or capillary Po_2 (67).

The National Conference on Oxygen Therapy (13) reported that transcutaneous oxygen electrode measurements were useful and commonly used in neonatal intensive care units but were not yet of proven benefit in adult patients. Also, transcutaneous oxygen electrode measurements may be useful for noninvasive exercise testing but ear oximetry may be preferable. Further clinical experience is necessary to show if measurements made with transcutaneous oxygen and carbon dioxide electrodes can reduce the need for arterial blood gas analysis.

INSPIRED AND EXPIRED GAS MEASUREMENTS

Monitoring the fraction of expired oxygen in patients on closed systems may readily be done with inexpensive devices. However, actually measuring the inspired and expired oxygen difference to calculate oxygen consumption is extremely difficult (13, 68).

Expired carbon dioxide can be measured by various methods but the two commonest methods of practical value are the rebreathing equilibration technique and rapid carbon dioxide analysis. Rapid carbon dioxide analysis uses infrared spectroscopy or mass spectrometry (13). Measuring expired carbon dioxide concentrations only approximates the arterial Pco_2. The correlation depends on many factors including cardiac output, respira-

Table 2. Recommendations for the Diagnostic Use of Arterial Blood Gas Analysis

1. In general, when adults are severely ill and in life-threatening situations due to conditions that produce gas exchange abnormalities or acid-base disturbances, arterial blood gas analysis should be done.

2. In general, when adults are chronically ill and stable, arterial blood gas analysis should only be done when a change in management is being considered or there is a change in clinical status. If the key question concerns oxygenation as compared to PCO_2 or acid-base disturbances, then noninvasive means such as oximetry should be considered. Unfortunately, there have been only few clinical situations where indications for arterial blood gas analysis have been studied.

3. Arterial blood gas analysis of patients with acute asthma in the emergency room can be decreased in frequency by the use of screening spirometry (peak expiratory flow rates [PEFR] or forced expiratory volume in 1 second [FEV_1]). If the PEFR or FEV_1 is adequate then this analysis will usually not be required. However, comparative costs need to be more carefully evaluated.

4. Stable patients in intensive care units have significant fluctuations in their PO_2. Therefore, physicians should not overreact and order unnecessary arterial blood gas analyses when confronted with predictable changes unaccompanied by alterations in clinical status.

5. By using standardized and well-studied weaning protocols, along with safe techniques for limiting mechanical ventilation time after surgery, the number of arterial blood gas measurements can be decreased. This has been shown in patients undergoing coronary artery bypass graft surgery.

6. In general, severely ill neonates can have carbon dioxide gas exchange effectively evaluated by transcutaneous PCO_2 electrode measurements. Oxygenation can be followed over time by PO_2 transcutaneous electrodes but individual values do not accurately predict true arterial or capillary PO_2 values.

7. Patients receiving prophylactic low-flow oxygen in the hospital usually do not need to have an arterial blood gas analysis done. For example, patients with acute uncomplicated myocardial infarctions do not need to have this analysis done before, during, or at the discontinuation of low-flow supplemental nasal oxygen.

8. Patients who are candidates for long-term supplemental oxygen therapy or who are undergoing sleep or exercise studies can have their oxygen gas exchange evaluated by finger or ear oximetry.

9. Although a normal PO_2 does not rule out pulmonary embolism, the presence of a normal alveolar-arterial oxygen difference makes it highly unlikely that a significant recent pulmonary embolism has occurred. Thus, arterial blood gas analyses are most useful in this setting when alveolar-arterial DO_2 values are calculated.

Table 2 (Continued)

10. Noninvasive arterial blood gas analysis using finger or ear oximetry, or transcutaneous electrodes in critically ill adults needs further clinical study. Comparative cost analysis between invasive and noninvasive analysis will be important. Finally, the usefulness of inspired-expired gas measurement, venous arterial blood gas analysis, tissue oxygen tension determination, and indwelling arterial blood gas measurement has yet to be verified.

tory exchange ratio, as well as ventilation-perfusion relationships (57). Although recent reports have supported the use of end-tidal PCO_2 measurements, it is not clear if the data are accurate, especially when the patient has pulmonary dysfunction (69). The usefulness of these measurements in replacing arterial blood gas analysis is yet to be verified.

SYSTEMS FOR CONTINUOUS INDWELLING
MEASUREMENT

An adaptation of a Clark PO_2 electrode for intravascular use was developed in 1958. Since that time there have been a number of continuous arterial measurement systems that have been developed and tested in patients (70, 71). Some of these systems use gas chromatography and others mass spectrometry. Difficulties with continuous indwelling measurement systems have been their questionable reliability and an increased risk for thromboembolism (72). These systems are expensive and require considerable expertise (73). More clinical investigation is necessary before this approach to arterial blood gas analysis will be accepted as standard practice.

Oximeters have been developed in pulmonary artery catheters to continuously monitor mixed venous oxygen saturation (74). Although continuous measurement of mixed venous oxygen saturation can give insight into overall cardiorespiratory status and trends, the impact of these data on patient care decisions has not been measured (75, 76).

Conclusions

The recommendations for the diagnostic use of arterial blood gas analysis derived from this review are listed in Table 2.

References

1. MOHLER JG. The basics for clinical blood gas evaluation. In: WILSON AF, ed. *Pulmonary Function Testing, Indications and Interpretations.* Orlando, Florida: Grune & Stratton; 1985:153-73.
2. CLARK LC. Monitor and control of blood and tissue oxygen tensions. *Trans Am Soc Artif Intern Organs.* 1956;**2:**41-8.
3. NATIONAL COMMITTEE FOR CLINICAL LABORATORY STANDARDS. *Percutaneous Collection of Arterial Blood for Laboratory Analysis.* 1985:1-24. (Publication code H11-A.)
4. HALL JR, SHAPIRO BA. Acute care/blood gas laboratories: profile of current operations. *Crit Care Med.* 1984;**12:**530-3.
5. HANSEN JE, STORE MF, ONG ST, VAN KESSEL AL. Evaluation of blood gas quality control and proficiency testing materials by tonometry. *Am Rev Respir Dis.* 1982;**125:**480-3.
6. SHOEMAKER WC. Monitoring of the critically ill patient. In: SHOEMAKER WC, THOMPSON WL, HOLBROOK PR, eds. *Textbook of Critical Care.* Philadelphia: W. B. Saunders; 1984:105-21.
7. CISSIK JH, SALUSTRO J, PATTON OL, et al. The effects of sodium heparin on arterial blood gas analysis. *CVP.* 1977;**5:**17-33.
8. ABRAMSON J, VERKAIK G, MOHLER JG. Blood gas stability in terumo plastic and glass syringes. *Respir Care.* 1978;**23:**63-4.
9. SHAPIRO BA, HARRISON RA, WALTON JR. *Clinical Applications of Blood Gases.* Chicago: Year Book Medical Publishers; 1982.
10. ALLEN EV. Thromboangitis obliterans: methods of diagnosis of chronic occlusive arterial lesions distal to the wrist with illustrative cases. *Am J Med Sci.* 1929;**178:**237-44.
11. SABIN S, TAYLOR JR, KAPLAN AL. Clinical experience using a small-gauge needle for arterial puncture. *Chest.* 1978;**69:**437-9.
12. HESS CE, NICHOLS AB, HUNT WB, SURATT PM. Pseudohypoxemia secondary to leukemia and thrombocytosis. *N Engl J Med.* 1979;**301:**361-3.
13. FULMER JD, SNIDER GL. ACCP-NHLBI National Conference on Oxygen Therapy. *Chest.* 1984;**86:**234-47.
14. DAVIS FM, STEWART JM. Radial artery cannulation: a prospective study in patients undergoing cardiothoracic surgery. *Br J Anaesth.* 1980;**52:**41-7.
15. ASHWOOD ER, KOST G, KENNY M. Temperature control of blood-gas and pH measurements. *Clin Chem.* 1983;**29:**1877-85.
16. SEVERINGHAUS JW. Blood gas concentrations. In: FENN WO, RAHN H, eds. *The Handbook of Physiology, Section 3: Respiration.* Baltimore: Williams & Wilkins, American Physiological Society; 1964:1475-87.
17. MOHLER JG, COLLIER CR, BRANDT W, ABRAMSON J, VERJAIK G, YATES S. Blood gases. In: CLAUSEN JL, ed. *Pulmonary Function Testing—Guidelines and Controversies.* New York: Academic Press; 1982:226-57.
18. SEVERINGHAUS JW. Measurements of blood gases: Po_2 and Pco_2. *Ann NY Acad Sci.* 1968;**148:**115-32.
19. MINTY BD, NUNN JF. Regional quality control survey of blood-gas analysis. *Ann Clin Biochem.* 1977;**14:**245-53.
20. FILLEY GF, GREGORIE F, WRIGHT GW. Alveolar and arterial oxygen tensions and the significance of the alveolar-oxygen tension difference in normal men. *J Clin Invest.* 1954;**33:**517-29.
21. MELLEMGAARD K. The alveolar-arterial oxygen difference: its size and components in normal man. *Acta Physiol Scand.* 1966;**67:**10-20.
22. SORBINI CA, GRASSI V, SOLINAS E, MUIESAN G. Arterial oxygen tension in relation to age in healthy subjects. *Respiration.* 1968;**25:**3-13.
23. EHRYMEYER SS, LAESSIG RH, GARBER CC. Monthly interlaboratory pH and blood-gas survey: establishing accuracy based on interlaboratory performance. *Am J Clin Pathol.* 1984;**81:**224-9.

24. FISHMAN AP. *Pulmonary Diseases and Disorders.* New York: McGraw-Hill; 1980.

25. MURRAY JF. Respiratory structure and function. In: WYNGAARDEN JB, SMITH LH, eds. *Cecil Textbook of Medicine.* Philadelphia: W. B. Saunders; 1982:339-49.

26. SNIDER GL. *Clinical Pulmonary Medicine.* Boston: Little, Brown & Co.; 1981.

27. NARDELL EA, SLATE JL, WESTPHAL DM, et al. Asthma. In: WILKINS EW, DINEEN JJ, MONCOURE AC, eds. *Massachusetts General Hospital Textbook of Emergency Medicine.* Baltimore: Williams & Wilkins; 1979:133-55.

28. UNGAR JR. Respiratory emergencies associated with bronchial asthma. In: SCHWARTZ GR, SAFER P, STONE JH, et al., eds. *Principles and Practices of Emergency Medicine.* Philadelphia: W. B. Saunders; 1979:855-89.

29. KELSEN SG, KELSEN DP, FLEEGER BF, JONES RC, RODMAN T. Emergency room assessment and treatment of patients with acute asthma. *Am J Med.* 1978;**64**:622-8.

30. MCFADDEN ER JR, LYONS HA. Arterial-blood gas tension in asthma. *N Engl J Med.* 1968;**278**:1027-32.

31. MARTIN TG, ELENBAAS RM, PINGLETON SH. Use of peak expiratory flow rates to eliminate unnecessary arterial blood gases in acute asthma. *Ann Emerg Med.* 1982;**11**:70-3.

32. NOWAK RM, TOMLANOVICH MC, SARKER DD, KVALE PA, ANDERSON JA. Arterial blood gases and pulmonary function testing in acute bronchial asthma: predicting patient outcomes. *JAMA.* 1983;**249**:2043-6.

33. FOSTER GH, CONWAY WA, PAMUKLOV N, LESTER JL, MAGILLIGAN DJ JR. Early extubation after coronary bypass: brief report. *Crit Care Med.* 1984;**12**:994-6.

34. KLINEBERG PL, GEER RT, HIRSH RA, AUKBURG SJ. Early extubation after coronary artery bypass graft surgery. *Crit Care Med.* 1977;**5**:272-4.

35. QUASHA AL, LOEBER N, FEELEY TW, ULLYOT DJ, ROIZEN MF. Postoperative respiratory care: a controlled trial of early and late extubation following coronary artery bypass grafting. *Anesthesiology.* 1980;**52**:135-41.

36. LICHETENTHAL PR, LEONARD WD, NIEMSKY PR, SHAPIRO BA. Respiratory management after cardiac surgery with inhalation anesthesia *Crit Care Med.* 1983;**11**:603-5.

37. WILSON JE III, PIERCE AK, JOHNSON RL JR, et al. Hypoxemia in pulmonary embolism: a clinical study. *J Clin Invest.* 1971;**50**:481-91.

38. The urokinase pulmonary embolism trial: a national cooperative study. *Circulation.* 1973;**47**(suppl 2):1-108.

39. DANTZKER DR, BOWER JS. Alterations in gas exchange following pulmonary thromboembolism. *Chest.* 1982;**81**:495-501.

40. LIPPMANN M, FEIN A. Pulmonary embolism in the patient with chronic obstructive pulmonary disease: a diagnostic dilemma. *Chest.* 1981;**79**:39-42.

41. THORSON SH, MARINI JJ, PIERSON DJ, HUDSON LD. Variability of arterial blood gas values in stable patients in the ICU. *Chest.* 1983;**84**:14-8.

42. MADIAS JE, MADIAS NE, HOOD WB JR. Precordial ST segment mapping: II. Effects of oxygen inhalation on ischemic injury in patients with acute myocardial infarction. *Circulation.* 1976;**53**:411-7.

43. MAROKO PR, RADVANY P, BRAUNWALD E, HALE SL. Reduction of infarct size by oxygen inhalation following acute coronary occlusion. *Circulation.* 1975;**52**:360-8.

44. MITHOEFER JC, KEIGHLEY JF, KARETZKY MS. Response of the arterial Po_2 to oxygen administration in chronic pulmonary disease: interpretation of findings in a study of 46 patients and 14 normal subjects. *Ann Intern Med.* 1971;**74**:328-35.

45. GILBERT R, KEIGHLEY JF. The arterial-alveolar oxygen tension ratio: an index of gas exchange applicable to varying inspiratory oxygen concentrations. *Am Rev Respir Dis.* 1974;**109**:142-5.

46. GROSS R, ISRAEL RH. A graphic approach for prediction of arterial oxygen tension at different concentrations of inspired oxygen. *Chest.* 1981;**79**:311-5.

47. GAMBINO SR. The clinical value of routine determination of venous plasma, pH and acid-base problems. *Am J Clin Pathol.* 1959;**32**:301-3.

48. JUNG RC, BALCHUM OJ, MASSEY FJ. The accuracy of venous and capillary blood for the prediction of arterial pH, Pco_2 and Po_2 measurements. *Am J Clin Pathol.* 1966;**45**:129-38.

49. PHILLIPS B, PERETZ DI. A computation of central venous and arterial blood gas values in the critically ill. *Ann Intern Med.* 1969;**70**:745-9.

50. SUTTON RN, WILSON RF, WALT AJ. Difference in acid-base levels and oxygen-saturation between central venous and arterial blood. *Lancet.* 1967;**2**:748-51.

51. KNIGHTON DR, SILVER IA, HUNT TK. Regulation of wound-healing angiogenesis—effective oxygen gradients in inspired oxygen concentrations. *Surgery.* 1981;**90**:262-70.

52. PAI MP, HUNT TK. Effect of varying oxygen tensions on healing of open wounds. *Surg Gynecol Obstet.* 1972;**135**:756-8.

53. CHANG N, GOODSON WH III, GOTTRUP F, HUNT TK. Direct measurement of wound and tissue oxygen tension in postoperative patients. *Ann Surg.* 1983;**197**:470-8.

54. MALENFANT AL, GAMBINO SR, WARAKSA AJ, ROE EI. Spectrophotometric determination of hemoglobin concentrations and percentage of oxyhemoglobin and carboxyhemoglobin saturation [Abstract]. *Clin Chem.* 1968;**14**:789.

55. TRASK CH, CREE EM. Oximeter studies on patients with chronic obstructive emphysema awakened during sleep. *N Engl J Med.* 1962;**266**:639-42.

56. CHAPMAN KR, D'URZO A, REBUCK AS. The accuracy and response characteristics of a simplified ear oximeter. *Chest.* 1983;**83**:860-4.

57. BURKI NK, ALBERT RK. Noninvasive monitoring of arterial blood gases: a report of the ACCP section on respiratory pathophysiology. *Chest.* 1983;**83**:666-70.

58. MIHM FG, HALPERIN BD. Noninvasive detection of profound arterial desaturations using a pulse oximetry device. *Anesthesiology.* 1985;**62**:85-7.

59. LUBBERS DW. Theoretical basis of the transcutaneous blood gas measurements. *Crit Care Med.* 1981;**9**:721-33.

60. EBERHART RC, WEIGELT JA. Continuous blood gas analysis: an elusive ideal [Editorial]. *Crit Care Med.* 1980;**4**:418.

61. Transcutaneous O_2 and CO_2 monitoring of the adult and neonate. *Crit Care Med.* 1981;**9**:689-760.

62. TREMPER KK, SHOEMAKER WC, SHIPPY CR, NOLAN LS. Transcutaneous Pco_2 monitoring in adult patients in the ICU and the operating room. *Crit Care Med.* 1981;**9**:752-5.

63. VENUS B, PATEL KC, PRATAP KS, KONCHIGERI H, VIDYASAGAR D. Transcutaneous PO_2 monitoring during pediatric surgery. *Crit Care Med.* 1981;**9**:714-6.

64. PACE NL, STANLEY TM, ANDRIANO KP, WILBRINK J, ZWAMKKEN P. Transcutaneous Po_2 poorly estimates arterial Po_2 in adults during anesthesia. *Int J Clin Monitor Comput.* 1985;**1**:227-32.

65. FALLET RJ. Respiratory monitoring. In: BONE RC, ed. *Critical Care— A Comprehensive Approach.* Park Ridge, Illinois: American College of Chest Physicians; 1984:189-205.

66. PEABODY JL, GREGORY GA, WILLIS MM, TOOLEY WH. Transcutaneous oxygen tension in sick infants. *Am Rev Respir Dis.* 1978;**118**:83-5.

67. VAN KESSEL AL, ARIAGNO RL, ROBIN ED. Clinical application of

transcutaneous g.. measurements in prematurely born infants [Abstract]. In: *Proceedings of the 11th Meeting of the International Federation of Clinical Chemistry*; 1985:33-43.

68. LEDINGHAM IM, MACDONALD AM, DOUGLAS IH. Monitoring of ventilation. In: SHOEMAKER WC, THOMPSON WL, HOLBROOK PR, eds. *Textbook of Critical Care.* Philadelphia: W. B. Saunders; 1984:121-36.

69. TAKKI F, AROMAA V, KAUSTE A. The validity and usefulness of the end-tidal Pco_2 during anesthesia. *Ann Clin Res.* 1972;**4**:278-84.

70. POLLITIZER MJ, SOUTTER LP, REYNOLDS EO. Continuous monitoring of arterial oxygen tension in infants: four years of experience with an intravascular oxygen electrode. *Pediatrics.* 1980;**66**:31-6.

71. RICHMAN KA, JOBES DR, SCHWALB AJ. Continuous in-vivo blood-gas determination in man: reliability and safety of a new device. *Anesthesiology.* 1980;**52**:313-7.

72. BRANTIGAN JW, GOTT VL, VESTAL ML, FERGUSSON GJ, JOHNSTON WH. A nonthrombogenic diffusion membrane for continuous in vivo measurements of blood gases by mass spectrometry. *J Appl Physiol.* 1970;**28**:374-7.

73. EBERHARD P, MINDT W, SCHAFER R. Cutaneous blood gas monitoring in the adult. *Crit Care Med.* 1981;**9**:702-5.

74. KRAUSS XH, VERDOUW PD, HUGENHOLTZ PG, NAUTA J. On-line monitoring of mixed venous oxygen saturation after cardiothoracic surgery. *Thorax.* 1975;**30**:636-43.

75. KANDEL G, ABERMAN A. Mixed venous oxygen saturation: its role in the assessment of the critically ill patient. *Arch Intern Med.* 1983;**143**:1400-2.

76. FAHEY PJ, HARRIS K, VANDERWARF C. Clinical experience with continuous monitoring of mixed venous oxygen saturation in respiratory failure. *Chest.* 1984;**86**:748-52.

The Erythrocyte Sedimentation Rate

Guidelines for Rational Use

HAROLD C. SOX, Jr., M.D.; and MATTHEW H. LIANG,
M.D., M.P.H.

AMONG THE MOST venerable of tests is the erythrocyte sedimentation rate (ESR). In 1918, Fahraeus (1) discovered that in pregnant women erythrocytes sedimented in plasma more rapidly than they did in nonpregnant women. Since then, with only minor modifications, the ESR has been used to detect and monitor a variety of diseases. Although a single measurement is inexpensive, the test is used frequently (1300 and 5400/month in two general hospitals [2, 3]) and is therefore expensive in the aggregate. In addition, the evaluation of a patient with an unexpectedly increased ESR may incur substantial costs.

Description

Because detailed descriptions and references are available in several reviews (4-6), the technical aspects of the ESR are summarized briefly.

An erythrocyte in plasma is subject to several forces. It is pulled down by gravitational force, which is directly proportional to the cell's mass. Upward forces include the buoyant force, which is proportional to the volume of the erythrocyte, and bulk plasma flow, which is due to currents established by downwardly moving cells. Erythrocytes normally settle slowly. When these cells become aggregated, they sediment rapidly because the proportional increase in their total mass (which determines the force exerted on them by gravity) exceeds the proportional increase in their volume.

▶ This chapter was originally published in *Annals of Internal Medicine.* 1986;**104**:515-23.

Erythrocyte aggregation is caused by electrostatic forces. These cells normally have a net negative charge and repel each other. Many plasma proteins are positively charged and neutralize the surface charge of erythrocytes, thereby reducing the repulsive forces and promoting aggregation (rouleaux formation). The plasma proteins known as acute-phase reactants include highly asymmetric molecules, such as fibrinogen, that are particularly effective facilitators of erythrocyte aggregation. The relative contribution of the plasma proteins to aggregation, on a scale of 10, is fibrinogen, 10; beta-globulin, 5; alpha-globulins, 2; gamma-globulins, 2; and albumin, 1. C-reactive protein in physiologic concentrations has no effect on the ESR. The rate is usually elevated in patients with proliferative diseases of immunoglobulin-producing cells (myeloma, macroglobulinemia, cryoglobulinemia, and cold agglutinin disease).

Disorders of erythrocytes also affect the ESR and may confuse the interpretation of the test. Anemia increases the ESR, probably because frictional forces between sedimenting aggregates are reduced. The ESR is directly proportional to the mass of the erythrocyte and inversely proportional to the area of its surface, which carries the negative charge that prevents aggregation. Large cells have a small surface-to-volume ratio and therefore less charge in relation to their mass than microcytes. Thus, macrocytes sediment more rapidly than normal cells, and microcytes sediment more slowly. In sickle cell disease, the abnormal shape of the erythrocyte interferes with rouleaux formation and retards sedimentation. These disorders and other conditions that affect the ESR are listed in Table 1.

TEST METHODS

The Westergren method for determining the ESR is recommended by the International Committee for Standardization in Hematology (7). Anticoagulated venous blood is diluted 4:1 with sodium citrate and put in a 200-mm glass tube with a 2.5-mm internal diameter. At the end of 1 hour, the distance from the meniscus to the top of the column of erythrocytes is recorded as the ESR. The modified Westergren method uses edetic acid (EDTA) rather than sodium citrate as an anticoagulant and is especially convenient because the same tube of blood can be used for the ESR and other hematologic

Table 1. Factors that Influence the Erythrocyte Sedimentation Rate (ESR)

Increase	Decrease	No Effect
Anemia	Sickle cell disease	Body temperature
Hypercholesterolemia	Anisocytosis	Recent meal
Female sex	Spherocytosis	Aspirin
Pregnancy	Acanthocytosis	Nonsteroidal
Tilted ESR tube	Polycythemia	anti-inflamma-
		tory drugs
High room	Extreme leukocytosis	
temperature		
Inflammatory disease	Bile salts	
	High doses of	
	adrenal steroids	
	Clotting of blood	
	sample	
	> 2-hour delay in	
	running the test	
	Low room tempera-	
	ture	
	Short ESR tube	
	Hypofibrinogenemia	
	Microcytosis	
	Congestive heart	
	failure	
	Cachexia	

studies. The modified and standard Westergren methods give essentially identical results. Some of the technical factors that influence the ESR are listed in Table 1. The Wintrobe method has been a popular technique for measuring the ESR but is less accurate than the Westergren method. All but one of the studies described in this article used the Westergren method.

THE RANGE OF NORMAL

The ESR is higher in women than in men and higher in older persons (Table 2) (8). Miller and colleagues (9) measured the ESR in 27 912 healthy adults between ages 20 and 65 years. They have derived an empirical formula for the value of the ESR that includes 98% of healthy persons: For men, age in years is divided by two, and for women, age in years plus ten is divided by two. The choice of an upper limit of normal is arbitrary. Some authors choose a value well above 2 SD above the mean in order to minimize false-positive results.

Asymptomatic Persons

Several issues should be considered in evaluating the role of the ESR in asymptomatic persons. First, in the studies being analyzed, how often was an elevated ESR the only finding that triggered a successful search for disease? Second, how often did an elevated ESR convince the clinician to start an ultimately successful investigation of another finding? Third, was the outcome of newly discovered diseases affected by the presymptomatic diagnosis?

Five studies of the effects of routinely performing an ESR are summarized in Table 3. In the only prospective study (10), women were randomly selected from the general population in Sweden. In the other studies, the rate was measured in subjects during a routine clinic visit (11, 12), on admission for elective surgery (13), or as part of an annual military examination (14). Three reports specified that a complete history and physical examination were done in addition to a few routine diagnostic tests (10, 12, 13). In three studies, all patients were reevaluated for disease that might have been overlooked at the index visit (10, 11, 14); in one study, only patients who had an unexplained increase in ESR were reevaluated periodically (13). Thus, although only one study design (10) was entirely satisfactory, these studies have provided reasonable assurance that all significant illnesses were detected.

INCREASED RATE AS THE SOLE CLUE TO SERIOUS DISEASE

Most patients with an increased ESR were easily diagnosed at the time of the initial history and physical exam-

Table 2. Upper Limit of Normal for the Erythrocyte Sedimentation Rate in Men and Women*

	Upper Limit of Normal
	mm/h
Age < 50 years	
Male	15
Female	20
Age > 50 years	
Male	20
Female	30

* Data from Bottiger and Svedberg (8).

Table 3. Effects of Doing the Erythrocyte Sedimentation Rate (ESR) as a Screening Procedure

Study Description (Reference)	Definition of Abnormal ESR	Patients with Increased ESR	ESR as Only Clue to Diagnosis
	mm/h	*n/n(%)*	*n(%)*
Random sample of Swedish women; 6-yr follow-up (10)	> 30	78/1462(5.3)	0
Clinic patients; 10-yr follow-up (11)	> 30 M > 35 W	790/9140(8.6)	5*(0.06)
Male clinic patients; no follow-up (12)	> 20	Not given	1†(0.05)
Surgical admissions; 6- to 42-mos follow-up (13)	‡	99/6148(6.0)	1§(0.06)
Israeli airmen aged 18 to 33; yearly follow-up for 15 yrs (14)	‖	44/1000(4.4)	10¶(1.0)

* Colonic cancer, pancreatic cancer, tuberculosis (in 2 patients) and systemic lupus erythematosus.

† Multiple myeloma.

‡ An abnormal ESR was defined as $\geq$ 15 mm/h for men < 50 years, $\geq$ 20 mm/h for women < 50, $\geq$ 20 mm/h for men > 50, and $\geq$ 30 mm/h for women > 50.

§ Patient died of prostate cancer 28 months after the index visit, at which there was no evidence of cancer and the ESR was 28 mm/h.

‖ An abnormal ESR was defined as one elevated to at least 2 SD above the mean for the same age group on at least three of four consecutive annual examinations.

¶ Ankylosing spondylitis (in 3 patients), myocardial infarction (in 4 patients), inflammatory bowel disease, psoriasis, and benign gammopathy were diagnosed several years after the abnormal ESR was first noted.

ination. When the test was included in a single screening examination, the ESR was the only clue to serious illness in 0.06% of patients. When the test was included in an annual screening examination in Israel of 1000 asymptomatic air crewmen, a persistently increased ESR (abnormal at three or more consecutive examinations) was present in 44 persons, of whom 10 subsequently developed disease (14). However, the yield of disease per ESR measurement was quite low, because 12 200 measurements were done during the 15-year study of 1000 men.

FREQUENCY OF FALSE-POSITIVE INCREASE

Two studies clearly indicated the number of patients with no detectable disease. Only 3 (0.2%) patients had an unexplainedly increased ESR among 1739 clinic patients (12). In the Israeli study, 3.5% of men without disease had an increased ESR at each of three or more consecutive yearly examinations (14). In the Swedish survey, 42 women (2.9%) had an unexplained increase.

INCREASED RATE LEADING TO INVESTIGATION OF ANOTHER FINDING

None of the studies was designed satisfactorily to assess the frequency with which an increased ESR led to investigation of another finding. However, one study (12) found eight patients (0.4%) in whom an increased ESR was said to be the clue that prompted a successful investigation of another finding.

OUTCOME OF DISEASES DETECTED SOLELY BY INCREASED RATE

Of 17 patients whose increased ESR was the sole initial clue to disease, 2 had tuberculosis and 1 had colonic cancer, both diseases in which the outcome is improved by early detection. One patient had systemic lupus erythematosus and 3 had ankylosing spondylitis, diagnoses that only became apparent after several years of observation. Four young men had a persistently elevated ESR several years before a myocardial infarction. The remaining patients had diseases whose outcomes are relatively unaffected by early detection: myeloma, prostate cancer, psoriasis, benign monoclonal gammopathy, and pancreatic cancer.

SUMMARY

The ESR makes a very small contribution to disease detection in asymptomatic persons. Fewer than 6 in 10 000 such persons will benefit from the test after a history and physical examination.

Symptomatic Patients

The ESR is sometimes used to provide confirmation when the history and physical findings point toward a diagnosis. The test is also used when the patient's chief complaint is not supported by evidence for a specific disease. In this situation, the physician uses the ESR to screen for any serious disease that may be present. Clinical studies have not provided sufficient information to define the role of the test in these two applications.

To evaluate the ESR in symptomatic patients, one must ask how well it predicts disease. The probability of a disease corresponding to an ESR result may be calculated with Bayes' theorem (15). Bayes' theorem requires that the pretest probability of the disease and the sensitivity and specificity of the ESR for the disease be known. Unless both sensitivity and specificity are known, a test cannot be interpreted in all situations.

The sensitivity of the ESR has been measured in many diseases, but its specificity has been measured accurately only a few times (16, 17). To understand why past studies are so limited, consider the design of an ideal study. The ESR is measured in all patients suspected of having a disease. All patients, regardless of the ESR results, undergo a definitive diagnostic procedure. Some study patients have the disease, and the sensitivity of the test is measured in them. The specificity of the ESR is measured in study patients who do not have the disease. In contrast to this ideal study design, the study populations in past studies have comprised only patients with a disease and not patients who were suspected of having the disease but did not. Because the specificity of the ESR for a disease has seldom been measured in the appropriate population, the frequency of a normal ESR in healthy persons is sometimes used as a proxy. This approach leads to error because the specificity of the ESR for a disease will be higher in healthy persons than in patients suspected of having the disease, who often have other diseases that increase the ESR.

The shortcomings of studies of the ESR affect only the interpretation of an abnormal ESR. As shown in Figure 1A, test specificity largely determines the probability of disease when the ESR is abnormal. Because the specificity of the ESR for most diseases is not known, the post-test probability when the ESR is abnormal cannot be calculated. When the ESR is normal, the sensitivity of the test determines the post-test probability of a disease (Figure 1B). Because the sensitivity of the ESR for many diseases is known, a normal ESR can be interpreted, even if its specificity is not known.

Patients with Vague, Unsubstantiated Illness

Patients whose history and physical findings do not suggest any cause for their illness are sometimes exam-

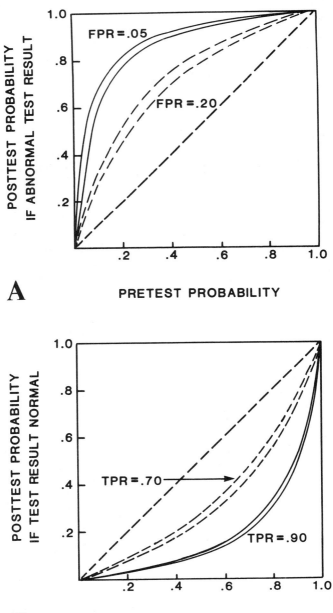

A PRETEST PROBABILITY

B PRETEST PROBABILITY

ined with the ESR. These patients' pretest probability of serious disease is presumably very low, perhaps nearly as low as that in asymptomatic persons. Although too little is known to be certain, several considerations suggest that the ESR is generally not useful in these patients.

In principle, either a normal or an increased ESR could be diagnostically useful. In practice, neither result is very useful. A normal ESR will exclude temporal arteritis, but the test is too often normal in other diseases to be of much value in excluding serious disease. An increased ESR is seldom a clue to unsuspected serious disease. As discussed in the introduction to this section, too little is known to interpret an increased ESR with confidence. However, when the pretest probability of disease is low, the post-test probability will be low unless the ESR is markedly elevated. The probability of some form of serious disease is probably relatively high when the ESR exceeds 50 mm/h, because in one population survey the ESR exceeded this rate in only 4 of 1462 women (16). However, the probability of a markedly increased ESR in a diseased person (a true-positive result) is very low when the pretest probability of disease is very low (15). This reasoning is substantiated by the very low frequency of an increased ESR in persons with unsuspected disease (Table 1).

These considerations suggest that the ESR is not very useful when the patient's symptom is unsubstantiated by the other clinical data. However, clinical studies of the ESR have not been done in such patients, and a precise recommendation cannot be made at present. Many diagnosticians will choose to focus on possible psychophysiologic explanations for symptoms and allow the evolution of the symptom over time to determine the need for diagnostic testing.

Figure 1. Relationship between pretest probability of disease and post-test probability. The post-test probability was calculated with Bayes' theorem. **Figure 1A.** The probability of disease in a patient with an abnormal test result. Two values for the false-positive rate (*FPR*) were assumed. For each value, the sensitivity of the test was assumed to be 0.9 (*top curve*) and 0.7 (*bottom curve*). **Figure 1B.** The probability of disease for a normal (or negative) test result. Two values for the sensitivity of the test (true-positive rate, *TPR*) were assumed. For each value, the false-positive rate of the test was assumed to be 0.2 (*top curve*) and 0.05 (*bottom curve*).

Cancer
OCCULT MALIGNANCY

Physicians often are concerned that patients with non-specific complaints have occult malignancy. Malignancy is quite common in symptomatic patients with an elevated ESR. In one study of 790 clinic patients with elevated rates, 70 (8.8%) had cancer (11). However, malignancy is seldom occult when the ESR is elevated: of the 70 patients with malignancy and an increased ESR, 68 had local signs that led directly to the diagnosis. Thus, occult malignancy was present in only 2 of 790 patients with an increased ESR. Malignancy develops infrequently in patients whose increased ESR cannot be explained. In a longitudinal study (10), no new cancers were detected in 6 years of surveillance of 42 women with an increased ESR that was unexplained after a thorough study at the start of the 6-year period.

INTERPRETATION OF THE RATE IN CANCER

The ESR is often normal in patients with cancer (Table 4). Peyman (18) measured the ESR in 300 patients within 6 weeks of establishing a histologic diagnosis of cancer. Only half of the patients had a rate of greater than 20 mm/h. Peyman's findings in patients with gastrointestinal cancer have been corroborated in two subsequent studies (19, 20). Furthermore, the ESR is seldom

Table 4. Prevalence of an Increased Erythrocyte Sedimentation Rate (ESR) in Patients with Cancer*

Type of Cancer	Patients	Prevalence of ESR > 10 mm/h	Prevalence of ESR > 20 mm/h
	n	*%*	*%*
Newly diagnosed cancer			
Myeloma	25	96	92
Colonic	27	89	63
Lung	101	82	61
Pancreatic	15	67	40
Gastric	51	65	31
Metastatic cancer			
To bone	38	87	74
To liver	58	79	57

* Adapted from Peyman (18).

the harbinger of malignancy in asymptomatic persons. In one longitudinal study, 0 of 11 women who developed cancer during a 6-year period of surveillance had an elevated ESR at the beginning of this period (10). In another study, 0 of 10 men who developed cancer during a 15-year period had a persistently increased ESR before developing clinical evidence of cancer (14).

As might be expected from Figure 1, a normal ESR has little effect on the probability of cancer in patients with vague symptoms. Bayes' theorem was used to calculate the probability of cancer if the ESR is 10 mm/h or less and the pretest probability of cancer is between 1% and 25%. The post-test probability of colonic cancer is 12% to 28% of its pretest value. The probability of gastric or pancreatic carcinoma, malignancies that present with few external clues, is reduced very little by a normal ESR (to 30% to 60% of the pretest probability). The lower bound of these ranges corresponds to an assumed specificity of 95% for an ESR of 10 mm/h or greater. The true specificity in patients who are suspected of having malignancy may be closer to 50%, which corresponds to the upper bound of these ranges.

METASTATIC CANCER

In patients with metastatic cancer, the ESR is usually elevated (Table 4). If these figures apply to patients with a low clinical suspicion of metastases, an ESR that is less than 10 mm/h reduces the probability of bone metastasis to 12% to 32% of its pretest value and that of liver metastasis to 22% to 48% of its pretest value (depending on whether the value assumed for specificity is 95% or 50%, as described earlier).

Extreme elevation of the ESR is a clue to metastatic cancer. In one study, all patients with cancer with a rate of greater than 100 mm/h also had metastases (2).

SUMMARY

The ESR is often normal in patients with cancer. Therefore, it is not a good test for excluding occult malignancy in patients with vague symptoms. The ESR can be useful in patients with known cancer: When the rate exceeds 100 mm/h in such a patient, metastases are usually present. However, a normal ESR does not exclude metastases.

Temporal Arteritis and Polymyalgia Rheumatica

Temporal arteritis (giant cell arteritis) and polymyalgia rheumatica are related syndromes that can occur alone or together. Both occur in older individuals and are associated with an increased ESR. The syndrome of polymyalgia rheumatica is characterized by severe aching and stiffness in the neck, shoulder girdle, or pelvic girdle areas. An increased ESR is a necessary criterion for the syndrome of polymyalgia rheumatica.

Patients with temporal arteritis almost always have an increased ESR (21, 22). In evaluating the ESR in the diagnosis of temporal arteritis, we included only studies in which the diagnosis was established by temporal artery biopsy (23-25). The findings were remarkably consistent (Table 5). The mean ESR exceeded 90 mm/h in all three studies and exceeded 30 mm/h in 136 of 138 patients (99%). These studies may underestimate the frequency of false-negative results, because patients with a normal ESR are not likely to undergo biopsy; nearly all patients with normal biopsy findings had an elevated ESR in one study (23). The false-positive rate of the ESR in patients who are suspected of having temporal arteritis is not known. In the studies summarized in Table 5, all but 1 patient with temporal arteritis had an ESR of greater than 50 mm/h, a rare finding in normal persons but probably common in persons who have diseases that may be confused with temporal arteritis.

INTERPRETATION OF A NORMAL RATE

The probability of temporal arteritis in a patient with a normal ESR is shown in Figure 2. Because the false-positive rate of the test in suspected temporal arteritis is unknown, two values (5% and 50%) were assumed. The probability of temporal arteritis is less than 1% for any

Table 5. The Erythrocyte Sedimentation Rate (ESR) in Patients with Proven Temporal Arteritis

Reference	Patients		Mean ESR
	ESR ≥ 30	ESR < 30	
	n	*n*	*mm/h*
Fauchald et al. (24)	60	1	93
Huston et al. (25)	42	0	96
Eshaghian and Goeken (23)	34	1	107

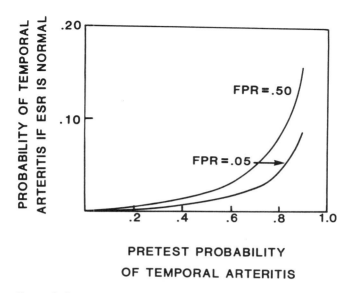

Figure 2. Probability of temporal arteritis if the erythrocyte sedimentation rate (*ESR*) is normal. The probability was calculated with Bayes' theorem. The sensitivity of the ESR in temporal arteritis is 0.99. Because the frequency of an increased ESR is not known in patients who are suspected of having temporal arteritis but do not, two values for the false-positive rate (*FPR*) were assumed: 0.5 (*top curve*) and 0.05 (*bottom curve*). The true value presumably lies within this range.

pretest probability up to 30%. Therefore, if there is little clinical evidence for temporal arteritis, a normal ESR excludes the diagnosis. However, if the clinical evidence is strong, temporal arteritis may be present despite a normal ESR (Figure 2). This conclusion has been substantiated by reports of temporal arteritis in patients with a normal ESR. Thus, if there is good clinical evidence for temporal arteritis, a normal ESR should be ignored, and the patient should have a temporal artery biopsy or an empirical trial of corticosteroids.

INTERPRETATION OF AN INCREASED RATE

When the ESR is increased, the interpretation depends on the clinician's pretest estimate of the probability of arteritis. The signs and symptoms of temporal arteritis, which include a tender, reddened, or nodular temporal artery, jaw claudication, and transient monocular blindness (26), are relatively specific. In patients with these findings, a very high ESR is almost certainly due to temporal arteritis and justifies initiation of high-dose corticosteroid therapy. Sometimes these findings are absent but temporal arteritis is suspected because of other findings (such as those of polymyalgia rheumatica). Using risk-benefit analysis, Chang and Fineberg (27) have shown that patients with polymyalgia rheumatica should receive high-dose corticosteroid therapy only if the probability of associated temporal arteritis is at least 50% and the physician is willing to accept the risk of up to 12 cases of severe corticosteroid toxicity to avoid 1 case of monocular blindness.

SUMMARY

The ESR is a cornerstone of diagnosis in patients with suspected temporal arteritis, a disease in which the rate is rarely normal. When the clinical evidence for temporal arteritis is weak, a normal ESR reduces the probability of the disease to less than 1%. When the clinical evidence is strong, the disease may be present despite a normal ESR.

Inflammatory Arthritis

The ESR is sometimes used to distinguish inflammatory arthritis from other causes of joint symptoms. An objective measure of the value of the test is its sensitivity and specificity for the diseases that cause inflammatory polyarthritis. The ideal population for measuring sensitivity and specificity should contain patients with undiagnosed joint symptoms whose diagnoses are determined independently of the ESR. A population survey of 1302 Scandinavian women is one of the few studies of the ESR that meets this criterion. Each woman had a careful joint examination, a Westergren ESR, and a serum rheumatoid factor assay (16). Thirty percent of the women reported joint symptoms in the preceding 6 years. In a subgroup with at least four symptoms or physical signs of rheumatoid arthritis, only 50% had an ESR that exceeded 30 mm/h. If one assumes that these women had rheumatoid arthritis, a normal ESR is scant evidence against the diagnosis.

An abnormal ESR may aid in the diagnosis of rheumatoid arthritis. The ESR is lower in women with signs of osteoarthritis (defined in the Scandinavian study as pain in the knees or hips and pain or crepitation on movement of the knees) than in women with signs of rheumatoid arthritis (16). Only 14% of women with signs of osteoarthritis had an ESR of greater than 30 mm/h, as compared with 50% of women with rheumatoid arthritis. Therefore, an abnormal ESR increases the probability of rheumatoid arthritis in women with joint symptoms, although not by a great deal.

The perceived role of the ESR in rheumatoid arthritis is reflected in the criteria for the classification of rheumatoid arthritis of the American Rheumatism Association (28), which are intended not for diagnosis but for classifying patients for clinical investigation. An increased ESR is used only in the classification of "possible" rheumatoid arthritis and then only as 1 of 20 findings that may be present in addition to clinical findings and at least 3 months of symptoms. An elevated ESR is not a criterion for "classic," "definite," or even "probable" rheumatoid arthritis. Although the ESR is sometimes used when other rheumatic diseases are suspected, its value as an independent diagnostic predictor of these diseases remains to be established.

In summary, the ESR has a limited role in diagnosing joint symptoms. A careful joint examination is far more important in confirming synovitis than is the ESR. A normal rate is very weak evidence against rheumatoid arthritis, whereas an increased rate in a patient with polyarthritis or polyarthralgia suggests inflammatory joint disease but is not diagnostic. The ESR is useful principally when the diagnosis is obscure and evidence for inflammation will affect therapy.

Suspected Infection

Clinicians sometimes use the ESR to confirm a suspicion of infection. Most studies of the ESR in patients with infectious diseases were done in the 1930s. Some used the Westergren method and are applicable to current practice. Wintrobe (29) noted that the ESR may be normal in the first several days after the onset of an infection and that the ESR returns to normal more slowly than the leukocyte count or body temperature. Thus, leukocytosis and fever are better indicators of an acute infection in its early stages than is an increased ESR. Bannick and colleagues (30) showed that only 2 of 25 patients with nonruptured appendicitis had an ESR of greater than 20 mm/h, in contrast to 67% of patients with ruptured appendixes and 86% of patients with pelvic inflammatory disease. Banyai and Anderson (31) characterized 128 patients who had tuberculosis and a normal ESR. Nearly one half had advanced cavitary disease, one third were febrile, and one half had hemoptysis. These patients were part of a series of 1730 consecutive admissions of patients with tuberculosis. Clearly, a normal ESR does not exclude pulmonary tuberculosis.

An Extreme or Unexplained Increase

Diagnostic searches prompted by extreme or unexplained ESR results can be extensive and are often futile and avoidable.

VERY HIGH RATE

Most patients with an ESR that exceeds 100 mm/h have malignancy, infection, or connective tissue disease, and in only 5% to 7% does the disease remain undiagnosed (2, 3, 32). Infection is the commonest cause, and malignancy is next in frequency (3). As noted earlier, nearly all patients with cancer and an ESR of greater than 100 mm/h have metastases (2). Because a significant number of patients with a rate that exceeds 100 mm/h have myeloma, the preliminary evaluation should include serum electrophoresis. A history, physical examination, and initial diagnostic tests were sufficient in one study to diagnose 94% of patients with cancer whose ESR was greater than 100 mm/h (3). Because only 15% of all patients with such an ESR will have cancer, an extensive search for cancer should not be undertaken until other, more likely diagnoses have been excluded.

UNEXPLAINED INCREASE

Many clinicians find an unexplained increase in the ESR difficult to ignore. In fact, most of these patients do not have serious disease. In one study (11), 790 patients with an increased ESR (> 35 mm/h in women and > 30 mm/h in men) were carefully evaluated. In 43 patients (5%), a disease remained undiagnosed and these patients were reexamined periodically for 10 years with repeated measurement of the ESR. The increased ESR was transitory in 32 of these patients (78%). Thus, the first step in evaluating an unexplained ESR is to repeat the test after a short interval. Two patients with a persistently elevated ESR were found eventually to have cancer; 1 had pancreatic cancer, and the other had colonic cancer. Other than a benign dysproteinemia, no diagnosis was ever established in the remaining 9 patients with a persistently elevated rate (33). These conclusions were confirmed when an ESR was obtained in asymptomatic Scandinavian women (10). None with an initially undiagnosed increase in ESR developed cancer, and the cause of the increase in over half remained undiagnosed during 6 years of observation. The ESR reverted to normal in 60% of these patients.

Thus, when the initial clinical evaluation does not explain an elevated ESR, the clinician should resist the temptation to search for a cause. The ESR will return to normal in most of these patients. Only a few will have occult malignancy, and most patients will have a benign dysproteinemia.

VERY LOW RATE

The causes of a very low ESR (0 to 1 mm/h) include polycythemia, hemoglobinopathy, hypofibrinogenemia, hereditary spherocytosis, hypochromic microcytic anemia, congestive heart failure, cachexia, and therapy with antiinflammatory drugs. In one study of patients with a low ESR, 38% had no evidence of disease and only 6% had one of the diseases commonly associated with a very low ESR (34). The remaining patients had a wide variety of diagnoses. An isolated finding of a very low ESR has little significance.

Monitoring Disease Activity

The ESR is used to monitor the activity of inflammatory diseases such as temporal arteritis, polymyalgia rheumatica, and rheumatoid arthritis.

TEMPORAL ARTERITIS AND POLYMYALGIA RHEUMATICA

Once a patient starts corticosteroid therapy for temporal arteritis or polymyalgia rheumatica, the ESR falls within a few days. Some authors recommend using the response of the ESR to a trial of corticosteroids as a diagnostic criterion for patients with polymyalgia rheumatica. However, rheumatoid arthritis, which can mimic polymyalgia, may also respond promptly to corticosteroids.

The ESR is the most widely used test for assessing disease activity in patients with temporal arteritis and polymyalgia rheumatica because these conditions have few specific clinical indicators of disease activity (35). In the typical response to treatment, the ESR falls to a level that is higher than normal, even when the patient's clinical status is dramatically improved (23, 24). Therefore, both the ESR and clinical status should be used as criteria for altering the dosage of corticosteroids. Because clinical relapse can occur when the ESR is normal (35), corticosteroid treatment should be resumed or the dosage increased when symptoms recur, even if the ESR is normal. Conversely, an elevated ESR in a patient with established temporal arteritis or polymyalgia rheumatica does not always mean active disease. Therefore, an elevated ESR should not be used as a rationale for maintaining or increasing high doses of corticosteroids in a patient who is clinically well.

RHEUMATOID ARTHRITIS

Although 5% to 10% of patients with definitely active rheumatoid arthritis will have a normal ESR, the ESR tends to parallel disease activity (36, 37). The ESR falls as clinical symptoms respond to the initiation of corticosteroid treatment and rises with recrudescence of active disease. The ESR does not fall in short-term therapy with aspirin or indomethacin (38). An isolated elevated ESR is not useful for prognosis, but sustained extreme elevation of the ESR is a predictor of worsening clinical status. Paradoxically, elevations of the ESR that exceed 80 mm/h in a patient with acute onset of symptoms are often followed by a good functional recovery.

The relationship between the ESR and disease activity in patients with rheumatoid arthritis has been evaluated in two studies. McConkey and associates (39) placed patients in three categories of disease activity and showed that the ESR increased as disease activity increased. Pinals and colleagues (40) evaluated the ESR as a predictor of overall disease activity. Without using the ESR as a criterion of disease activity, they classified patients as in remission, partial remission, or relapse. A multivariate analysis identified six predictors of disease inactivity: less than 15 minutes of morning stiffness, no morning stiffness, no fatigue, no joint pain, no joint tenderness, no joint or tendon sheath swelling, and a normal ESR. A normal ESR did not exclude active disease, because 38% of those patients with a partial remission and a slightly higher proportion of those with a relapse had an ESR of less than 30 mm/h. The rate that best distinguished those in remission from those with active disease was 20 mm/h for men and 30 mm/h for women.

In summary, the ESR is sometimes useful in monitoring disease activity in patients with rheumatoid arthritis. The rate generally confirms the findings of joint examination and parallels symptoms (morning stiffness, fatigue, and arthritis). The joint examination is far more useful than the ESR in assessing synovitis. When active synovitis cannot be distinguished from synovial thickening alone, an increased ESR may be used as additional evidence of disease activity. An elevated rate does not necessarily connote disease activity, nor does a normal rate exclude disease activity. Therefore, the ESR is never the sole basis for altering therapy.

HODGKIN'S DISEASE

The ESR may have a role in monitoring for relapse of Hodgkin's disease. In a prospective study (17), the sensitivity of the test in active Hodgkin's disease was measured in newly diagnosed, untreated patients. Overall, 87% of untreated patients had an elevated ESR (63% in patients with stage I disease; 89% in those with stage II; 91% in those with stage III; and 100% in those with stage IV). The specificity of the test was measured in treated patients at the start of a 1-year period in which these patients had no evidence of recurrence. Only 21% of treated, disease-free patients had an elevated ESR. Thus, the sensitivity and specificity of the ESR as a measure of relapse are 87% and 79%, respectively. When clinical evidence indicates that the probability of relapse is 10%, the probability of relapse if the ESR is normal is 2%. If the pretest probability of relapse is high (50%) and the ESR is normal, the probability of relapse is 14%.

The data suggest that the ESR may be underused as an indicator of relapse in patients with Hodgkin's disease. A normal ESR is reassuring if there is minimal evidence for relapse but is of little value if the suspicion of relapse is high. An increased rate is evidence for relapse but would not be used as the sole pretext for aggressive diagnostic or therapeutic measures (17).

Table 6. Recommendations for the Diagnostic Use of the Erythrocyte Sedimentation Rate (ESR)

1. The ESR should not be used to screen asymptomatic persons for disease.

2. The ESR should be used selectively and interpreted with caution when the history and physical examination fail to provide any evidence for a specific diagnostic hypothesis in a symptomatic person.

> Significant infectious, inflammatory, or neoplastic disease is unlikely in such patients, and the ESR must be markedly elevated to be diagnostically useful. Extreme elevation of the ESR seldom occurs in patients with no evidence of serious disease.

3. If there is no immediate explanation for an increased ESR, the physician should repeat the test in several months rather than search for occult disease.

> A careful history and physical examination will generally disclose the cause of an elevated ESR. An increased ESR in the setting of a normal examination is usually transitory and is infrequently the harbinger of serious occult disease.

4. The ESR is indicated for diagnosis and monitoring of temporal arteritis and polymyalgia rheumatica.

> A normal ESR excludes the diagnosis of temporal arteritis in most patients who are suspected of having the disease. However, when the ESR is normal despite other strong clinical evidence for temporal arteritis, aggressive diagnostic or therapeutic intervention is still indicated.

> Although the ESR is an indicator of disease activity in temporal arteritis and polymyalgia rheumatica, the patient's clinical status must be taken into account in adjusting the dosage of corticosteroids.

5. In diagnosing and monitoring patients with rheumatoid arthritis, the ESR should be used principally to help resolve conflicting clinical evidence. The role of the ESR in other rheumatic diseases has not been studied.

6. The ESR may be helpful in monitoring patients with treated Hodgkin's disease.

OTHER DISEASES

The ESR is sometimes used to monitor the course of other diseases that are characterized by an inflammatory response. The test may be perceived as particularly useful when specific measures of disease activity cannot be obtained. However, the value of the ESR as a measure of disease activity is unknown, precisely because independent confirmation of disease activity is so difficult. Clinical studies of the ESR as a measure of the response to therapy are also needed.

Conclusions

The recommendations derived from the analyses in this article are listed in Table 6.

ACKNOWLEDGMENTS: The authors thank Fred Wolfe, M.D.; Earl Steinberg, M.D.; and Elazer Edelman, M.D., Ph.D., for helpful criticism.

Grant support: in part by a contract from the Blue Cross-Blue Shield Association, and by grants AM20580 and RR05669 from the National Institutes of Health.

References

1. FAHRAEUS R. The suspension-stability of the blood. *Acta Med Scand.* 1921;**55**:1-228.
2. ZACHARSKI LR, KYLE RA. Significance of extreme elevation of erythrocyte sedimentation rate. *JAMA.* 1967;**202**:264-6.
3. WYLER DJ. Diagnostic implications of markedly elevated erythrocyte sedimentation rate: a reevaluation. *South Med J.* 1977;**70**:1428-30.
4. LASCARI AD. The erythrocyte sedimentation rate. *Pediatr Clin North Am.* 1972;**19**:1113-21.
5. GIBBS D. Symptomless abnormalities: ESR. *Br J Hosp Med.* 1982;**27**:493-6.
6. BEDELL SE, BUSH BT. Erythrocyte sedimentation rate: from folklore to facts. *Am J Med.* 1985;**78**(6 pt 1):1001-9.
7. INTERNATIONAL COMMITTEE FOR STANDARDIZATION IN HEMATOLOGY. Recommendation of measurement of erythrocyte sedimentation rate of human blood. *Am J Clin Pathol.* 1977;**68**:505-7.
8. BOTTIGER LE, SVEDBERG CA. Normal erythrocyte sedimentation rate and age. *Br Med J.* 1967;**2**:85-7.
9. MILLER A, GREEN M, ROBINSON D. Simple rule for calculating normal erythrocyte sedimentation rate. *Br Med J [Clin Res].* 1983;**286**:266.
10. RAFNSSON V, BENGTSSON C, LENNARTSSON J, LINDQUIST O, NOPPA H, TIBBLIN E. Erythrocyte sedimentation rate in a population sample of women, with special reference to its clinical and prognostic significance. *Acta Med Scand.* 1979;**206**:207-14.
11. LILJESTRAND A, OLHAGEN B. Persistently high erythrocyte sedimentation rate: diagnostic and prognostic aspects. *Acta Med Scand.* 1955;**155**:425-39.
12. PINCHERLE G, SHANKS J. Value of the erythrocyte sedimentation rate as a screening test. *Br J Prev Soc Med.* 1967;**21**:133-6.
13. NIELSEN SE, ANDERSEN B, BADEN H. Value of routine estimation of erythrocyte sedimentation rate in surgical patients. *Acta Chir Scand.* 1976;**142**:97-8.
14. FROOM P, MARGALIOT S, CAINE Y, BENBASSAT J. Significance of erythrocyte sedimentation rate in young adults. *Am J Clin Pathol.* 1984;**82**:198-200.
15. SOX HC. Probability theory in the use of diagnostic tests: an introduction to critical study of the literature. *Ann Intern Med.* 1986;**104**:60-6.
16. RAFNSSON V, BENGTSSON C, LURIE M. Erythrocyte sedimentation rate in women with different manifestations of joint disease. *Scand J Rheumatol.* 1982;**11**:87-95.

17. RAY GR, WOLF PH, KAPLAN HS. Value of laboratory indicators in Hodgkin's disease: preliminary results. *Natl Canc Inst Monogr.* 1973;**36**:315-23.
18. PEYMAN MA. The effect of malignant disease on the erythrocyte sedimentation rate. *Br J Cancer.* 1962;**16**:56-71.
19. DEYOUNG NJ, ASHMAN LK, LUDBROOK J, MARSHALL VR. A comparison of three blood tests for cancer. *Surg Gynecol Obstet.* 1980;**150**:12-6.
20. SALTER RH. Gastrointestinal malignancy and the ESR. *Practitioner.* 1981;**225**:566-8.
21. HAMILTON CR JR, SHELLEY WM, TUMULTY PA. Giant cell arteritis: including temporal arteritis and polymyalgia rheumatica. *Medicine (Baltimore).* 1971;**50**:1-27.
22. GOODMAN BW JR. Temporal arteritis. *Am J Med.* 1979;**67**:839-52.
23. ESHAGHIAN J, GOEKEN JA. C-reactive protein in giant cell (cranial, temporal) arteritis. *Ophthalmology.* 1980;**87**:1160-6.
24. FAUCHALD P, RYGVOLD O, OYSTESE B. Temporal arteritis and polymyalgia rheumatica: clinical and biopsy findings. *Ann Intern Med.* 1972;**77**:845-52.
25. HUSTON KA, HUNDER GG, LIE JT, KENNEDY RH, ELVEBACK LR. Temporal arteritis: a 25-year epidemiologic, clinical, and pathologic study. *Ann Intern Med.* 1978;**88**:162-7.
26. HEALEY LA, WILSKE KR. *The Systemic Manifestations of Temporal Arteritis.* New York: Grune & Stratton; 1978;120.
27. CHANG RW, FINEBERG HV. Risk-benefit considerations in the management of polymyalgia rheumatica. *Med Decis Making.* 1983;**3**:459-76.
28. ROPES MW, BENNETT GA, COBBS S, JACOX R, JESSAR RA. 1958 revision of diagnostic criteria for rheumatoid arthritis. *Bull Rheum Dis.* 1958;**9**:175-6.
29. WINTROBE MM. The erythrocyte sedimentation rate. *Int Clin.* 1936;**2**:34-61.
30. BANNICK EG, GREGG RO, GUERNSEY CM. The erythrocyte sedimentation rate. *JAMA.* 1937;**109**:1257-62.
31. BANYAI AL, ANDERSON SV. Erythrocyte sedimentation test in tuberculosis. *Arch Intern Med.* 1930;**46**:787-96.
32. FORD MJ, INNES JA, PARRISH FM, ALLAN NC, HORN DB, MUNRO JF. The significance of gross elevations of the erythrocyte sedimentation rate in a general medical unit. *Eur J Clin Invest.* 1979;**9**:191-4.
33. OLHAGEN B, LILJESTRAND A. Persistently elevated erythrocyte sedimentation rate with good prognosis. *Acta Med Scand.* 1955;**151**:441-9.
34. ZACHARSKI LR, KYLE RA. Low erthrocyte sedimentation rate: clinical significance in 358 cases. *Am J Med Sci.* 1965;**250**:208-11.
35. PARK JR, JONES JG, HAZLEMAN BL. Relationship of the erythrocyte sedimentation rate to acute phase proteins in polymyalgia rheumatica and giant cell arteritis. *Ann Rheum Dis.* 1981;**40**:493-5.
36. DOBSON MH, SIA RHP, BOOTS RH. The differential diagnosis of rheumatoid and osteoarthritis: the sedimentation reaction and its value. *J Lab Clin Med.* 1930;**15**:1065-71.
37. RICHARDSON AT. Routine clinical pathology in rheumatoid arthritis. *Proc R Soc Med.* 1957;**50**:466-9.
38. MCCONKEY B, CROCKSON RA, CROCKSON AP, et al. The effects of some anti-inflammatory drugs on the acute-phase proteins in rheumatoid arthritis. *Q J Med.* 1973;**42**:785-91.
39. MCCONKEY B, CROCKSON RA, CROCKSON AP. The assessment of rheumatoid arthritis: a study based on measurements of the serum acute-phase reactants. *Q J Med.* 1972;**41**:115-25.
40. PINALS RS, MASI AT, LARSEN RA. Preliminary criteria for clinical remission in rheumatoid arthritis. *Arthritis Rheum.* 1981;**24**:1308-15.

The Complete Blood Count and Leukocyte Differental Count

An Approach to Their Rational Application

MARTIN F. SHAPIRO, M.D., Ph.D.; and SHELDON GREENFIELD, M.D.

THE COMPLETE BLOOD COUNT and the leukocyte differential count are two of the commonest clinical laboratory tests obtained in medical practice. These tests should not be accepted as routine studies for persons who are sick or for screening those who are well without critical appraisal of available empirical evidence (1). The tens of millions of tests done annually contribute to health care costs (2, 3). Today, there are few patients who are hospitalized who do not have a complete blood count and leukocyte differential count done once or several times. In ambulatory care, the complete blood count and leukocyte differential count are common components of screening batteries in asymptomatic patients. There is little doubt that these tests provide information useful to the care of some patients. Nevertheless, like all tools in medicine, they should be applied rationally and selectively, in situations in which there is a reasonable prospect of some demonstrable benefit to patients (4).

We review the evidence that these tests can contribute to patient care in four clinical situations: screening in ambulatory care; case finding on admission to the hospital; testing in patients suspected of having an abnormality; and monitoring the response to treatment of those with an abnormal test.

Description of Test Methods

A complete blood count is generally done with a Coulter counter that measures the hemoglobin level, hemato-

▶ This chapter was originally published in *Annals of Internal Medicine*. 1987;**106**:65-74.

crit, total leukocyte count, erythrocyte count, mean cellular volume, and mean cellular hemoglobin concentration. The test does not include the platelet count, reticulocyte count, or leukocyte differential count (5). Manual hematocrits and total leukocyte counts are done separately in some settings. The leukocyte differential count is a manual test involving the estimation (based on counting 100 cells) of the percentages of leukocytes that are mature neutrophils, band neutrophils, lymphocytes, monocytes, eosinophils, basophils, or other cell types (5). Automated equipment to perform the differential count has recently begun to be used in hospital practice (6, 7). There is no evidence that this equipment performs better than the manual test (8). The issues regarding the utility of the automated test are similar to those concerning the manual test.

NORMAL VALUES

Complete Blood Count: The normal ranges reported in the literature differ widely (9). For example, 95% confidence limits for the total leukocyte count and the leukocyte differential count were different in important respects among three studies (10-12), one of which (10) is cited in a leading textbook of hematology (13) (Table 1).

There is considerable variation in the "normal" range for the complete blood count in various demographic groups. A number of studies have noted differences in hemoglobin values between blacks and whites. Blacks have hemoglobin levels approximately 1 g/dL lower than those of whites. These differences hold up throughout life and for all socioeconomic levels (14, 15) and during pregnancy (16). Leukocyte counts are also lower among blacks throughout life (9). The meaning of these differences remains controversial. Although some authors recommend "that race specific norms for hemoglobin concentration be developed, published and utilized" (17), others attribute the lower hemoglobin levels in blacks to a higher prevalence of iron deficiency anemia (18). Similarly, differences have been reported between men and women that are not solely due to menstrual blood loss. Studies of white men and women in their 60s or older have found that the men have higher hemoglobin levels (approximately 1 g/dL) (19, 20) hematocrit levels, and leukocyte counts (9, 19).

Table 1. The 95% Confidence Limits for the Leukocyte Count and Differential in Various Studies

	Orfanakis and associates (10)	Zacharski and coworkers (11)
	←——————— *cells/mm³* ———————→	
Total leukocytes	4300 - 10 000	4100 - 10 900
Total neutrophils	1830 - 7250	2266 - 7676
Lymphocytes	1500 - 4000	832 - 3140
Eosinophils	0 - 700	0 - 492
Monocytes	200 - 950	123 - 804
Basophils	0 - 150	0 - 156

	Bain and England (12)	
	Male	Female
Total leukocytes	3487 - 9206*	3839 - 10 135*
Total neutrophils	1539 - 5641*	1861 - 6821 *
Lymphocytes	1168 - 3262	1149 - 3664
Eosinophils	30 - 592	20 - 582
Monocytes	217 - 849	225 - 836
Basophils	0 - 131 *	0 - 138 *

* Morning values; afternoon values were slightly higher for total neutrophils and total leukocytes.

It is important to understand whether a definition of anemia as a hemoglobin value more than two standard deviations below the mean has clinical utility. If conventional definitions for a normal hematocrit are used, the following prevalences for anemia are found: all males, 1%; all females, 10%; pregnant women, 10% to 60%; elderly men, 10%; and elderly women, 15% (21). Such "anemia" could represent one of four situations: mild abnormalities for which no cause can be identified; mild abnormalities due to a specific pathophysiologic deficiency (such as iron, folate, or vitamin B_{12}) or metabolic abnormality; severe anemia from any cause that requires treatment because it poses a cardiovascular or other risk to health; or anemia that is a manifestation of a serious underlying disease.

Leukocyte Differential Count: Do "abnormal" values (Table 1) for the components of the leukocyte differential count represent disease or unreliable reading of the test? Unreliability is a critical problem with the test, due to both random variation in small samples (22, 23) and observer error (24, 25). Variations in the frequency distribution of cell lines occur frequently by chance, because of the large number of cell lines and the small number of cells that are usually counted (22). In the usual test, in which 100 cells are counted, the percentage of cells attributed to a particular cell line can differ by as much as 15% in each direction due to chance variation in the cells selected for counting when the smear is read (23). With respect to the second source of error, observer reliability, a test that is read as normal in one laboratory may be judged to be abnormal in another (26). Much variability appears to occur because perceptions of what constitutes a band neutrophil (as compared to a mature neutrophil) or a monocyte (as compared to a lymphocyte or atypical lymphocyte) can differ (24, 26).

Finally, in addition to these sources of unreliability, physiologic variations can occur in subjects without the conditions of interest, thereby reducing the test's specificity. Such deviations from normal in the leukocyte differential count in healthy populations can be considerable (11). Some of this variation may be due to physiologic factors, such as cigarette smoking (27) and childbirth (28), that depress certain cell lines. Surgery can increase the neutrophil count by 160% to 350% (29). Extreme values clearly represent disease most of the time. However, it is important to recognize that smaller deviations from "normal" may be nonspecific.

The impact of unreliability and nonspecificity on the leukocyte differential can be substantial. In one study of 117 000 tests over 18 months, 30% of variance in the neutrophil count was due to unreliability of the test, as was evident in paired, repeated specimens; 50% was due to physiologic variation (nonspecificity) and only 20% was due to disorders thought to be associated with neutrophil abnormalities (30). Because of physiologic variation and unreliability of the test due to sampling variation and observer error, increases or decreases in the percentage of a particular cell line may not correlate with a meaningful change in the patient's condition, or even with a real change in the concentration of that particular line of cells (8, 31).

Will the advent of more precise technologies eliminate the variations described? Some authors contend that automated technologies that can count 500 cells will increase precision (32) and will improve the clinical efficiency and utility of the test (33). Clearly, these technologies require thorough evaluation. Although these technologies may reduce errors due to random variation by counting more cells, they may increase errors due to systematic misclassification of cell types (8, 31).

Clinical Applications

OUTPATIENT SCREENING

Complete Blood Count: Screening is "the presumptive identification of unrecognized disease or defect by the application of tests, examinations, or other procedures which can be applied rapidly" (34). Screening tests "sort out apparently well persons who have a disease from those who probably do not" (34). *Mass screening* involves application of screening tests to large, unselected populations, whereas *case finding* is the application of these tests to patients with unrelated symptoms (35).

There are three possible reasons to use the complete blood count for screening in ambulatory medical practice: to enable early identification and treatment of an underlying illness, of which anemia or an abnormal leukocyte count is a manifestation; to prevent adverse outcomes from the consequences of anemia in patients who are currently asymptomatic; or to identify a specific, treatable cause of asymptomatic, mild anemia.

One study evaluated the utility of the test in the identification of serious, underlying illnesses in a largely community-based sample of 1080 nonpregnant women aged 20 to 64. Although 120 (11.1%) women had hemoglobin levels less than 12 g/dL and 44 (4.1%) had hemoglobin levels below 10 g/dL, only 1 woman had a serious illness detected: a bronchial carcinoid found by chest radiography. Among 91 of the 120 women with hemoglobin levels below 12 g/dL who submitted stool specimens for occult blood testing, only 4 (all with histories of bleeding hemorrhoids) were positive on repeat testing. Although not all subjects with occult blood in their stools had exhaustive investigations, the study suggests that the complete blood count is not an efficient means of detecting serious underlying disorders (36). Although further studies might reasonably be done, the complete blood count currently cannot be recommended for this purpose (37, 38).

Is there value in detecting anemia unrelated to underlying disease? If a specific etiologic factor for anemia can be identified (such as iron, folate, or vitamin B_{12} deficiency) or if the anemia is severe, treatment might reasonably be undertaken. It is recognized that profound, symptomatic anemia merits treatment (39). Similarly, even less severe anemia associated with symptoms, such as pernicious anemia causing peripheral neuropathy, requires treatment (40). Such anemia is rare in community-based samples. In one study, 19 of 533 persons over 65 years of age had vitamin B_{12} levels of less than 100 pg/mL, but none had macrocytic anemia, and there was no evidence of an association of these low values to abnormal cerebral function (41).

Are less severe degrees of anemia that are asymptomatic worthy of early detection? The most comprehensive study of the consequences of anemia was a 3-year prospective study of 18 740 Welsh women by Elwood and colleagues (42). They examined the question of whether anemia itself (as opposed to the underlying diseases with which it can be associated) contributes to mortality. Mortality was highest for subjects with high hematocrits, apparently due to pulmonary disease. When patients with malignancies were excluded, there was no difference in mortality between normal persons and those with hematocrits of less than 36%. In fact, cardiovascular mortality was lower in the anemic group. Because this study was not designed to evaluate the ability of the complete blood count to identify serious, underlying diseases, no data are presented on whether the malignancies had been recognized previously (42).

These investigators also found no morbid effects of mild anemia when it was not associated with an underlying disease. In a comprehensive community survey, 7.3% of 91.5% of 1005 women aged 20 to 64 had hemoglobin levels between 10 and 11.9 g/dL. There was no relationship between symptoms and hemoglobin level among women not previously diagnosed as anemic, or between treatment with iron and relief of symptoms (43, 44). Another study (45) attempted to evaluate the clinical importance of lower hemoglobin levels in some women by determining the range of hemoglobins in three groups of women: those who were symptom-free; those who had normal laboratory findings (including blood smears) but had anxiety, tension, or fatigue; and those with gynecologic complaints such as menstrual irregularity. There were no differences in hemoglobin level between the groups, but many women in each group were anemic, according to conventional definitions (the 95% confidence limits were 10.2 to 14.8 g/dL) (45).

Symptoms do not correlate with hemoglobin level, and a rise in hemoglobin level does not produce beneficial effects on cardiorespiratory symptoms or on psychomotor function when the initial hemoglobin level is above 8 g/dL (44). Hemoglobin levels lower than this are uncommon: in one survey only 0.6% of nearly 3000 women screened had hemoglobin levels below 8 g/dL, and two thirds were already receiving treatment because the diseases associated with anemia had brought them to medical attention (43, 46). Studies of physical function have not shown a consistent correlation with hemoglobin level, and its relationship to functional status and sense of well-being remains unclear (44, 47). Nonetheless, these findings suggest the need to identify possible patients with anemia who have impaired exercise tolerance.

Even the treatment of specific deficiency states causing mild anemia may not improve the patient's well-being. There is little evidence to suggest that the treatment for iron deficiency anemia is beneficial when the patient is asymptomatic (43, 44, 48-50). Vitamin B_{12} deficiency may have serious neurologic sequelae but is rare. It should be considered in the differential diagnosis of any patient with neurologic symptoms or signs (51).

There is no evidence to support the use of the complete blood count for screening for anemia in asymptomatic members of the general population (Table 2). Values in many subjects differ from what are generally called "normal" values of the hemoglobin level, hematocrit, and leukocyte count for physiologic or statistical reasons. Most cases of anemia are asymptomatic and mild in degree, and the patients have no adverse effects of their condition; studies have identified no benefit from treating such persons.

Are there specific subgroups of the population in whom the prevalence of anemia is so high or the consequences so serious that a convincing case can be made to screen for and treat anemia? Such screening has been proposed for infants, pregnant women, the institutionalized elderly, and immigrants from Third World countries. The Committee on Iron Deficiency of the American Medical Association's Council on Foods and Nutrition

advocates nutritional supplementation, rather than
screening for anemia, for groups with a high prevalence
of iron deficiency, such as infants and pregnant women
(52). When sensitive indices such as serum iron and
iron-binding capacity are used, the prevalence of iron deficiency anemia is 15% to 58% among pregnant women
and 8% to 64% among infants in the first year of life
(the latter rate being inversely related to birth weight)
(52). The relationship of iron deficiency in these populations to morbidity or mortality has not been adequately
studied (52). Nevertheless, it would be appropriate to
screen for anemia in pregnant women if the clinician suspects that iron supplementation or nutrition has been inadequate.

Mild anemia is common in the elderly (53, 54). However, severe asymptomatic anemia is uncommon among
elderly in the community. In two British studies, 0.9%
and 2.4% of elderly persons had hemoglobin levels less
than 10.4 g/dL and 10.0 g/dL, respectively (20, 55).
Most investigators have found no morbid effects of anemia in the elderly when it is not associated with an underlying disease (41). In nursing homes, the prevalence
of mild anemia may be higher: it was 40% in one study
(56). The authors (56) reported that mortality was related more closely to underlying disease processes than to
the presence or absence of anemia, but did not present
the data on which they based that conclusion. It is unclear whether the benefits of screening the elderly for anemia outweigh the costs (37). Nevertheless, the utility of
screening for anemia among the elderly in North America should be studied.

Immigrants from Third World countries may have a
higher prevalence of various anemias, but most persons
with clinically significant abnormalities in hemoglobin
levels are symptomatic (57). The value of screening in
asymptomatic immigrants is unclear and should be studied by clinics that care for large numbers of such persons.

It may be reasonable to use the complete blood count
to identify persons who are severely anemic because of
inadequate nutrition or undiagnosed chronic illness in
four populations: infants during the first year of life; institutionalized elderly persons (75 or older); pregnant
women; and recent immigrants from underdeveloped
countries. It must be emphasized that no randomized,
controlled trials have been done to evaluate the effect of

screening and treating these subgroups. However, these populations are those likeliest to benefit from screening because the relatively high prevalences of disease (particularly among subjects of low social class at greater risk of being malnourished), increases the probability of serious disease if the patient is anemic.

Leukocyte Count: Although there have been no prospective studies of the leukocyte count as a screening test in patients not suspected of having an infection or a hematologic disorder, there is no reason to suspect that it would be useful. There is no evidence, for example, that earlier diagnosis affects the outcome of chronic or acute leukemia in asymptomatic patients (58, 59). Bone marrow transplantation may be effective in the chronic phase of chronic myelogenous leukemia (58), and transfusion requirements may be decreased in symptomatic patients with preleukemia, but the care of asymptomatic patients will not be affected (59).

Leukocyte Differential Count: Evidence that the leukocyte differential count is not useful as a routine test in outpatients comes from a study by Rich and associates (60). Among 59% of 799 outpatients at a teaching hospital who had leukocyte differential counts, 13% had unsuspected abnormalities, but none had a clinical disorder that could be identified (60). In another study (61), 51% of healthy subjects had leukocyte differential counts that were abnormal by percentage criteria for normal values for cell lines. Even the 10% of subjects that had abnormalities in the absolute count in a cell line were mostly instances of lymphocytopenia. No clinical disease was evident in this population, although it is unclear how thoroughly the investigators looked for it (61).

The leukocyte differential count has no value in ambulatory screening (Table 3), because it is unreliable (due to random variation in the populations of cells counted and observer error), the prevalence of disease is very low, and abnormalities are nonspecific. Among outpatients, it should be done in only those with symptoms that may be associated with abnormalities of the test. Many unnecessary work-ups will ensue if this test is commonly done in outpatients and abnormalities are investigated.

ADMISSION CASEFINDING

In hospitalized patients, it is often appropriate to do an initial complete blood count, leukocyte differential count, or both because of suspicion of an infection or of a hematologic disorder. Is it also appropriate to do these tests on admission in patients who show no reason to suspect a disorder associated with abnormalities of these tests?

Complete Blood Count: When patients are admitted for major surgery that may involve more than minor blood loss, or if an infection or a hematologic disorder is suspected, a complete blood count is clearly indicated. However, in patients who are otherwise well and will be undergoing surgical procedures in which bleeding is minimal, the test is not necessary for the management of the patient through surgery. Kaplan and associates (62) found that the test almost never contributed to patient care in these circumstances. They reviewed the results from 610 preoperative tests of which 48% had no specific indication. Only results from two of these unindicated tests were abnormal, and neither abnormality (one case of mild, unsuspected anemia, and another of leukocytosis for which no treatment was initiated) was judged to be clinically important (62).

No study to date has evaluated the complete blood count as a routine admission test for patients hospitalized on nonsurgical services. A useful inquiry would be one that examined both the test's overall yield on admission to the medical service, and its yield among patients with each of the commonest admitting diagnoses or clinical presentations, and with or without a clinical suspicion of an important abnormality in the test. Besides counting abnormalities, the study should determine the proportion of abnormal results that lead to new diagnoses, to changes in treatment, and, at least potentially, to changes in the patients' status. A patient with a terminal malignancy and who eventually dies of cachexia will not benefit from the diagnosis of unsuspected, mild iron deficiency anemia. On the other hand, a patient found to be leukopenic after chemotherapy, and placed in isolation until his or her blood counts recover, may well benefit.

The complete blood count is rarely useful on admission when no abnormality in the test is suspected, but it has not been studied adequately on nonsurgical services. The test should not be done on admission in any situation in which the probability of an abnormality is very low and in which the information obtained from it will not affect diagnosis or therapy. Examples of such situations are patients admitted for minor surgical procedures in which substantial blood loss is not anticipated; patients admitted for procedures such as gastrointestinal endoscopy who have not been bleeding; and patients admitted for exacerbations of dermatologic diseases when infection is not suspected. In these and similar situations, minor abnormalities in a "routine" test will not affect management.

Leukocyte Differential Count: The leukocyte differential count can also be a valuable test when done on admission to confirm an infectious process, or to detect patients who are at risk of infection due to granulocytopenia caused by a treatment or a disease already identified. Apart from these situations, the test appears to be of limited benefit for newly admitted patients.

Connelly and colleagues (63) studied the utility of the leukocyte differential count among 287 randomly selected inpatients from all services. Twenty-three percent of tests were obtained in patients in whom no abnormality was suspected. Of these patients, half had an abnormal result. Only one third of abnormalities were recorded in the medical record by the physician. In no instance did an abnormality of the leukocyte differential count have clinical significance (63).

A study of 390 random preoperative leukocyte differential counts in patients undergoing elective surgery in a university hospital found no specific indication for 83% of tests. Only one of the tests not indicated (0.3%) yielded an abnormality in any of the three aspects of the test that were analyzed. Even that single abnormality (two nucleated erythrocytes that resolved without any change in management of a patient admitted for a neurosurgical procedure) was not acted on by the clinicians (62).

Finally, in a study that provided generous criteria of justifiability for the leukocyte differential count (64), the authors found that 52% of initial surgical tests and 13% of initial medical tests in a university hospital were not indicated. None of these 295 unindicated tests led to otherwise inapparent diagnoses or to changes in therapy.

There is no evidence to support doing the leukocyte differential count on admission to the hospital unless there is clinical reason to suspect either an infection or a hematologic disorder, and such a diagnosis has not already been confirmed by other clinical data; or unless therapy will be affected by the results of the test. The leukocyte differential count is not indicated in most patients admitted for elective surgery.

TESTS FOR SUSPECTED ABNORMALITIES

Hemoglobin Level and Hematocrit: A complete blood count should be obtained in any situation in which there are clinical findings suggestive of anemia (such as fatigue, conjunctival pallor, and peripheral neuropathy) (65), abnormal bleeding, or findings suggestive of polycythemia (66) or any other primary hematologic disorder. In addition, this test is useful in conditions that may be associated with severe anemia, such as chronic renal insufficiency (67) and malignancy (68). However, the test will be most useful in these situations if it affects management (by leading to transfusions in the patient with end-stage renal disease or by modifying the work-up in newly diagnosed cancer). In patients with well-established conditions with no symptoms or signs of anemia, there may be less to be gained by obtaining the test and documenting mild anemia of chronic disease. At the same time, both patients and their physicians may be anxious to know whether anemia is present, even if effective therapy is unavailable.

Leukocyte, Neutrophil, and Band Neutrophil Counts: There are many clinical situations in which abnormalities of these tests correlate with clinically important disease. The utility of each test in specific situations depends on its ability to contribute information (including the ability of the leukocyte differential count to contribute new information beyond that obtainable from the leukocyte count), and on whether the test results enable the clinician to cross a diagnostic or therapeutic threshold (4).

The total leukocyte count generally is an index of the neutrophil count, except in hematologic malignancies. In the setting of acute infections, the total leukocyte and differential counts both can be abnormal, due to neutrophilia or neutropenia (69-81) but may not provide sufficient information either to confirm or to exclude the presence of disease.

Many patients with sepsis can have normal total leukocyte counts (69-71). Most patients with sepsis have an abnormality of the leukocyte count alone, the leukocyte differential count alone, or both (69-71); however, in one study, 7% of patients with blood cultures positive for bacteria or fungi had normal leukocyte counts (< 10 000 cells/mm³) and leukocyte differential counts. Because of the seriousness of the disorder being studied, this may be an unacceptably high false-negative rate (72). Furthermore, requiring an abnormality in only one of the two tests improves sensitivity, but specificity and, therefore, the probability of disease if either test is abnormal, are lower than if abnormalities in both tests were required for the diagnosis (69-71, 73). Requiring abnormalities in both tests is no more satisfactory. In one study, bacterial infections in children would have been missed in 25% of cases, had both criteria (more than 10 000 leukocytes/mm³ and more than 500 band neutrophils/mm³) been required (73). Yet, each test alone is both insensitive and nonspecific for the diagnosis of bacterial infections (74).

Situations that diminish the specificity of the leukocyte count for infection, by generating "false" abnormal results, include administration of epinephrine, corticosteroids and other medications, exercise, hemorrhage, hemolysis, trauma, diabetic ketoacidosis, and sickle-cell crisis (72, 75, 76). Some of these factors are germane to many situations in which the diagnosis of sepsis is suspected.

Appendicitis is a useful model for understanding the value and limitations of these tests. In one study, leukocytosis (defined as greater than 15 000 leukocytes/mm³ in children and greater than 9000/mm³ in adults) had a sensitivity of only 84% and a specificity of 66% in patients suspected of having acute appendicitis (77). In another study, the sensitivity increased from 87% to 96% when the diagnosis was based on the presence of either an abnormal differential, and abnormal leukocyte count or both, but at the cost of specificity and positive predictive value: one or both tests were abnormal in 59% of subjects with negative laparotomies (78).

In a study of 252 patients with acute abdominal pain, the leukocyte count had a sensitivity of only 60% and a specificity of 70% for the need for surgical intervention, when 11 000/mm³ was used as the upper limit of normal. The differential count did not increase the discriminatory value of the test: the receiver-operating characteristic curves for the leukocyte count and neutrophil count were virtually identical (79). The available data suggest that these tests may not be useful in deciding the need for surgical intervention in patients with abdominal pain (79-81).

None of the studies cited examined the frequency with which the test contributed new information. It would be necessary to ask physicians, both before and after the test was obtained, what they considered the likelihood of appendicitis to be and whether they were inclined to operate on the patient on the basis of the information available at that time. If positive tests resulted in increased estimations of the likelihood of disease and led to more decisions to operate, and negative tests decreased estimates of disease and diminished the rate of operation, then the test could be judged to have affected clinical decision making in those cases. Patients could then be followed prospectively, to determine how often the decision that was affected by the test results was a good one (that is, how often a patient with a positive test who underwent surgery as a result of the test actually had appendicitis, and how often a patient with a negative test who did not undergo surgery as a result of the test did not later prove to have appendicitis). Finally, it would be important to know if the information provided altered the patient's outcome.

The leukocyte count may provide useful confirmatory information when an infection is suspected, but when the diagnosis is clear from other data, documentation of leukocytosis is less likely to affect management. The leukocyte differential count is most useful in the diagnostic work-up of a patient in the following situations: a newly suspected infection or fever (when the complete blood count is normal); suspicion of a disorder associated with secondary abnormalities of the cell lines if the results of the test can affect diagnosis or treatment; any suspicion of a primary hematologic disorder (such as anemia, leukemia, or thrombocytopenia); or any other indication to examine the smear. The test has limited value within 36 hours after surgery, because it is often abnormal in this situation. The test generally is not necessary to confirm the presence of bacterial infection when leukocytosis has been documented. The leukocyte differential count may be justified in the diagnostic evaluation of a patient with an abnormal leukocyte count, if there is uncertainty about the cause of the abnormality, or if the results (such as the neutrophil count in a neutropenic patient) may affect diagnosis or management. The leukocyte differential count will not exclude sepsis when the suspicion is high, nor confirm it when the suspicion is low. For example, even management of most patients admitted with the clinical diagnosis of acute pyelonephritis, confirmed by urinalysis and culture, will not be affected by the results of the differential.

Other Cell Lines: Eosinophilia (82-93), monocytosis (94-96), basophilia (97, 98), and lymphocytosis or lymphopenia (99-101) have been reported to correlate with the presence, severity or prognosis of numerous disorders, although the sensitivity and specificity of these abnormalities generally are not high. Detailed discussion of those conditions in which the test may provide useful confirmatory information when the diagnosis is otherwise unclear, such as eosinophilia in allergic reactions (82), is beyond the scope of this article.

REPEAT TESTS TO MONITOR THE COURSE OF ILLNESS

Hemoglobin Level and Hematocrit: There have been no adequate studies of the utility of repeat hemoglobin level and hematocrit measurements in patients with identified abnormalities that are being treated. There is, however, no reason to repeat these tests until after several days of iron therapy for anemia to look for evidence of a response, because peak reticulocytosis does not occur for 7 days (102), and only 20% of a total increase in hemoglobin on iron therapy occurs in the first week (103). There is no information about the appropriate frequency for repeat testing for other indications in patients who are not bleeding, but it is difficult to envision clinical scenarios in which daily testing would be appropriate.

The major cost savings from complete blood counts done on inpatients would be realized from the elimination of unnecessary repeat testing. A patient who responds to treatment does not require a repeat test unless there is concern that the treatment has not been curative, transfusions are anticipated in an anemic or bleeding patient, or dramatic changes in the result are anticipated that might affect management. The interval between tests in patients for whom a repeat complete blood count is indicated needs to be studied. Until such data are available, it would be reasonable not to test patients daily unless clinically important changes in the result are anticipated. A repeat test is not indicated in patients in whom no abnormality is suspected.

Leukocyte and Leukocyte Differential Counts: Neutrophilia and band neutrophilia are markers of infection. How often should a patient who is being treated for an infection have these tests repeated? The repeat leukocyte differential count has little value in many of the clinical situations in which it is ordered. In one inpatient study in a university hospital (64), 73% of 347 medical and 53% of 211 surgical leukocyte differential counts were repeat tests. With the exception of one leukopenic patient, a subsequent test never affected patient care. Using criteria for clinically justifiable use of the leukocyte differential count that clinicians could accept, the authors found that 60% of subsequent medical counts and 71% of repeat surgical leukocyte differential counts were unjustifiable. Another study (104) found that the sensitivity of the leukocyte count to changes in the neutrophil count was 99%. These findings were confirmed in a more recent study (8). Thus, even in the patient who is not recovering from an infection associated with neutrophilia, it may not be necessary to repeat the leukocyte differential count (105).

In patients who are improving clinically, the tests have no value. In patients deteriorating clinically, or in whom the infection is disseminating, as shown by physical examination or imaging studies, the tests are unlikely to change management from that dictated by more accurate data. Only in the patient in whom it is unclear that the treatment will be effective, for whom alternative treatments are available, and in whom the course is difficult to discern, is there potential value for a repeat total leukocyte count or differential count (106).

In the patient at risk for leukopenia because of chemotherapy or disease of the bone marrow, leukocyte counts are often done. The frequency with which the test should be obtained has never been studied. If the leukocyte count is greater than 4500/mm^3, a leukocyte differential count is not necessary to screen for granulocytopenia because the neutrophil count correlates linearly with the leukocyte count (107). Among 1260 patients undergoing chemotherapy who had leukocyte counts of 5000 cells/mm^3 or greater, none had fewer than 1500 neutrophils/mm^3 (108). In patients who are isolated because of granulocytopenia, leukocyte counts are necessary, but it may not always be necessary to obtain a leukocyte differential count as well. When the total leukocyte count is less than 500 or 1000/mm³ (depending on the cutoff point used for decisions regarding isolation), the granulocyte count will be too low to protect against hospital-acquired infection, and repeated differential counts will not be helpful.

A repeat leukocyte or leukocyte differential count is justified in monitoring a patient with an infection who is not improving clinically, and in patients with new symptoms raising suspicion of an infection or a hematologic process. In addition, a repeat leukocyte differential count is justified in a patient with leukopenia, a patient on cytotoxic therapy if leukopenia is developing, a patient with another reason to monitor the smear, or a patient with previous abnormalities of the leukocyte differential count to assure that they have resolved. How soon should an indicated repeat test be done? Data are lacking on this subject and should be gathered prospectively in studies assessing the way in which the information is used.

Until such studies are done, it would be reasonable not to repeat the leukocyte differential count every day in the nonleukopenic patient, or in the mildly leukopenic patient whose counts are stable, unless a precipitous decline is anticipated (such as due to chemotherapy that is particularly toxic to bone marrow). Often, it will be appropriate not to repeat the count for several days or weeks. If the patient is more than mildly leukopenic, or the count is unstable, the frequency of testing should differ with the clinical situation. In a patient receiving chemotherapy that is particularly toxic to bone marrow, or in whom the count is falling rapidly, it may be appropriate to repeat the test daily if clinical decision making will be affected by the results. The leukocyte differential count need not be repeated in a patient who has been placed in protective isolation if the total leukocyte count is too low to take the patient out of isolation.

Conclusions

The complete blood count is a widely used diagnostic procedure in many practice settings. Although the test provides important information in some clinical situations, there is no evidence that it is useful as a "routine" test in patients who are otherwise well. Many patients may be anxious to know their blood count. Physicians

Table 2. Applications of the Complete Blood Count

Indication, *Usefulness*	Rationale
Ambulatory screening General population, *not useful*	Specificity and prevalence of disease too low; no evidence of benefit from detection of mild asymptomatic abnormalities
Specific subgroups (pregnant women, institutionalized elderly, immigrants from underdeveloped countries), *possibly useful*	Higher prevalence may improve predictive value; studies needed of effect of screening on outcomes
Admission to hospital No abnormality suspected, *rarely useful*	Not useful in many situations in which it is often ordered, such as elective minor surgery when major blood loss is not anticipated, minor diagnostic procedures such as endoscopy, and exacerbation of dermatologic disease when infection is not suspected; unsuspected minor abnormalities will not affect management
Abnormality suspected, *useful*	May have confirmatory value when abnormality is primary hematologic disorder or is otherwise likely to affect management
Repeat tests, *useful in some patients at appropriate intervals*	Test should only be repeated if: there is concern that treatment has not been effective; transfusions are anticipated in anemic or bleeding patients; dramatic changes in the complete blood count are anticipated that might affect management (such as chemotherapy) Appropriate testing interval needs to be studied but is unlikely to be daily in most clinical situations

Table 3. Applications of the Leukocyte Differential Count

Indication, *Usefulness*	Rationale
Ambulatory screening, *not useful*	Test unreliable; prevalence of disease very low; abnormalities nonspecific
Admission to hospital No abnormality suspected, *not useful*	Test unreliable; prevalence of disease very low; abnormalities nonspecific
Abnormality suspected Newly suspected infection or new fever, *useful in some patients*	Only useful when other data are inconclusive; may have confirmatory value in borderline cases; usually will not contribute diagnostic information when leukocytosis is present; will not exclude diagnosis of infection strongly suggested by other data; rarely abnormal when leukocyte count normal
Suspicion of a primary hematologic disorder, *useful*	Primary means of making diagnosis
Leukocytosis or leukopenia, *useful in some patients*	May be useful when cause is unclear or when management may be affected (that is, isolation of leukopenic patient)
Repeat tests, *useful in some patients at appropriate intervals*	Repeat test may have diagnostic value when infection not improving; new symptoms suggest developing infection or hematologic disorder; patient is severely leukopenic; or to assure that previous abnormalities have resolved, if results would affect management Appropriate testing interval needs to be studied, but is unlikely to be daily in nonleukopenic patients in most instances

need to respond to these concerns, but may be able to teach patients to think probabilistically as well. Likewise, the leukocyte differential count can be helpful in the diagnosis of infectious and hematologic disorders, but sometimes the former can be diagnosed without the benefit of the test. The leukocyte differential count is not useful as a "routine" test in asymptomatic persons. Much research remains to be done on specific uses for these two tests and on the appropriate frequency for testing. Conclusions regarding the clinical usefulness of the complete blood count and leukocyte differential count, derived from the analyses in this article, are shown in Tables 2 and 3.

References

1. BRESLOW L, SOMERS AR. The lifetime health-monitoring program: a practical approach to preventive medicine. *N Engl J Med.* 1977;**296**:601-8.
2. MOLONEY TW, ROGERS DE. Medical technology—a different view of the contentious debate over costs. *N Engl J Med.* 1979;**301**:1413-9.
3. ANGELL M. Cost containment and the physician. *JAMA.* 1985;**254**:1203-7.
4. SOX HC. Probability theory in the use of diagnostic tests: an introduction to critical study of the literature. *Ann Intern Med.* 1986;**104**:60-6.
5. WINTROBE MM, LEE GR, BOGGS DR, et al., eds. *Clinical Hematology.* 8th ed. Philadelphia: Lea & Febiger; 1981:2-32.
6. GRISWOLD DJ, CHAMPAGNE VD. Evaluation of the Coulter S-Plus IV three-part differential in an acute care hospital. *Am J Clin Pathol.* 1985;**84**:49-57.
7. LEWIS SM. Automated differential leukocyte counting: present status and future trends. *Blut.* 1981;**43**:1-6.
8. CHARACHE S, NELSON L, KEYSER E, METZGER P. A clinical trial of three-part electronic differential white blood cell counts. *Arch Intern Med.* 1985;**145**:1852-5.
9. VAN ASSENDELFT OW. Reference values for total and differential leukocyte count. *Blood Cells.* 1985;**11**:77-90.
10. ORFANAKIS NG, OSTLUND RE, BISHOP CR, ATHENS JW. Normal blood leukocyte concentration. *Am J Clin Pathol.* 1970;**53**:647-51.
11. ZACHARSKI LR, ELVEBACH LR, LINMAN JW. Leukocyte counts in healthy adults. *Am J Clin Pathol.* 1971;**56**:148-50.
12. BAIN BJ, ENGLAND JM. Normal haematological values: sex differences in neutrophil counts. *Br Med J.* 1975;**1**:306-9.
13. WINTROBE MM, LEE GR, BOGGS DR, et al., eds. *Clinical Hematology.* 8th ed. Philadelphia: Lea & Febiger; 1981:1885-8.
14. GARN SM, SMITH NJ, CLARK DC. The magnitude and the implications of apparent race differences in hemoglobin values. *Am J Clin Nutr.* 1975;**28**:563-6.
15. GARN SM, CLARK DC. Lifelong differences in hemoglobin levels between blacks and whites. *J Natl Med Assoc.* 1975;**67**:91-6.
16. GARN SM, SHAW HA, McCABE K. Black-white hemoglobin differences during pregnancy. *Ecol Food Nutr.* 1976;**5**:99-100.
17. OWEN GM, YANOCHIK-OWEN A. Should there be a different definition of anemia in black and white children? *Am J Public Health.* 1977;**67**:865-6.
18. REEVES JD, DRIGGERS DA, LO EY, DALLMAN PR. Screening for anemia in infants: evidence in favor of using identical hemoglobin criteria for blacks and caucasians. *Am J Clin Nutr.* 1981;**34**:2154-7.
19. MILNE JS, WILLIAMSON J. Hemoglobin, hematocrit, leukocyte count, and blood grouping in older people. *Geriatrics.* 1972;**27**:118-26.
20. HOBSON W, BLACKBURN EK. Haemoglobin levels in a group of elderly persons living at home alone or with spouse. *Br Med J.* 1953;**1**:647-9.

21. FRAME PS, CARLSON SJ. A critical review of periodic health screening using specific screening criteria. Part 4: Selected miscellaneous diseases. *J Fam Pract.* 1975;2:283-9.
22. RUMKE CL. The statistically expected variability in differential leukocyte counting. In: KOEPKE JA, ed. *Differential Leukocyte Counting.* Skokie, Illinois: College of American Pathologists; 1979:40-5.
23. BARNETT CW. The unavoidable error in the differential count of the leukocytes of the blood. *J Clin Invest.* 1933;12:77-85.
24. KOEPKE JA, DOTSON MA, SHIFMAN MA. A critical evaluation of a manual/visual differential leukocyte counting method. *Blood Cells.* 1985;11:173-86.
25. BACUS JW. The observer error in peripheral blood cell classification. *Am J Clin Pathol.* 1973;59:223-30.
26. RAJAMAKI A. Interlaboratory variation of leukocyte differential counts: results from the Finnish proficiency testing programme in haematological morphology, 1974-1977. *Scand J Clin Lab Invest.* 1979;39:613-7.
27. WINKEL P, STATLAND BE. The acute effect of cigarette smoking on the concentrations of blood leukocyte types in healthy young women. *Am J Clin Pathol.* 1981;75:781-5.
28. TAYLOR DJ, PHILLIPS P, LIND T. Puerperal haematological indices. *Br J Obstet Gynaecol.* 1981;88:601-6.
29. KIROV SM, SHEPHARD JJ, DONALD KD. Intraoperative and postoperative changes in peripheral white blood cell counts: the contribution of stress. *Aust NZ J Surg.* 1979;49:738-42.
30. BULL B, KORPMAN RA. Characterization of the WBC differential count. *Blood Cells.* 1980;6:411-9.
31. RUMKE CL, BEZEMER PD, KUIK DJ. Normal values and least significant differences for differential leukocyte counts. *J Chronic Dis.* 1975;28:661-8.
32. KINGSLEY TC. The automated differential: pattern recognition systems, precision, and the spun smear. *Blood Cells.* 1980;6:483-7.
33. ROSS DW. WBC differential counts [Letter]. *JAMA.* 1983;250:483-4.
34. COMMISSION ON CHRONIC ILLNESS. *Chronic Illness in the United States.* Cambridge, Massachusetts: Harvard University Press; 1957.
35. FLETCHER RH, FLETCHER SW, WAGNER EH. *Clinical Epidemiology—the Essentials.* Baltimore: Williams & Wilkins; 1982:67-73.
36. ELWOOD PC, WATERS WE, GREEN WJ, WOOD MM. Evaluation of a screening survey for anemia in adult non-pregnant women. *Br Med J.* 1967;4:714-7.
37. CANADIAN TASK FORCE ON THE PERIODIC HEALTH EXAMINATION. The periodic health examination. *Can Med Assoc J.* 1974;121:1193-254.
38. MEDICAL PRACTICE COMMITTEE, AMERICAN COLLEGE OF PHYSICIANS. Periodic health examination: a guide for designing individualized preventive health care in the asymptomatic patient. *Ann Intern Med.* 1981;95:729-32.
39. LAWSON DH, MURRAY RM, PARKER JL. Early mortality in the megaloblastic anemias. *Q J Med.* 1971;41:1-14.
40. PANT SS, ASBURY AK, RICHARDSON EP. The myelopathy of pernicious anemia. *Acta Neurol Scand.* 1968;44(suppl 5):1-36.
41. ELWOOD PC, SHINTON NK, WILSON CI, SWEETNAM P, FRAZER AC. Haemoglobin, vitamin B_{12} and folate levels in the elderly. *Br J Haematol.* 1971;21:557-63.
42. ELWOOD PC, WATERS WE, BENJAMIN IT, SWEETNAM PM. Mortality and anemia in women. *Lancet.* 1974;1:891-4.
43. ELWOOD PC, WATERS WE, GREENE WJ, SWEETNAM P, WOOD MM. Symptoms and circulating haemoglobin level. *J Chronic Dis.* 1969;21:615-28.
44. ELWOOD PC. Evaluation of the clinical importance of anemia. *Am J Clin Nutr.* 1973;26:958-64.

45. JUDY HE, PRICE NB. Hemoglobin level and red blood cell count findings in normal women. *JAMA*. 1958;**167**:563-6.
46. COCHRANE AL, HOLLAND WW. Validation of screening procedures. *Br Med Bull*. 1971;**27**:3-8.
47. VITERI FE, TORUN B. Anaemia and physical work capacity. *Clin Haematol*. 1974;**3**:609-27.
48. ELWOOD PC. Anaemia. *Lancet*. 1974;**2**:1364-5.
49. HOLLAND WW. Taking stock. *Lancet*. 1974;**2**:1494-7.
50. ELWOOD PC. The clinical evaluation of circulating haemoglobin level. *Clin Haematol*. 1974;**3**:705-19.
51. VICTOR M, LEAR AA. Subacute combined degeneration of the spinal cord. *Am J Med*. 1956;**20**:896-911.
52. Iron deficiency in the United States. *JAMA*. 1968;**203**:119-24.
53. HILL RD. The prevalance of anaemia in the over-65s in a rural practice. *Practitioner*. 1976;**217**:963-7.
54. GRIFFITHS HJ, NICHOLSON WJ, O'GORMAN P. A haematological study of 500 elderly females. *Gerontol Clin (Basel)*. 1970;**12**:18-32.
55. MCLENNAN WJ, ANDREWS GR, MACLEOD C, CAIRD FI. Anemia in the elderly. *Q J Med*. 1973;**42**:1-13.
56. KALCHTHALER T, TAN ME. Anemia in institutionalized elderly patients. *J Am Geriatr Soc*. 1980;**28**:108-13.
57. BRITT RP, HARPER C, SPRAY GH. Megaloblastic anaemia among Indians in Britain. *Q J Med*. 1971;**40**:499-520.
58. SPECK B, GRATWOHL A, OSTERWALDER B, NISSEN C. Bone marrow transplantation for chronic myeloid leukemia. *Semin Hematol*. 1984;**21**:48-52.
59. GRIFFIN JD, SPRIGGS D, WISCH JS, KUFE DW. Treatment of preleukemic syndromes with continuous intravenous infusion of low-dose cytosine arabinoside. *J Clin Oncol*. 1985;**3**:982-91.
60. RICH EC, CROWSON TW, CONNELLY DP. Effectiveness of differential leukocyte count in case finding in the ambulatory care setting. *JAMA*. 1983;**249**:633-6.
61. WESSON SK, MERCADO T, AUSTIN M, SCHUMACHER HR. Differential counts and overuse of the laboratory [Letter]. *Lancet*. 1980;**1**:552.
62. KAPLAN EB, SHEINER LB, BOECKMANN AJ, et al. The usefulness of preoperative laboratory screening. *JAMA*. 1985;**253**:3576-81.
63. CONNELLY DP, MCCLAIN MP, CROWSON TW, BENSON ES. The use of the differential leukocyte count for inpatient casefinding. *Hum Pathol*. 1982;**13**:294-300.
64. SHAPIRO MF, HATCH RL, GREENFIELD S. Cost containment and labor-intensive tests: the case of the leukocyte differential count. *JAMA*. 1984;**252**:231-4.
65. DALLMAN PR. Manifestations of iron deficiency. *Semin Hematol*. 1982;**19**:19-30.
66. WASSERMAN LR. The management of polycythaemia vera. *Br J Haematol*. 1971;**21**:371-6.
67. DESFORGES JF. Anemia in uremia. *Arch Intern Med*. 1970;**126**:808-11.
68. FRIEDELL GH. Anaemia in cancer. *Lancet*. 1965;**1**:356-9.
69. AKENZUA GI, HUI YT, MILNER R, ZIPURSKY A. Neutrophil and band counts in the diagnosis of neonatal infections. *Pediatrics*. 1974;**54**:38-42.
70. ZIPURSKY A, PALKO J, MILNER R, AKENZUA GI. The hematology of bacterial infections in premature infants. *Pediatrics*. 1976;**57**:839-53.
71. MANROE BL, ROSENFELD CR, WEINBERG AG, BROWNE R. The differential leukocyte count in the assessment and outcome of early-onset neonatal group B streptococcal disease. *J Pediatr*. 1977;**91**:632-7.
72. WEITZMAN M. Diagnostic utility of white blood cell and differential cell counts. *Am J Dis Child*. 1975;**129**:1183-9.
73. TODD JK. Childhood infections: diagnostic value of peripheral white blood cell and differential cell counts. *Am J Dis Child*. 1972;**127**:810-6.

74. RASMUSSEN NH, RASMUSSEN LN. Predictive value of white blood cell count and differential cell count to bacterial infections in children. *Act Paediatr Scand.* 1982;**71**:775-8.

75. BWIBO NO, DAWA B. White blood cell (WBC) counts in children with sickle cell anaemia. *East Afr Med J.* 1981;**58**:412-7.

76. MANROE BL, WEINBERG AG, ROSENFELD CR, BROWNE R. The neo-natal blood count in health and disease: I. Reference values for neutro-philic cells. *J Pediatr.* 1979;**95**:89-98.

77. MISKOWIAK J, BURCHARTH F. The white cell count in acute appendi-citis: a prospective blind study. *Dan Med Bull.* 1982;**29**:210-1.

78. BOWER RJ, BELL MJ, TERNBERG JL. Diagnostic value of the white blood cell count and neutrophil percentage in the evaluation of abdom-inal pain in children. *Surg Gynecol Obstet.* 1981;**152**:424-6.

79. PATRICK GL, STEWART RJ, ISBISTER WH. Patients with acute ab-dominal pain: white cell and neutrophil counts as predictors of the surgical acute abdomen. *NZ Med J.* 1985;**98**:324-6.

80. LEE PW. The leukocyte count in acute appendicitis. *Br J Surg.* 1973;**60**:618.

81. HUBBELL DS, BARTON WK, SOLOMON OD. Leukocytosis in appendi-citis in older persons. *JAMA.* 1961;**175**:139-41.

82. FAUCI AS, HARLEY JB, ROBERTS WC, FERRANS VJ, GRALNICK HR, BJORNSON BH. The idiopathic hypereosinophilic syndrome: clinical, pathophysiologic, and therapeutic considerations. *Ann Intern Med.* 1982;**97**:78-92.

83. SPRY CJF. Eosinophilia. *Practitioner.* 1982;**226**:79-88.

84. ELLUL-MICALLEF R, MOHAMMED DE, FENECH FF. The hypereosi-nophilic syndrome—a diagnostic enigma. *Postgrad Med J.* 1980;**56**:506-8.

85. CASTLEMAN B, MCNEELY BU. Case records of the Massachusetts General Hospital: weekly clinicopathological exercises: case 36-1970. *N Engl J Med.* 1970;**283**:476-85.

86. UHRBRAND H. The number of circulating eosinophils: normal figures and spontaneous variations. *Acta Med Scand.* 1958;**160**:99-104.

87. MUNAN L, KELLY A. Eosinophil counts in women: epidemiologic data. *Hum Biol.* 1980;**52**:279-87.

88. BURROWS B, FAYSAL MH, BARBEE RA, HALONEN M, LEBOWITZ MD. Epidemiologic observations on eosinophilia and its relation to respiratory disorders. *Am Rev Respir Dis.* 1980;**122**:709-19.

89. AGARWAL MB. Eosinophilia—a review. *Indian J Med Sci.* 1980;**34**:203-8.

90. BHAT AM, SCANLON JW. The pattern of eosinophilia in premature infants: a prospective study in premature infants using the absolute eosinophil count. *J Pediatr.* 1981;**98**:612-6.

91. MONTOLIU J, LOPEZ-PEDRET J, ANDREU L, REVERT L. Eosinophilia in patients undergoing dialysis. *Br Med J.* 1981;**282**:2098.

92. KAJOSAARI M, SAARNEN UM. Evaluation of laboratory tests in child-hood allergy: total serum, IgE, blood eosinophilia and eosinophil and mast cells in nasal mucosa of 178 children aged 3 years. *Allergy.* 1981;**36**:329-35.

93. LAWRENCE R JR, CHURCH JA, RICHARDS W, LIPSEY AI. Eosino-philia in the hospitalized neonate. *Ann Allergy.* 1980;**44**:349-52.

94. MEE AS, BERNEY J, JEWELL DP. Monocytes in inflammatory bowel disease: absolute monocyte counts. *J Clin Pathol.* 1980;**33**:917-20.

95. WARD PCJ. The myeloid leukocytoses. *Postgrad Med.* 1980;**67**:219-29.

96. KOIVUNEN E, GRONHAGEN-RISKA C, KLOCKARS M, SELROOS O. Blood monocytes and serum and bone marrow lysozyme in sarcoidosis. *Acta Med Scand.* 1981;**210**:107-10.

97. CHARLES TJ, WILLIAMS SJ, SEATON A, BRUCE C, TAYLOR WH. His-tamine, basophils and eosinophils in severe asthma. *Clin Sci.* 1979;**57**:39-45.

98. ANTHONY HM. Blood basophils in lung cancer. *Br J Cancer.* 1982;**45**:209-16.
99. GOSKE J, ASKARI A, DICKMAN E, FORMAN WB, CRUM ED. Granulocytopenia with marked lymphocytosis manifesting Sjogren syndrome. *Am J Hematol.* 1980;**9**:435-7.
100. MACLENNAN KA, HUDSON BV, JELLIFE AM, HAYBITTLE JL, HUDSON GV. The pretreatment peripheral blood lymphocyte count in 1100 patients with Hodgkins disease: the prognostic significance and the relationship to the presence of systemic symptoms. *Clin Oncol.* 1981;**7**:333-9.
101. DELLON AL, POTVIN C, CHRETIEN PB. Prognostic value of pre-treatment lymphocyte count and T cell levels in localized bronchogenic carcinoma. *J Surg Oncol.* 1979;**12**:253-61.
102. MINOT GR, HEATH CW. The response of the reticulocytes to iron. *Am J Med Sci.* 1932;**183**:110.
103. SWAN HT, JOWETT GH. Treatment of iron deficiency with ferrous fumarate: assessment by a statistically accurate method. *Br Med J.* 1959;**2**:782-7.
104. BRECHER G, ANDERSON RE, MCMULLEN PD. When to do diffs: how often should differential counts be repeated? *Blood Cells.* 1980;**6**:431-54.
105. JUUL S, PLISKIN JS, FINEBERG HV. Variation and information in white blood cell differential counts. *Med Decis Making.* 1984;**4**:69-80.
106. LENNARD ES, DELLINGER EP, WERTZ MJ, MINSHEW BH. Implications of leukocytosis and fever at conclusion of antiobiotic therapy for intra-abdominal sepsis. *Ann Surg.* 1982;**195**:19-24.
107. BENSON AB III, READ TR, GOEBEL SL, KOELLER JM, TORMEY DC. Correlations between leukocyte count and absolute granulocyte count in patients receiving cancer chemotherapy. *Cancer.* 1985;**56**:1350-5.
108. LI FP, DANAHY J, GELMAN R. Utility of differential leukocyte counts in cancer management. *JAMA.* 1984;**252**:1312-4.

Diagnostic Uses of the Activated Partial Thromboplastin Time and Prothrombin Time

ANTHONY L. SUCHMAN, M.D.; and
PAUL F. GRINER, M.D.

OF THE MANY tests available to assess blood coagulation, clinicians use the activated partial thromboplastin time (APTT) and prothrombin time (PT) most frequently, and for good reason. These tests are relatively inexpensive and accurate, yet their use varies considerably among practitioners and institutions. Often, they are ordered unnecessarily. In this review, we briefly describe the tests and then consider their value in four common clinical situations: screening patients preoperatively to reduce the risk of postoperative hemorrhage; screening nonsurgical patients for coagulation disorders and liver disease; evaluating abnormal bleeding; and monitoring treatment with anticoagulants. Table 1 summarizes our recommendations and their justifications.

Description

ACTIVATED PARTIAL THROMBOPLASTIN TIME

The APTT measures the activity of the intrinsic system and common pathway of the coagulation system (Table 2). The result, expressed in seconds, reflects the time required for a fibrin clot to form after calcium and an activating agent are added to the patient's citrated, platelet-poor plasma. The result is compared either to the time obtained simultaneously on a normal control plasma sample or to a distribution of normal values (4).

False-positive test results may occur in patients with polycythemia, when an inadequate volume of blood is obtained, or when blood is drawn from an intravenous or

▶ This chapter was originally published in *Annals of Internal Medicine.* 1986;**104**:810-6.

Table 1. Recommendations on Use of the Activated Partial Thromboplastin Time and Prothrombin Time

Screening
    Neither test indicated for screening asymptomatic patients.
    Clinical assessment is equally sensitive.
    Low prevalence of clinically unsuspected coagulopathies results in a high ratio of false-positive to true-positive test results.
Evaluating abnormal bleeding
    Both tests are indicated.
    Both tests are sensitive and have low false-positive rates.
    The pattern of results guides further investigation.
Monitoring anticoagulation therapy
    Activated partial thromboplastin time and prothrombin time are indicated to monitor heparin and warfarin therapy, respectively.
    Monitoring appears to enhance safety and effectiveness.

intra-arterial catheter containing heparin. False-negative results may occur when a minor deficiency of one clotting factor is masked by high levels of another, particularly factor VIII (an acute phase reactant) (5).

PROTHROMBIN TIME

The PT assesses the function of the extrinsic system and common pathway (Table 2). In particular, the test measures the activity of factor VII, a vitamin-K-dependent factor that is synthesized in the liver and has a short half-life. Thus, the PT yields evidence about the current synthetic capacity of the liver, the adequacy of vitamin K (hence, fat) absorption, and the inhibition of clotting factor synthesis by warfarin.

The result, expressed in seconds, reflects the time required for fibrin strands to appear after the addition of tissue thromboplastin and calcium to a patient's platelet-poor plasma (2). False-positive tests result from under-filling of the test tube or other improper handling of the blood sample (6, 7). At usual therapeutic doses, heparin has little effect on the PT (8).

Preoperative Screening for Coagulation Disorders

ACTIVATED PARTIAL THROMBOPLASTIN TIME

Effect of Disease Detection on Outcome: In using the APTT as a screening test, clinicians want to identify asymptomatic patients who are at increased risk for postoperative hemorrhage so that they may take appropriate preventive action. (The evaluation of symptomatic patients is not considered screening.) However, screening cannot affect the course in the large majority of patients with postoperative hemorrhages because the bleeding is caused not by coagulation abnormalities but by problems of anatomy, concurrent treatments, or surgical technique which the test cannot detect (Suchman AL, Mushlin AI. Unpublished observations). As will be discussed later, serious hemorrhages caused by coagulopathies are extremely unlikely in adults with no clinical evidence of bleeding risk. Thus, in asymptomatic patients, there are virtually no such events to prevent. At best, screening might reduce the perioperative transfusion requirements of patients with occult minor coagulopathies, but even this small gain would be offset by the additional fresh frozen plasma that would have to be given prophylactically.

Table 2. Concentrations of Plasma Coagulation Factors Needed for Normal Coagulation

Factor		Percent Normal Concentration Needed for Normal Coagulation*
Intrinsic system only		
XII	Hageman factor	. . .
XI	Plasma thromboplastin antecedent	20
IX	Christmas factor†	40
VIII	Antihemophilic factor	30
Extrinsic system only		
VII	Proconvertin†	25‡
Common pathway (intrinsic and extrinsic systems)		
X	Stuart factor†	40
V	Proaccelerin	40
II	Prothrombin†	40
I	Fibrinogen	(100 mg/dL§)

* Disorders of the intrinsic system may lead to prolongation of the activated partial thromboplastin time; disorders of the extrinsic system may lead to prolongation of the prothrombin time; and disorders of the common pathway may lead to prolongation of both. Data on normal concentrations are from Colman and colleagues (1).
† Vitamin K dependent.
‡ Data from Hougie (2) and Britten and Salzman (3).
§ Because the fibrinogen concentration is so variable, the actual concentration is more useful than a percentage to indicate adequacy of coagulation.

Some physicians order an APTT test before surgery to have a "baseline" value in the chart, reasoning that if a postoperative hemorrhage were to occur, an APTT drawn at the time of the hemorrhage would be uninterpretable because of transfused blood, consumption of clotting factors, or other confounding circumstances. However, to the extent that this "uninterpretable" test reflects the current competence of the coagulation system, it is the only test that matters in planning immediate treatment. A baseline study would not influence treatment, and although it might hasten the definitive diagnosis of the bleeding disorder, no harm results from delay.

Studies of Test Performance: Several studies have addressed the clinical usefulness of screening with the APTT test. Robbins and Rose (9) retrospectively reviewed the charts of all inpatients (surgical and nonsurgical) with abnormal APTT results from a series of 1000 consecutive determinations (none of the tests in this series was ordered to monitor heparin therapy because their hospital used the activated clotting time rather than the APTT for that purpose). Of the 143 patients with elevated values, 82% had historical findings (known before the screening test was ordered) that raised the suspicion of a clotting disorder. These findings included history of anticoagulant administration, hemophilia, liver disease, and malabsorption. The remaining 18% either had values that were only slightly elevated (within 10 seconds of normal) or had a second APTT determination that was normal. In none of the 143 patients did the test offer new information or alter clinical management. The authors suggested that clinical assessment suffices and that the APTT test is not necessary. However, because their study group was small, did not include any "target" outcomes (that is, unsuspected bleeding disorders or postoperative hemorrhages), and did not compare patients with abnormal results to those with normal results, it cannot help us assess quantitatively the value of screening.

Eisenberg and coworkers (10) monitored the clinical courses of 750 patients admitted consecutively to three surgical and obstetric/gynecologic services. Of these 750 patients, 611 had no clinical evidence to suggest increased risk of postoperative hemorrhage (no history of anticoagulant administration, liver disease, or abnormal bleeding in the patient or a relative and no ecchymosis, hematoma, purpura, or petechiae on physical examination). Four hundred eighty of these patients, in turn, had preoperative PT or APTT determinations done, or both. Among the 13 patients who had prolongation of one or more of these screening tests, only 1 had a postoperative hemorrhage (she had bleeding from a single small artery after an emergency cesarean section). Thus, of the 480 low-risk patients, only 1 might have benefited from the information gained from a preoperative APTT and none from a preoperative PT. As with the study by Robbins and Rose (9), the number of "target" outcomes was small and patients with normal test results were not evaluated.

In a recent study, we used hospital management and laboratory computer files to review the records of all adult inpatients who had invasive procedures at Strong Memorial Hospital in 1981 (11). Of these 12 338 patients, 1827 could not be identified as being at increased risk of hemorrhage on clinical grounds (no concurrent liver disease, malabsorption, malnutrition, or previously documented coagulation disorder) but had a screening APTT test performed. In this low-risk group, only 7.7% of the patients who had postoperative hemorrhages had an abnormal test result (sensitivity, 7.7%). Thirteen percent of the patients who did not have a postoperative hemorrhage had abnormal screening results (false-positive rate, 13%). In contrast, among patients with clinical evidence to suggest increased risk of bleeding, the sensitivity of the APTT test was 57% and the false-positive rate was 33%.

Pretest Probability (Prevalence): The incidence of postoperative hemorrhage varies considerably with the type of procedure. Many departments of surgery calculate hemorrhage rates for each type of procedure. Such data, if available, would give the best estimate of a particular patient's risk. As a global estimate, we found that the probability of postoperative hemorrhage was 0.22% among patients at low risk (on clinical grounds) and 1.7% among patients at high risk (11).

Post-test Probability: In our study (11), the post-test probability of hemorrhage (risk of hemorrhage when the APTT is known) in the low-risk group after an abnormal test (0.41%) was actually lower than (the pretest probability (0.71% for patients who had an APTT measured). After a normal test, the probability was 0.75%. In the high-risk group, the probability of hemorrhage after an abnormal test was 7.69% and after a negative test, 2.95% (the pretest probability in patients who had an APTT done was 4.5%). Thus, the APTT could not predict hemorrhages in the low-risk group. (This finding should not be surprising, because most hemorrhages occur for reasons other than coagulation defects.) In the high-risk group, the APTT was a predictor of weak magnitude but appropriate direction.

Using published estimates of disease prevalence and APTT performance, Clarke and Eisenberg (12) have found that the probability of hemophilia in an asymptomatic man after an abnormal screening test would be only 0.11%, not large enough to warrant additional action. Their analysis shows that although the sensitivity and false-positive rate of the APTT test in detecting hemophilia are quite good (as we shall see below), the prevalence of clinically inapparent coagulopathies is so low that false-positive results greatly outnumber true-positive results, making screening pointless.

PROTHROMBIN TIME

The PT adds little to the APTT in preoperative screening. The only condition predisposing to bleeding that the PT can detect and the APTT cannot is an isolated deficiency of factor VII. The prevalence of this condition is 2 to 3/1 000 000 (13, 14). Consequently, the post-test probability of factor VII deficiency after an abnormal PT will be even lower than that in hemophilia screening, as described above. Furthermore, homozygous factor VII deficiency imparts a much lower risk of hemorrhage than do homozygous deficiencies of factors VIII or IX, and then only after procedures that leave raw surfaces, such as dental extraction and tonsillectomy (3).

Asymptomatic patients need not be screened with a PT determination for acquired factor VII deficiency, such as occurs in hepatic disease, malabsorption, and malnutrition, because the test result is abnormal only in the presence of advanced, obvious disease (15). However, when such conditions are present, the PT may be prolonged even when the APTT is not (16).

Table 3. Elements of the Preoperative Assessment of Bleeding Risk*

History
    Personal or family history of known bleeding disorder.
    Personal or family history of prolonged bleeding after an injury, dental extraction, or other surgical procedure.
    Personal or family history of frequent or severe nosebleeds or spontaneous bleeding at other sites.
    Personal history of liver disease, malabsorption, or malnutrition.
    Recent use of anticoagulants (although not related to coagulation defects, history of recent aspirin use should also be sought).
Physical findings
    Inspection of the skin and mucous membranes for petechiae, echymoses, and hematomas.

---

* Patients with one or more of these findings or for whom these elements cannot be adequately assessed should have preoperative screening with the activated partial thromboplastin time and prothrombin time. Patients who do not have these findings do not require screening coagulation tests. Data on history from Rapaport (17).

RECOMMENDATIONS

An adequate clinical assessment (Table 3)—which includes a properly obtained medical history, such as that outlined by Rapaport (17), and an examination for evidence of purpura, liver disease, malabsorption, and malnutrition—is sufficiently sensitive in detecting congenital and acquired coagulopathies as to obviate laboratory testing of persons with normal findings (9, 10, 13, 18). Therefore, we do not recommend preoperative screening with either the APTT or PT test for patients without clinical evidence of a coagulation disorder. We do recommend preoperative testing with both the APTT and PT tests for patients in whom adequate clinical assessment is not possible; for patients with clinical evidence to suggest a bleeding disorder, liver disease, malabsorption, or malnutrition; and for patients whose normal coagulation may be disrupted by the planned procedure (for example, insertion of a peritoneovenous shunt, prostatectomy, or procedures involving extracorporeal circulation). Abnormal test results warrant repetition and, if results are still abnormal, more detailed evaluation with second-order tests (for example, factor assays and correction studies).

Screening Nonsurgical Patients for Coagulation Disorders

The screening of inpatients not undergoing surgical or other invasive procedures does not seem warranted, because the APTT and PT tests are no more sensitive than clinical assessment in detecting coagulation disorders (or liver disease) (15). In addition, there is not a pressing need to identify patients at risk for bleeding.

Nonsurgical patients (both in and out of the hospital) who do not have specific indications for coagulation testing do not require screening. The practice of ordering the APTT or PT or both routinely for all admitted patients should be abandoned.

Evaluation of Abnormal Bleeding

Patients who develop spontaneous bleeding or prolonged bleeding after an injury or surgical procedure may have a hereditary or acquired coagulation defect. Appropriately, the APTT and PT tests are universally recommended as the initial studies in the evaluation of such patients (1, 19, 20).

Detection and categorization of a coagulation disorder in a bleeding patient allows administration of the most specific treatment available, which, in turn, maximizes both therapeutic benefit and efficiency in the use of blood products. Also, preventive measures may be taken before doing subsequent elective procedures in a patient so identified.

ACTIVATED PARTIAL THROMBOPLASTIN TIME

Studies of Test Performance: Eight years after Langdell and colleagues (21) introduced the partial thromboplastin time, Proctor and Rapaport (22) reported their experience with a refined version, the APTT, and evaluated its performance in 37 patients with known deficiencies of intrinsic clotting factors. The APTT was abnormal in all patients with moderate and severe deficiency but failed to detect 1 patient with mild factor VIII deficiency (factor VIII levels were 47% of normal) and 3 with mild factor XI deficiency (levels were 36% to 43% of normal). However, they defined normal as within 3 SD of the mean. Had they used a cutoff of 2 SD, as is the practice today, only 2 patients with mild factor XI deficiency (levels of 40% and 43% of normal) would have gone undetected.

Using test samples of known factor VIII concentration, Poller (23) found a 99% sensitivity in the detection of factor VIII levels of 10% of normal and a sensitivity of 90% for levels of 24% of normal. Nye and coworkers (16) found an overall sensitivity of 99% in detecting deficiencies of any intrinsic factor among 618 patients referred for evaluation of abnormal bleeding. In that study, the investigators used the partial thromboplastin time, which may be less sensitive than the APTT in detecting minor factor deficiencies. Offsetting this potential underestimation of sensitivity is the potential overestimation resulting from a detection bias, a problem that arises when some patients are not evaluated as fully as others. In this case, patients with abnormal test results would have been more likely to receive complete testing than those with normal results. Therefore, some patients classified as having true-negative results may actually have had factor deficiencies and should have been classified as having false-negative results. Such misclassification makes the sensitivity appear better than it is.

Estimates of the performance of the APTT test in detecting deficiencies of each of the intrinsic coagulation factors are presented in Table 4. In each case, the false-positive rate is shown as a range. The lower limit, 2%, represents the statistical definition of the cutoff, 2 SD above the mean in a population of normal patients. However, when the test is used in patients who do not have normal clinical findings, the false-positive rate will be higher. Nye and associates (16) found a false-positive rate of 11% among patients undergoing evaluation for abnormal bleeding. Variability in the false-positive rate may also result from technical factors such as nonstandardized reagents, instrumentation, and specimen handling (24).

Pretest Probability of Coagulopathy: The pretest probability (prevalence) of coagulopathy depends heavily on the clinical setting. In the general population, the prevalence of congenital defects is approximately 17/100 000 among men (primarily factor VIII deficiency, factor IX deficiency, and von Willebrand's disease) and 5/100 000 among women (primarily von Willebrand's disease) (14, 20, 26). However, among patients who have abnormal bleeding, the prevalence can be as high as 40% (16). The prevalence of acquired coagulopathies depends on the

Table 4. Test Characteristics of the Activated Partial Thromboplastin Time (APTT) in Detecting Deficiences of the Intrinsic and Common Pathway Factors

Deficient Factor (Reference*)	Sensitivity	False-Positive Rate†
	%	%
XII (16, 22, 24)	100	2-11
XI (16, 22, 24)	100	2-11
IX (12, 22,24)	100	2-11
VIII		
Severe (0% to 5% normal) (16, 22,24)	100	2-11
Moderate (6% to 15% normal) (22-24)	99	2-11
Mild (16% to 30% normal) (22-24)	90	2-11
von Willebrand's disease (16, 25)	48-100	2-11
X (16)	100	2-11
V (16)	100	2-11
Any intrinsic factor (16, 24)	98	2-11

* Data from reference 16 was obtained with the partial thromboplastin time, which may be less sensitive than the APTT in detecting mild deficiencies.
† Eleven percent for patients being evaluated for abnormal bleeding; 2% for clinically normal patients.

prevalence of the underlying conditions and is difficult to summarize with a single statistic.

Post-test Probability of Coagulopathy: If the prior probability of a coagulation defect in a symptomatic patient is 40% and the sensitivity and false-positive rate of the APTT test are 99% and 11%, respectively, the probability of disease after an abnormal test result is 86% (justifying additional studies) and after a normal test is 0.7% (effectively ruling out coagulopathy). Even at a pretest probability as low as 5%, the post-test probability of 32% is sufficiently high to warrant further testing.

PROTHROMBIN TIME

The PT contributes to the evaluation of abnormal bleeding in two ways. First, it is highly sensitive in detecting factor VII deficiency. Two extensive reviews have shown that the sensitivity of the PT test in detecting both severe (< 5% of normal) and moderate (5% to 25% of normal) factor VII deficiency is 100% (27, 28). Thus, a normal test result rules out the possibility of disease. Second, the PT in combination with the APTT directs attention to factors of the intrinsic, extrinsic, or common pathway (Table 1), allowing selective use of expensive second-order tests (1, 19, 20).

RECOMMENDATIONS

Both the APTT and PT tests, along with the platelet count and bleeding time, are useful in investigating patients with suspected coagulation abnormalities. Normal APTT and PT results essentially rule out a significant coagulation defect. Abnormal results of one or both tests focus further attention on limited segments of the coagulation sequence.

Monitoring Anticoagulation
ACTIVATED PARTIAL THROMBOPLASTIN TIME

Effect of Disease Detection on Outcome: When giving heparin anticoagulation therapy to a patient, clinicians would like to prevent unwanted clotting without increasing the risk of hemorrhage. Because these two consequences of treatment cannot be separated, clinicians try to balance them by keeping the degree of anticoagulation within a therapeutic range (APTT between 1.5 and 2.5 times control) (29). It is assumed that an APTT less than 1.5 times control indicates insufficient anticoagulation (hence, an unacceptable risk of recurrent thrombosis), and that an APTT greater than 2.5 times control indicates an unacceptably increased risk of hemorrhage. It is further assumed that restoring the APTT to the proper range reduces the excess risk. Testing these assumptions quantitatively is difficult because of the nonlinear relationship between heparin concentrations in the blood and APTT values and because instruments and reagents vary in their sensitivity to heparin-induced anticoagulation (prompting suggestions that other tests be used instead) (24, 30, 31). Nonetheless, although there are no prospective controlled studies, some observational studies offer qualitative evidence that monitoring is useful.

Studies of Test Performance: In a retrospective study, Norman and Provan (32) have found a relationship between persistent excessive prolongation of the APTT and major hemorrhage. Five of ten patients whose APTT values were prolonged beyond the therapeutic range in more than 50% of their determinations developed major hemorrhages as compared with 1 of 40 patients having more than 50% of their determinations within the therapeutic range. Several other retrospective studies, reviewed in detail by Kelton and Hirsh (30), have shown similar results. In the only prospective study of hemorrhagic complications of continuous heparin infusion (which was nevertheless uncontrolled), Basu and colleagues (29) found no difference in APTT values between patients who bled and those who did not. However, the anticoagulation of their 234 patients was so well regulated that they had little opportunity to observe an increase in the risk of hemorrhage.

Kelton and Hirsh (30) caution against the overreliance on observational data (comparing patients who bleed with those who do not), because "factors that influence the results of the blood test [may] influence bleeding independently." They conclude that in the absence of randomized studies, evidence on the association between the APTT and risk of hemorrhage is suggestive but not conclusive.

Similarly, the association between subtherapeutic APTT values and recurrent thrombosis is suggested but not firmly established. In the study by Basu and colleagues (29), five patients developed recurrent thromboembolism while receiving heparin. All five had had subtherapeutic APTT values just before their recurrences. Although it is not clear whether the recurrences resulted from peculiarities of the patients' coagulation systems or simply insufficient therapy, the APTT test did appear to identify successfully the patients at risk. There have been no studies of optimal timing of APTT determinations in monitoring patients on heparin therapy.

PROTHROMBIN TIME

Effect of Disease Detection on Outcome: Just as with heparin, clinicians wish to keep oral anticoagulation within a therapeutic range (defined according to the PT) to maximize efficacy and minimize the risk of bleeding. This range has recently been revised from 2 to 2.5 down to 1.3 to 1.4 times control (using rabbit brain thromboplastin, the most widely used reagent in North America) (33).

Studies of Test Performance: Hull and associates (34) randomly assigned 96 patients with proximal deep vein thrombosis to receive warfarin and monitored them with either the Simplastin time (General Diagnostics, Scarborough, Ontario, Canada) (resulting in more intensive anticoagulation) or the Manchester (England) comparative reagent (resulting in less intensive anticoagulation). No differences were seen in the rates of recurrent thrombosis (2.0% and 2.1%, respectively) or major bleeding complications (4.1% and 4.3%, respectively) between the two groups. Each of the 4 patients (2 in each group) who had major hemorrhages had both predisposing factors for bleeding and excessively prolonged PT values. Minor hemorrhages occurred in 18.4% of the more intensively anticoagulated group but in no patients from the less intensively anticoagulated group. None of the patients with minor bleeding had underlying causes. The mean warfarin dosages in the more intensely and less intensely anticoagulated groups were 5.8 and 4.9 mg/d, respectively. The study did not assess monitoring per se, in that it did not compare administration of warfarin according to PT values with administration according to some other basis (for example, body weight). However, it does show that greater and lesser degrees of PT elevation identify intensities of anticoagulation with greater and lesser risk of hemorrhagic complications.

An earlier randomized study and several retrospective studies reviewed by Kelton and Hirsh (30) suggest that the PT test can discriminate between ranges of adequate and inadequate anticoagulation. Therefore, although there is considerable controversy regarding reagents, technique, and exact definitions of the therapeutic range, the PT test appears to be useful in monitoring treatment with oral anticoagulants.

In current practice, the PT is measured daily during the first week of therapy, then weekly, and eventually monthly, provided that frequent adjustments in anticoagulant dosage are not required. More frequent determinations may be needed when therapy is started with a new drug that may interact with warfarin. Although formal proof is lacking, the low cost of the test as compared with the high costs engendered by hemorrhagic complications and recurrent thrombosis would seem to justify this practice (Figure 1).

RECOMMENDATIONS

Although definitive evidence is lacking, we recommend that heparin anticoagulation therapy be monitored with daily APTT measurements (with more frequent mea-

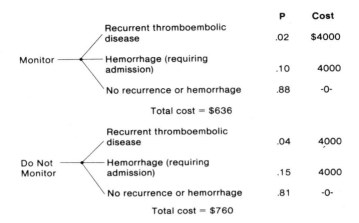

Figure 1. A decision tree comparing weekly monitoring to no monitoring over a 3-month course of warfarin therapy. Estimates for costs and reduction in rates of recurrent thromboembolic disease and hemorrhage are deliberately conservative and are based on 1982 charges at Strong Memorial Hospital and event rates cited by Hull and colleagues (34) and Kelton and Hirsh (30). Figures in the cost column represent the average cost of hospitalization for thromboembolic disease or hemorrhage. Total cost of monitoring ($636) includes charges for weekly prothrombin time (PT) determinations for 3 months ($156). Charges decrease as the frequency of PT determinations decreases from weekly to monthly. We have used a "worst-case" example in which the anticoagulant dose does not remain stable, necessitating weekly PT measurements. In less extreme cases, the cost of monitoring will be even less.

surements during the initiation of therapy) and that warfarin anticoagulation therapy be monitored with PT measurements (daily during the first week of therapy, weekly for the next few weeks, and then monthly if the values are stable). There is no reason to order both tests simultaneously, except to monitor a change from one type of anticoagulation to the other. The prophylactic use of low-dose, subcutaneous heparin injections does not require monitoring (35).

Conclusions

We have reviewed the three main uses of the APTT and PT tests: screening, evaluating abnormal bleeding, and monitoring anticoagulation therapy. We have presented evidence that clinical assessment constitutes adequate screening of surgical and nonsurgical patients alike, and that the APTT and PT do not perform well as screening tests. It is probably in routine admission and preoperative screening that most unnecessary coagulation tests are ordered (the other circumstance being the ordering of both tests when only one is needed). We recommend that these tests be used only to follow up patients with abnormal clinical findings, to screen patients who cannot be adequately evaluated clinically (for example, if the history is unavailable), and to screen patients having procedures that will interfere with hemostasis (for example, insertion of a peritoneovenous shunt, transurethral prostatectomy, and procedures requiring extracorporeal circulation).

For the evaluation of abnormal bleeding, we conclude that both the APTT and PT measurements constitute an appropriate first step in the laboratory investigation. If results of both tests are normal, no further study of the coagulation system is needed. If results of either or both tests are abnormal, the subsequent evaluation can be highly focused. The APTT and PT appear to be useful in monitoring anticoagulation therapy with heparin and warfarin, respectively, to reduce the risks of recurrent thrombosis and hemorrhagic complications.

ACKNOWLEDGMENTS: The authors thank Dr. Victor Marder for his comments during the preparation of this manuscript.

Grant support: By the Blue Cross/Blue Shield Association Medical Necessity Program in cooperation with the Technology Assessment Committee of the Society for Research and Education in Primary Care Internal Medicine (SREPCIM). Part of this work was done while Dr. Suchman was a Henry J. Kaiser Family Foundation Fellow in General Internal Medicne.

References

1. COLMAN RW, HIRSH J, MARDER VJ, SALZMAN EW. Approach to the bleeding patient. In: COLMAN RW, HIRSH J, MARDER VJ, SALZMAN EW, eds. *Hemostasis and Thrombosis: Basic Principles and Clinical Practice.* Philadelphia: J. B. Lippincott Company; 1982:694-700.
2. HOUGIE C. One-stage prothrombin time. In: WILLIAMS WJ, BEUTLER E, ERSLEV AJ, LICHTMAN MA, eds. *Hematology.* 3rd ed. New York: McGraw-Hill Book Co.; 1983:1665-7.
3. BRITTEN AFH, SALZMAN EW. Surgery in congenital disorders of blood coagulation. *Surg Gynecol Obstet.* 1966;**123:**1333-58.
4. HOUGIE C. Recalcification time test and its modifications (partial thromboplastin time, activated partial thromboplastin time and expanded partial thromboplastin time). In: WILLIAMS WJ, BEUTLER E, ERSLEV AJ, LICHTMAN MA, eds. *Hematology.* 3rd ed. New York: McGraw-Hill Book Co.; 1983:1662-5.
5. EDSON JR, KRIVIT W, WHITE JG. Kaolin partial thromboplastin time: high levels of procoagulants producing short clotting times or masking deficiencies of other procoagulants or low concentrations of anticoagulants. *J Lab Clin Med.* 1967;**70:**463-70.

6. PETERSON P, GOTTFRIED EL. The effects of inaccurate blood sample volume on prothrombin time (PT) and activated partial thromboplastin time. (APTT). *Thromb Haemost.* 1982;**47**:101-3.

7. PALMER RN, KESSLER CM, GRALNIK HR. Warfarin anticoagulation: difficulties in interpretation of the prothrombin time. *Thromb Res.* 1982;**25**:125-30.

8. SALZMAN EW, DEYKIN D, SHAPIRO RM, ROSENBERG R. Management of heparin therapy: a controlled prospective trial. *N Engl J Med.* 1975;**292**:1046-50.

9. ROBBINS JA, ROSE SD. Partial thromboplastin time as a screening test. *Ann Intern Med.* 1979;**90**:796-7.

10. EISENBERG JM, CLARKE JR, SUSSMAN SA. Prothrombin and partial thromboplastin times as preoperative screening tests. *Arch Surg.* 1982;**117**:48-51.

11. SUCHMAN AL, MUSHLIN AI. Preoperative screening with the activated partial thromboplastin time. *JAMA.* 1986. (In press).

12. CLARKE JR, EISENBERG JM. A theoretical assessment of the value of the PTT as a preoperative screening test in adults. *Med Decis Making.* 1981;**1**:40-3.

13. BACHMANN F. Diagnostic approach to mild bleeding disorders. *Semin Hematol.* 1980;**17**:292-305.

14. HOUGIE C. Hemophilia and related conditions—congenital deficiencies of prothrombin (factor II), factor V, and factors VII to XII. In: WILLIAMS WJ, BEUTLER E, ERSLEV AJ, LICHTMAN MA, eds. *Hematology.* 3rd ed. New York: McGraw-Hill Book Co.; 1983:1381-99.

15. EISENBERG JM, GOLDFARB S. Clinical usefulness of measuring prothrombin time as a routine admission test. *Clin Chem.* 1976;**22**:1644-7.

16. NYE SW, GRAHAM JB, BRINKHOUS KM. The partial thromboplastin time as a screening test for the detection of latent bleeders. *Am J Med Sci.* 1962;**243**:279-87.

17. RAPAPORT SI. Preoperative hemostatic evaluation: which tests, if any? *Blood.* 1983;**61**:229-31.

18. BEVAN DH. A field guide to the bleeding disorders for the general practitioner. *Practitioner.* 1982;**226**:25-32.

19. PASMANTIER MW, COLEMAN M. Current concepts in fibrin clot formation. In: DONOSO E, HAFT JI, eds. *Thrombosis, Platelets, Anticoagulation, and Acetylsalicylic Acid.* New York: Stratton Intercontinental Medical Book Corp.; 1976:1-15.

20. MCKEE PA. Disorders of blood coagulation. In: WYNGAARDEN JB, SMITH LH, eds. *Cecil Textbook of Medicine.* 17th ed. Philadelphia: W. B. Saunders Company; 1985:1040-58.

21. LANGDELL RD, WAGNER RH, BRINKHOUS KM. Effect of antihemophilic factor on one-stage clotting tests. *J Lab Clin Med.* 1953;**41**:637-47.

22. PROCTOR RR, RAPAPORT SI. The partial thromboplastin time with kaolin: a simple screening test for first stage plasma clotting factor deficiencies. *Am J Clin Pathol.* 1961;**36**:212-9.

23. POLLER L. Severe bleeding disorders in children with normal coagulation screening tests [Letter]. *Br Med J [Clin Res].* 1982;**285**:377.

24. HATHAWAY WE, ASSMUS SL, MONTGOMERY RR, DUBANSKY AS. Activated partial thromboplastin time and minor coagulopathies. *Am J Clin Pathol.* 1979;**71**:22-5.

25. LIAN EC, DEYKIN D. Diagnosis of von Willebrand's disease: a comparative study of diagnostic tests on nine families with von Willebrand's disease and its differential diagnosis from hemophilia and thrombocytopathy. *Am J Med.* 1976;**60**:344-56.

26. WEIS HJ. Von Willebrand's disease. In: WILLIAMS WJ, BEUTLER E, ERSLEV A, LICHTMAN M, eds. *Hematology.* 3rd ed. New York: McGraw-Hill Book Co.; 1983:1413-20.

27. MARDER VJ, SHULMAN NR. Clinical aspects of congenital factor VII deficiency. *Am J Med.* 1964;**37**:1982-94.

28. OWEN CA, AMUNDSEN MA, THOMPSON JH, et al. Congenital deficiency of factor VII (hypoconvertinemia). *Am J Med.* 1964;**37**:71-91.
29. BASU D, GALLUS A, HIRSH J, CADE J. A prospective study of the value of monitoring heparin treatment with the activated partial thromboplastin time. *N Engl J Med.* 1972;**287**:324-7.
30. KELTON JG, HIRSH J. Bleeding associated with antithrombotic therapy. *Semin Hematol.* 1980;**17**:259-91.
31. BRANDT JT, TRIPLETT DA. Laboratory monitoring of heparin: effect of reagents and instruments on the activated partial thromboplastin time. *Am J Clin Pathol.* 1981;**76**(4 suppl):530-7.
32. NORMAN CS, PROVAN JL. Control and complications of intermittent heparin therapy. *Surg Gynecol Obstet.* 1977;**145**:388-42.
33. HIRSH J. Therapeutic range for the control of oral anticoagulant therapy [Editorial]. *Arch Intern Med.* 1985;**145**:1187-8.
34. HULL R, HIRSH J, JAY R, et al. Different intensities of oral anticoagulant therapy in the treatment of proximal-vein thrombosis. *N Engl J Med.* 1982;**307**:1676-81.
35. TURPIE AG, HIRSH J. Prophylaxis and therapy of venous thromboembolism. *CRC Crit Rev Clin Lab Sci.* 1979;**10**:247-74.

Blood Cultures

MARK D. ARONSON, M.D.; and DAVID H. BOR, M.D.

SINCE THE EARLIEST application, when *Streptococcus viridans* was diagnosed as the cause of "malignant endocarditis" (1), blood cultures have been used whenever physicians suspect the presence of clinically significant bacteremia. Although several other assays and methods can be used to detect evidence of bacteremia (2), the blood culture remains the "gold-standard" test for defining that condition.

Although more than 200 000 cases of septicemia occur annually (3), controversy exists around the optimal number of cultures necessary to ensure the detection of this condition. This article reviews the literature on the performance of the blood culture as a diagnostic test and examines the data on the optimal number of cultures to draw. An extensive literature, much of it recent, describes the methods and role of the clinical microbiology laboratory, epidemiologic patterns of bacteremias of hospital and community origin, and clinical characteristics of patients with bacteremia (3-11). We discuss these data only as they pertain to the interpretation of the results of the blood culture and as they help to improve understanding of the test's sensitivity and specificity.

Test Description

In order to detect clinically "significant bacteremia," a patient's blood must be sampled at one or more points in time and then incubated in culture media. Bacterial growth is detected by various techniques, a specific organism(s) identified, and antimicrobial susceptibility tested. A single sampling is termed a blood culture. Fre-

▶ This chapter was originally published in *Annals of Internal Medicine*. 1987:**106**:246-253.

quently, several samples are collected, thereby constituting a blood culture series.

Optimal functioning of this test depends on timing, the number of samplings, sterile technique in drawing and handling the blood samples, the volume of blood sampled, the growth characteristics of the medium, the system for detection of growth in culture, and the clinician's ability to interpret the results. In the Appendix, we describe some details of blood culture methods. More comprehensive descriptions have been published by the American Society for Microbiology (6, 12) and the Mayo Clinic (4).

Clinical Application

Detection of bacteremia has great clinical significance in establishing the primary diagnosis for certain high-risk populations (for example, febrile hospitalized patients, febrile neutropenic patients, and patients with nosocomial infections); ascertaining or confirming the bacteriologic cause of a focal infection; providing prognostic information and alerting the physician to potential complications of a focal infection (for example, osteomyelitis or meningitis); providing a means to exclude serious illness (for example, infective endocarditis); and monitoring therapy. In many situations, the positive result in a blood culture directly establishes the diagnosis (for example, infective endocarditis or spontaneous pneumococcal bacteremia); in other situations, when the organism causing the infection is difficult to isolate from the primary source, a positive blood culture provides indirect evidence (for example, osteomyelitis).

Bacteremias are classified as transient, intermittent, or continuous (6, 13). Transient bacteremias may occur early in the course of many localized infections or after manipulation of infected tissue or colonized mucosal surfaces (such as during surgical drainage of an abscess or during dental procedures) (14). Activities of daily living, such as bowel movements or teeth brushing, also cause transient bacteremias. These bacteremias usually resolve spontaneously. Intermittent bacteremia is typical of undrained abscesses. Continuous bacteremia is the *sine qua non* of endovascular infections like infective endocarditis, septic thrombophlebitis, and mycotic aneurysms and of the early phases of typhoid fever and brucellosis.

Definitions

"GOLD-STANDARD" TEST

The blood culture is the only test used to define bacteremia; there is no independent "gold-standard" test with which to evaluate the blood culture. Ideally, ascertaining whether the conventional blood culture is a valid gold-standard test for clinically significant bacteremia would require sampling blood continuously; identifying and quantifying bacteria by an independent technique, perhaps one that does not require microbial growth; and following untreated patients to ascertain the significance of the bacteremia. These cannot be done. Instead, small quantities of blood are sampled and cultured at a limited number of intervals. A series of these cultures become a surrogate for a true gold-standard test. Any single culture yielding microbial growth defines the series as positive. This surrogate standard is interpreted in the context of clinical and other laboratory data.

The analysis of the sensitivity and specificity of the blood culture in the absence of an independent gold-standard test creates several distortions. First, the surrogate standard and the individual tests that it comprises rely on identical sampling and culturing methods. Therefore, an individual test will always appear to perform well, regardless of technique—a self-fulfilling prophesy.

SENSITIVITY

Without an independent gold-standard test, sensitivity cannot be expressed. Sensitivity, or the true-positive rate, is defined as the likelihood of a positive test result in a person with bacteremia or as the number of true-positive results divided by the sum of the true-positive plus false-negative results (TP/[TP + FN]) (15). Because there is no independent standard, false-negative results cannot be identified, and sensitivity cannot be calculated. Instead, what can be calculated, and what is emphasized in this article, is the rate of positive blood culture sets among all blood cultures obtained from patients known to have bacteremia as defined by the surrogate gold-standard procedure (blood culture series). This ratio overestimates sensitivity. It will most closely approximate sensitivity when the number of false-negative results is reduced by employing a large number of individual cultures in the blood culture series or by studying a population with continuous bacteremia. On the other hand, when fewer tests are included in the surrogate standard, the correlation of the result of one test with that of the surrogate standard will appear higher, even when the two results are related only by chance. For example, in establishing the operating characteristics of this test, its sensitivity would be judged to be 100% if only one blood culture were studied. Yet, a single sampling may well miss transient or intermittent bacteremia.

SPECIFICITY

Similarly, the lack of an independent gold-standard test confounds the calculation of specificity. Specificity, or the true-negative rate, is defined as the likelihood of a negative test result in a patient without disease or as the number of true-negative results divided by the sum of true-negative plus false-positive results (TN/ [TN + FP]) (15).

Ultimately, false-positive blood cultures are differentiated from true-positive ones on clinical grounds: the cultured organism is not consistent with the infection in question. Because the same skin and mouth flora cause transient nonsignificant bacteremia and contaminate blood cultures, cultures yielding these organisms are probably lumped together as false positives.

Most studies of blood cultures investigate populations of hospitalized patients considered, by their physicians, to be at high enough risk for bacteremia to warrant culturing the blood. Clinical investigators subsequently determine whether these patients are not bacteremic through nonblinded, retrospective chart review. False-negative results are probably underdiagnosed, particularly among patients with intermittent bacteremia, and thus specificity is overestimated.

A larger problem with specificity calculations is one of nomenclature. Most investigators derive their study populations from the records of the bacteriology laboratory. The denominator is expressed as the number of blood cultures rather than as the number of patients. This practice probably causes an overestimation of the true specificity. Without information about the number of cultures drawn on each patient (surrogate gold-standard test), specificity cannot be calculated. Despite these problems with past evaluations of the operating characteristics of the blood culture as a diagnostic test, much information can be gleaned from the literature.

Test Performance: Literature Review

SENSITIVITY

The sensitivity of blood cultures has been analyzed most thoroughly in a study that evaluated laboratory, epidemiologic, and clinical features of patients with at least one positive blood culture (7). Patients were identified by positive culture reports from microbiology laboratories at a university and a Veterans Administration hospital. Investigators used multiple clinical and laboratory criteria to distinguish between true-positive and false-positive results. This method, similar to that used in an earlier study by MacGregor and Beaty (16), is necessarily subjective and based on an assessment of patients' records by a reviewer who knows that at least one blood culture was positive. The two studies (7, 16) are the best available in adhering strictly to standard methods of extracting and interpreting data from medical records (17). Table 1 lists factors, modified from the criteria in these two studies, that help in interpreting the results of a positive blood culture. The results of Weinstein and colleagues (7) are worth considering in some detail, because

Table 1. Guidelines Useful in Identifying False-Positive Blood Cultures

Test characteristics
  Skin flora are usually contaminants: diphtheroids, *Staphylococcus epidermidis, Bacillus* species.
  Enterobacteriaceae isolates, gram-negative anaerobes, *Streptococcus pyogenes*, or *Streptococcus pneumoniae* are rarely contaminants.
  Contaminants are rarely isolated in subsequent cultures.
  Multiple organisms isolated from one culture suggests contamination (polymicrobial bacteremia is unusual).
  Delayed detection of bacterial growth is commoner for contaminants.
Clinical findings
  Clinical course is not consistent with sepsis.
  Primary infection with the same flora is not found.
  Predisposing factors that would lead to bacteremia are absent, such as prosthetic devices, intravenous drug abuse, immunosuppression, and recent hospitalization.
  There is no leukocytosis or left shift in the differential count.

they are based on the most carefully performed study to date of positive blood cultures.

In that study (7), 282 patients from whom at least three sets of blood cultures were obtained had "true septicemia." Of the bacteremic episodes, 91.5% were detected by the first culture, 99.3% by the first two cultures, and 99.6% by at least one of the first three cultures. Only 1 of the 282 patients with true septicemia had negative results on the first three cultures.

The constancy of bacteremia was striking even among those 259 patients without infective endocarditis. The likelihood that a subsequent culture would be positive after the first positive culture was 75% to 80%. By contrast, in the set of 23 patients with endocarditis, the likelihood that a subsequent culture would be positive after an initial positive result was 95% to 100%.

A smaller study from the Mayo Clinic yielded similar results (18). Eighty patients with clinical and culture-proven bacteremia were evaluated. Unfortunately, in this study, the definition of true bacteremia was not provided. Eighty percent of cultures were positive with the first set, 89% after the first two sets, and 99% by the third set. Other series did not report the data in this way (9, 10).

Several factors may affect the sensitivity of a culture. The volume of blood is particularly important, especially in settings of low-level bacteremia. The majority of blood samples from patients with streptococcal and staphylococcal endocarditis bacteremia contain less than 30 colony-forming units per millilitre (19). More than half of 464 patients with gram-negative bacteremias studied by DuPont and Spink (20) were not identified by pour plates containing only 1 mL of blood. Hall and coworkers (21) showed that 10-mL blood samples per culture yielded significantly better recovery of gram-negative bacilli than did 5-mL blood samples. Weinstein and colleagues (7) have suggested that the reason their series reports a higher sensitivity than the Mayo Clinic series (18) is that they used 15-mL samples per culture rather than the 10-mL samples used in the Mayo Clinic series. A recent review by Washington and Ilstrup (3), from the Mayo Clinic, has recommended that at least 10-mL—and preferably 20 to 30 mL—of blood be obtained for each culture. (See the Appendix for further discussion of blood volume.)

Several observations challenge the conclusion that three blood cultures detect nearly all cases of bacteremia. "Nonsignificant" transient bacteremias probably occur frequently but, owing to their brevity, are usually missed. Studies of bacteremia that occur after manipulative procedures illustrate this problem. Reported rates of transient bacteremia vary from a low of 18% to a high of 85% after dental extractions (14, 22). The bacteremia occurs 1 to 5 minutes after a procedure and is usually cleared within 15 minutes. Transient bacteremia also follows bowel movements and teeth brushing. (Patients with bacteremia of this type would not have been included as having true septicemia in the studies of Weinstein and colleagues [7] and MacGregor and Beaty [16].) Patients with classical pneumococcal pneumonia typically have a rigor and almost certainly have transient bacteremia; yet, bacteremia is detected in only 25% to 30% of patients hospitalized with this disease (23, 24).

Detecting Continuous Bacteremia—The Special Problem of Endocarditis: The premortem diagnosis of infective endocarditis is usually defined, in large part, by the presence of continuous bacteremia. As with bacteremia in general, the rate of positive blood cultures is highly dependent on the criteria used to define the condition. Beeson and colleagues (25) used quantitative cultures to show that the magnitude of bacteremia is relatively constant. They concluded that the timing and number of cultures were not as important in patients with infective endocarditis as in those with intermittent forms of bacteremia because cultures were generally all positive or all negative.

Werner and colleagues (19) tested this notion in their landmark study of bacteremia in 206 patients with endocarditis at the New York Hospital-Cornell Medical Center. This study reviewed the cases of all patients with endocarditis at that hospital from 1944 through 1960. During that time, the technique of handling blood cultures did not change. Although strict diagnostic criteria were not provided, it is likely, given the expertise of the authors, that the diagnosis of endocarditis was rarely incorrect. The authors investigated the frequency with which blood cultures would be positive in patients with infective endocarditis and showed that, in the absence of antimicrobial therapy within the 2 weeks before hospitalization, 97% of cultures were positive in 129 patients with streptococcal infective endocarditis. For the 49 patients who had received antibiotics, the rate was lowered to 91%. For staphylococcal infective endocarditis, the same trend appeared: 41 of 43 blood cultures were positive in 17 patients with this condition. The 2 negative cultures occurred in 2 patients treated with antibiotics within the 2 weeks before the blood cultures.

Some studies have reported variable rates of bacteremia ranging from 53% to 99% in patients with infective endocarditis (26-29). There are several possible explanations for the lower rates of positive blood cultures reported by some authors. One frequently cited study (26) used only a 5-mL inoculum of blood. The magnitude of bacteremia may be quite low in infective endocarditis (19), and a 5-mL inoculum may be too small. Use of antibiotics and failure to do anaerobic cultures may have also resulted in lower rates. Other studies, before and since Werner and colleagues report (19), have corroborated the high sensitivity reported by this group. Barritt and Gillespie (27), using methods similar to those of Werner and colleagues, reported 99% of their cultures to be positive, and Cates and Christie (29) isolated the causative organism from 98% of cultures.

Since the 1970s, other factors have tended to reduce the very high rate of positive blood cultures in patients with infective endocarditis. Patients with prosthetic valves appear to have a slightly lower frequency of positive cultures than do patients with native valve endocarditis. Prosthetic-valve infective endocarditis accounted for 12% to 21% of cases in a recent series of patients with infective endocarditis (30-32). Positive rates as low as 68% have been reported (30). In Pelletier and Petersdorf's study (32), blood cultures were drawn from 162 of 165 patients with infective endocarditis. In only 3 patients with positive cultures were more than three cultures required to isolate the causative organism, and 2 of those patients had prosthetic valves. Another review did not distinguish between native and prosthetic-valve infective endocarditis in describing the constancy of bacteremia (33). Finally, prior use of antibiotics appears to lower the rate of positivity (19, 30).

Endocarditis in patients with drug addiction is more likely to escape diagnosis. Diverse and unexpected organisms may be involved, and self-administration of antibiotics is a common practice (32). Also, right-sided valvular lesions are more likely (22), and peripheral signs of infective endocarditis are rarer in these patients.

Culture-Negative Endocarditis: The term culture-negative endocarditis has caused confusion in the literature on infectious disease. Reported rates of this entity vary from 5% to 24% of all endocarditis cases (30). Improved microbiologic techniques and rigid definitions for infective endocarditis suggest that the high rates reported in the early literature reflected an inadequate technology (by current standards). Most cases of culture-negative infective endocarditis in early studies would now be identified as being caused by various organisms with unusual growth characteristics. They include fastidious, slow-growing, gram-negative organisms (such as *Haemophilus aphrophilus, H. parainfluenzae,* and *Cardiobacterium hominis*), diphtheroids, *Brucella* species, anaerobic microorganisms, flora having special growth requirements (such as certain nutritionally dependent viridans streptococci), and those organisms that cannot be expected to grow at all (organisms that cause Q fever, psittacosis, histoplasmosis, tuberculosis, and so on). A review of organisms that cause culture-negative infective endocarditis has been presented by Van Scoy (34). With current methods, culture-negative endocarditis is an infrequent diagnosis and should account for less than 5% of cases (30). In many of these cases, patients have received prior antimicrobial therapy.

SPECIFICITY OF BLOOD CULTURES

The problem of the false-positive result was first evaluated systematically by MacGregor and Beaty (16). In their study of 1707 cultures taken from 857 patients, 18.9% of cultures were positive. Forty-seven percent of the positive cultures were falsely positive, and 8.9% of all blood cultures were falsely positive. Rates of contamination were highest among specimens collected in the "interns' laboratory" and in the emergency-night laboratory.

Several authors have noted that the spectrum of organisms causing true septicemia is very different from that associated with false positives. In MacGregor and Beaty's series, 61% of 152 isolates from false-positive tests were coagulase-negative staphylococci and 8% were diphtheroids. Weinstein and colleagues (7) found 55% of 276 false-positive tests to yield *Staphylococcus epidermidis* and 36% yielded diphtheroids. Ninety-two percent of the diphtheroids, 94% of the *S. epidermidis,* and 94% of the *Bacillus* isolates were contaminants. Conversely, all pneumococci, 97% of groups A and B streptococci, 98% of *Enterobacteriaceae* isolates, 91% of yeast, and all *H. influenzae, Neisseria gonorrhoeae,* and anaerobic gram-negative bacilli were judged to be true positives.

The false-positive rate may depend, in part, on patient characteristics. Many infections today are nosocomial—65% of blood isolates in Weinstein and colleagues' study (7)—and affect persons who are immunocompromised or have prosthetic devices. In these settings, commensual microbial flora, which ordinarily do not infect healthy adults and thus are usually considered contaminants, may cause true septicemia. Weinstein and colleagues reported that 21% of their corynebacterial isolates and 6% of both *S. epidermidis* and *Bacillus* isolates represented true infection. Thus, in high-risk patients with suspected bacteremia, these organisms should be considered pathogens (35).

Review of the other cultures within a series provides crucial data for distinguishing between true-positive and false-positive results. For patients with bacteremia in Weinstein and colleagues' series (7), the probability of a subsequent culture being positive after an initial true-positive result was greater than 75%. On the other hand, after an initial false-positive result, subsequent positive blood cultures were rare and had different flora.

Another factor distinguishing false-positive from true-positive cultures is the increased time of incubation required by contaminants growing in the microbiology laboratory (36). This observation may not be useful in an individual patient, however, because there is considerable overlap between the growth rate of contaminants and true pathogens.

Wilson and coworkers (37) studied the frequency of false-positive blood cultures in 240 outpatients with no known infection. Only 5 patients had positive cultures with organisms thought not to represent true bacteremia, for a false-positive rate of 2%. This study is the only modern one that evaluated the rate of contamination in healthy adults. (An early series reported much higher rates of contamination [38].) The low false-positive rate among healthy adults probably does not represent what one would expect in sick, hospitalized patients. Such persons would be more likely to have specimens that were contaminated while being drawn by weary house officers than would healthy outpatients whose blood cultures were drawn in a standardized manner.

Between 1% and 4.5% of blood cultures have been reported to be falsely positive (7, 10, 11). The variation may be explained by technique: study protocols yield lower rates than routine hospital practice, and houseofficer-staffed services in public hospitals have higher rates. Again, physician behavior with respect to sterile techniques greatly influences test performance. Rates of contamination are much higher in neonates (4).

These data allow some conclusions about false-positive tests. The likelihood of a false-positive culture result increases as the number of cultures in a series increases. However, because individual blood culture results are reviewed within the context of a series and not independently, correct interpretation improves as the size of the series increases. Thus, we conclude that drawing additional cultures may improve the specificity of the series despite increasing the risk of individual false-positive results.

The Diagnosis of Bacteremia: Use and Interpretation of the Blood Culture

PRETEST PROBABILITY

Data on the pretest probabilities of bacteremias in their various settings are, by nature, incomparable, as shown in Table 2. Procedure-induced bacteremias show the highest incidence rates because blood drawing can be timed and standardized optimally. The rates of crucially

Table 2. Pretest Probability of Bacteremia for Selected Conditions

	Probability	Reference
	%	
Transient bacteremia		
After a dental extraction	18-85	14
After childbirth	0-11	14
Intermittent bacteremia		
Fever and neutropenia	22	39
Pneumococcal pneumonia	20-30	24
Suppurative thrombophlebitis	60	40

Table 3. Operating Characteristics of the Blood Culture Series: Effect of Varying Pretest Probability, Sensitivity, and Specificity

Example	Pretest Probability of Bacteremia*	Test Sensi- tivity†	Test Speci- ficity‡	Post-test Probability of Bacteremia§	
				Positive Test	Negative Test
			%		
A	50	80	95	94	17
B	50	99	95	95	2
C	22	80	95	82	6
D	22	99	95	84	0.3
E	5	80	95	46	1
F	5	99	95	51	0.1
G	5	80	99	81	1
H	5	99	99	84	0.1

* Pretest probabilities of 5%, 22%, and 50% correspond to the incidence of bacteremia among unselected febrile inpatients on a medical service (see text), febrile neutropenic patients (39), and febrile intravenous drug abusers with multiple pulmonary infiltrates, respectively.

† Values of 80% and 99% correspond to the sensitivity of blood culture series consisting of one and three culture sets, respectively (18).

‡ Values of 95% and 99% represent a best estimate for the range of blood culture specificity.

§ Post-test probabilities are calculated with Bayes' theorem (15).

important transient or intermittent bacteremias associated with focal infections are undoubtedly underestimated. Studies of associated bacteremias using appropriate protocols have not been reported, in part because the appropriate timing of these cultures (ostensibly before the onset of rigor or fever) is so difficult to arrange. The rate of bacteremia among patients with fever and neutropenia is probably the most accurate (39). In most cases, the clinician can only make a subjective estimate of the pretest probability of bacteremia (Table 2 can be a guide).

INFLUENCE OF PRETEST PROBABILITY ON POST-TEST PROBABILITY

Table 3 illustrates the use and interpretation of the blood culture test using Bayes' theorem under various hypothetical situations. A 5% pretest probability of bacteremia corresponds to the incidence among febrile patients on a medical service (Bor and colleagues. Unpublished data), 22% corresponds to the rate among febrile neutropenic patients (39), and 50% corresponds to the rate for febrile intravenous drug abusers with multiple pulmonary infiltrates. The sensitivity of the blood culture series is taken to be 80% and 99% for one and three blood cultures, respectively, as observed at the Mayo Clinic (18).

Interpretation of a Negative Test Result: When the pretest probability of bacteremia is high and the test result positive, changes in test sensitivity have little effect on the post-test probability (examples A and B). However, if the test result were negative, changes in sensitivity would profoundly influence the post-test probability. Hence, a physician confronted with an intravenous drug abuser with fever, dyspnea, myalgias, confusion, and bilateral nodular pulmonary infiltrates might treat this patient with vancomycin and an aminoglycoside for right-sided endocarditis despite one or two negative blood cultures. However, three negative cultures should suggest the probability of other diagnoses, such as pneumocystis pneumonia. On the other hand, when the pretest probability of bacteremia is moderate or low, as in febrile neutropenic patients (examples C and D) or febrile patients on a medical service (examples E and F), changes in test sensitivity (within the range considered) have little effect on the post-test probability for either positive or negative test results.

Interpretation of a Positive Test Result: Table 3 illustrates the importance of a highly specific test. When the pretest probability of bacteremia is low, only a positive result from a very specific test will establish a high post-test likelihood of bacteremia (examples G and H compared with E and F). Even tests with a moderately high specificity (95%) will yield similar numbers of true-positive and false-positive results in situations with a low prevalence (examples E and F).

Interpretation of a Series of Blood Cultures: The blood culture series, comprising several single blood culture sets, should be viewed as a single diagnostic test. In two hypothetical cases presented in Table 4, we explore the operating characteristics of this diagnostic test as we increase the number of component blood culture sets. These cases show the high degree of clinical sophistication required of physicians: they must estimate the pretest probabilities of bacteremia as well as predict the microbial species to be isolated.

Case 1 is that of an elderly diabetic patient with pain in the right upper abdomen and fever. The clinician anticipates cholangitis or diverticulitis giving rise to bacteremia with enteric flora. The clinician would not be misled by the isolation of *S. epidermidis* or other common skin or mouth flora which make up approximately 80% of blood culture contaminants. Thus, the false-positive rate of 3% based on all contaminating flora can be reduced to 0.6

Table 4. Operating Characteristics of the Blood Culture Series: Effect on Post-test Probability of Increasing the Number of Blood Culture Sets

	Number of Blood Culture Sets in One Series*			
	1	2	3	4
	←———— % ————→			
Case 1: Fever and abdominal pain†				
False-positive rate	6	1.2	1.8	2.4
False-negative rate	20	4	0.8	0.1
Pretest probability of bacteremia = 1%				
Post-test probability‡ with positive test	57	44	35	30
Post-test probability with negative test	0.2	0.1	0.1	0.1
Pretest probability of bacteremia = 20%				
Post-test probability‡ with positive test	97	95	93	91
Post-test probability with negative test	5	0.5	0.3	0.1
Case 2: Fever and emboli following aortic valve replacement§				
False-positive rate	3	0.09	0.25	0.34
False-negative rate	20	36	10	2.7
Pretest probability of bacteremia = 10%				
Post-test probability‡ with positive test	...‖	99	98	97
Post-test probability with negative test	...‖	4	1	1
Pretest probability of bacteremia = 80%				
Post-test probability‡ with positive test	...‖	99	99	99
Post-test probability with negative test	...‖	59	29	1

* A series is defined as a cluster of blood culture sets obtained to evaluate one episode of bacteremia.

† Assumptions include 80% sensitivity of a single culture (18); 0.6% false-positive rate of a single culture (20% of usual contaminants are potential enteric pathogens and usual contamination rate is 3%: that is, 0.006 = 0.2 × 0.03); positive series defined as at least one positive blood culture set.

‡ Post-test probabilities are calculated with Bayes' theorem (15).

§ Assumptions include 80% sensitivity of a single culture (30); 3% false-positive rate of single culture; positive series defined as at least two positive blood culture sets.

‖ Values cannot be calculated because, in this example, a positive series is defined as at least two positive blood culture sets.

because only 20% of contaminants are likely to mislead the physician.

In this case of intermittent bacteremia, most clinicians would regard the blood culture series as positive if enteric flora were isolated even from only one culture set. Therefore, the false-negative rates expressed in Table 4 are the likelihoods of failing to detect any positive cultures among patients with bacteremia. The false-positive rates are the probabilities of finding at least one positive culture set within a blood culture series obtained from a patient without bacteremia.

At the predicted 20% pretest probability of abdominal sepsis, even a single blood culture significantly alters the post-test probability of sepsis. However, 5% of patients with one negative culture will actually have undiagnosed bacteremia and perhaps go untreated. Adding a second blood culture set to the series reduces these missed bacteremias to less than 1% but at the cost of increasing the proportion of false-positive tests. Obtaining more than two blood cultures in this example is counterproductive: the post-test probability with a positive test decreases (because of more false-positive results), and the post-test probability with a negative test decreases negligibly.

When the predicted pretest probability of abdominal sepsis is as low as 1%, the example illustrates the dangers of drawing any blood cultures. The physician's ability to exclude the diagnosis of bacteremia is increased trivially by obtaining blood cultures, and in culture series comprising greater than one blood culture set, more nonbacteremic than bacteremic patients would be diagnosed and perhaps treated for sepsis.

Case 2 is that of a patient with fever and systemic emboli several weeks after aortic valve replacement. The clinician considering prosthetic valve endocarditis anticipates a diverse assortment of causative organisms, including many that commonly contaminate cultures; the clinician cannot exclude any isolates as potential pathogens. In addition, diagnosis relies on documentation of continuous bacteremia, defined in this model by at least two positive blood culture sets within a series. A false-positive series is defined by finding at least two individual positive culture sets obtained from a patient without endocarditis; a false-negative series is one in which only one or zero positive cultures are obtained from a patient with endocarditis.

Table 5. Guidelines for the Use of Blood Cultures to Diagnose Bacteremia

1. The blood culture is a test that is unusually dependent on physician behavior (that is, use of sterile techniques, and choice of the number, volume, and timing of culture sets) and on their clinical judgment (that is, estimating the pretest probability of septicemia, anticipating the causative bacterial pathogens, and interpreting the results).

2. Sensitivity of the blood culture series can be maximized by drawing multiple cultures containing at least 10 mL of blood per set and beginning at the onset of a febrile episode. Blood obtained from one venipuncture site defines one blood culture set, regardless of the number of bottles it fills.

3. A highly sensitive test (that is, culture series) is indicated for excluding a diagnosis of bacteremia that is thought to be highly likely, for documenting bacteremia that is continuous rather than transient or intermittent, or for detecting bacteremia in a patient who has received antimicrobials recently.

4. Specificity of the blood culture series can be maximized by adhering strictly to aseptic techniques, by never sampling from an indwelling venous catheter, and by requiring that multiple sets be positive with the same organism for the series to be considered positive when the anticipated isolates are also common contaminants.

5. A highly specific test is necessary to establish the diagnosis of bacteremia when the pretest probability of disease is low or when the expected pathogen is one of the organisms that commonly contaminate cultures.

6. Continuous bacteremia can be documented by requiring that two or more cultures be positive with the same organism within a blood culture series containing multiple samplings.

7. Strict guidelines cannot be formulated about the number of cultures to be drawn within each series. Further studies must first accurately define the sensitivity and specificity of modern blood culture systems. The following suggestions are our best estimates.

One blood culture set is rarely, if ever, sufficient.

Two blood culture sets are necessary and sufficient to rule out or establish a diagnosis of bacteremia when the anticipated pathogen is different from the usual contaminating flora and when the pretest probability of bacteremia is low to moderate (for example, in a patient with pneumonia, gastrointestinal sepsis).

Three blood culture sets should be obtained to rule out bacteremia when the pretest probability of bacteremia is high or when continuous bacteremia is the diagnosis being pursued.

Four or more blood culture sets should be obtained to rule out bacteremia when the pretest probability of bacteremia is high *and* either the anticipated pathogens are also common contaminants (as in prosthetic-valve endocarditis) or the patient with suspected endocarditis has received antimicrobials within the prior 2 weeks.

Table 5. (Continued)

8. Changes in the blood culture growth and detection system used by the diagnostic microbiology laboratory will obviously affect the performance of the test. Physicians should familiarize themselves with the characteristics of the system used in their clinical setting and work closely with the microbiology staff.

When the pretest probability of endocarditis is 10%, 4% of the patients with negative tests will have endocarditis if only two culture sets are drawn. Three culture sets would be optimal, reducing the post-test probability to 1%. On the other hand, if the series consists of three blood cultures and the pretest probability of endocarditis is estimated to be as high as 80%, the test (blood culture series) shows a surprisingly high post-test probability with a negative test. Nearly one third of the patients with negative test results (defined in this example as zero or one out of three positive cultures sets) would have undiagnosed bacterial endocarditis. Because the utility of diagnosing endocarditis strongly outweighs the risk of missing that diagnosis, the physician should perform four or more blood cultures.

Conclusions

Guidelines for the use of blood cultures are summarized in Table 5.

Appendix: Blood Culture Methods

TIMING AND NUMBERS OF SAMPLINGS

In one of the earliest analyses of blood cultures, Weiss and Ottenberg (41) suggested that the optimal time to culture the blood was before the onset of fever and chills. Bennett and Beeson (13) showed that rigors and fever often followed bacteremia by an hour, and others showed that they followed endotoxemia by about 90 minutes. Hence, blood should be cultured as early as possible in the course of a febrile episode. Subsequent samplings should be spaced at wide intervals, if practicable, to detect transient or intermittent bacteremia. To minimize the risk of contamination, multiple specimens should never be drawn from the same venipuncture site. Samples may be obtained at much longer intervals to document continuous bacteremia.

STERILE TECHNIQUE IN DRAWING AND HANDLING THE BLOOD CULTURES

An optimal venipuncture site should be selected, and the skin prepared and disinfected concentrically with alcohol, followed by 2% iodine or the less allergenic iodophor solution. Sterilization does not occur immediately, so it is preferable to allow 1 minute before drawing blood. After skin preparation, the clinician should palpate the vein while wearing a sterile glove. Blood should not be sampled through indwelling catheters but may be drawn through a closed-collection system and inoculated directly into evacuated culture bottles or collected with a syringe and needle. After the rubber stoppers are disinfected, the blood should be inoculated into both aerobic and anaerobic culture bottles or into collection tubes containing sodium polyanetholesulfonate and then sent directly to the laboratory.

THE VOLUME OF BLOOD SAMPLED

The volume of blood may be more important than medium or atmosphere, especially in settings of low-level bacteremia. Weinstein and colleagues (7) have suggested that the reason their series had a higher than 99% positivity rate with two cultures, as opposed to a similar rate with three cultures in the Mayo Clinic series (18), was that 15-mL of blood per culture were required at the University of Colorado hospitals whereas only 10 mL/culture was required at the Mayo Clinic. After that report, Washington (4), of the Mayo Clinic, recommended collection of larger volumes of blood for each set of cultures. It seems safe to conclude that at least 10 mL/culture is optimal in most instances. Lesser amounts should not be considered sufficient. Some automated detection systems supply culture bottles that accommodate smaller volumes of blood. Some centers may prefer to use multiple sets of blood cultures with smaller volumes or to inoculate blood drawn from one venipuncture into three or more bottles (still evaluated as one set) rather than one or two sets with larger volumes. Washington and Ilstrup (3) recommend drawing at least 10 mL and preferably 20 to 30 mL of blood for each culture. They have shown a direct relationship between blood volume and culture yield.

THE GROWTH CHARACTERISTICS OF THE MEDIUM

Special processing of media may be required to support growth of fastidious flora: *Brucella* and *Leptospira* species, nutritionally deficient streptococci, cell-wall-deficient forms, and so on. If these flora are expected, or in situations in which bacteremia is considered likely but conventional blood cultures are negative, it is reasonable to attempt isolation with a different culture system. Sensitivity may be enhanced by new systems of detecting microbial growth (biphasic media, radiometric systems), of inactivating or removing antimicrobials, and of lysing eukaryotic cells (5). Some centers have begun to combine two or more isolation systems to maximize sensitivity.

Most aerobic and facultatively anaerobic bacteria can be recovered from commercially available, nutritionally enriched liquid media. Comparison of recovery broths is beyond the scope of this paper. Sodium polyanetholesulfonate, a polyanionic anticoagulant, is added to most commercial broths. In addition to inactivating aminoglycosides, this agent interferes with phagocytosis and inhibits lysozyme activity and complement formation. Its presence in blood culture media improves the recovery of most microorganisms, although some (for example, *N. meningitidis*) can be inhibited.

The optimal blood-to-broth ratio of 1:5 to 1:10 neutralizes the bactericidal effects of blood and has the added effect of diluting out most antimicrobial agents to noninhibitory concentrations. An alternate approach to the neutralization of antimicrobials is the absorption of antimicrobials with mixed resin systems before inoculation of blood into culture media. Several commercial mixed resin systems are available. Unfortunately, these trials have shown conflicting results.

Other systems may enhance the detection of bacteremia, fungemia, and polymicrobial septicemia. By the "lysis-centrifugation" staining method, blood is drawn directly into a tube that contains lysing agents, anticoagulants, and an inert fluorochemical to cushion microorganisms during centrifugation. Lysis of eukaryotic cells occurs rapidly, and the tube is then centrifuged to concentrate microorganisms that might be present. The concentrate is subcultured on solid media; thus the time to detection is equivalent to the time to isolation. This system enables quantitation of microorganisms and removal of the microorganisms from toxic effects of antimicrobial agents and bactericidal effects of blood. Its disadvantage is a high rate of contamination.

THE SYSTEM FOR DETECTION OF GROWTH

Blood culture bottles should be examined daily for at least 1 week for turbidity, hemolysis, gas production, or formation of discrete colonies. Some fastidious organisms that may cause endocarditis may require longer incubation.

New systems for early detection of bacteremia include biphasic medium and radiometric methods. In a biphasic system an agar slant is immersed within the broth culture. Subcultures are made by allowing the broth to wash over the slant. Generally, time to detection and time to isolation are equivalent. The system's main disadvantages seem to be its inhibition of growth of some organisms and a higher rate of contamination.

Automated systems are now widespread. This approach identifies CO_2 that is produced by bacterial metabolism in a broth media. The CO_2 produced by metabolism is released from the medium and measured in an ionization chamber (as $^{14}CO_2$ in the radiometric version of this test or by an infrared spectrometer in newer versions of this method). A growth index is then generated. This system appears to be able to detect bacteremia more quickly than conventional systems and, despite the smaller volume of blood used, has an equivalent sensitivity to conventional methods. The automated methods also decrease the laboratory workload.

ACKNOWLEDGMENTS: The authors thank Harold Sox, whose suggestions went beyond the usual editorial assistance; and Philip Hanff, Thomas Delbanco, Marilyn Spellmeyer, and the three anonymous reviewers for their many helpful suggestions.

References

1. FOSTER WD. *A History of Medical Bacteriology and Immunology.* London: William Heinemann Medical Books, Ltd.; 1979:172.
2. FUNG JC, TILTON RC. Detection of bacterial antigens by counterimmunoelectrophoresis, coagglutination and latex agglutination. In: LENNETTE EH, BALOWS A, HAUSER WJ JR, SHADOMY HJ, eds. *Manual of Clinical Microbiology.* 4th ed. Washington, D.C.: American Society for Microbiology; 1985:883-90.
3. WASHINGTON JA II, ILSTRUP DM. Blood cultures: issues and controversies. *Rev Infect Dis.* 1986;**8**:792-802.
4. WASHINGTON JA. Conventional approaches to blood culture. In: WASHINGTON JA II, ed. *The Detection of Septicemia.* West Palm Beach, Florida: CRC Press, Inc.; 1978:41-87.
5. RELLER LB. Laboratory procedures in the management of infective endocarditis. In: BISNO AL, ed. *Treatment of Infective Endocarditis.* New York: Grune & Stratton; 1981:235-68.
6. RELLER L, MURRAY P, MCLOWRY J, CUMITECH LA. *Blood Cultures II.* Washington, D.C.: American Society for Microbiology; 1982:1-11.
7. WEINSTEIN MP, RELLER LB, MURPHY JR, LICHTENSTEIN KA. The clinical significance of positive blood cultures: a comprehensive analysis of 500 episodes of bacteremia and fungemia in adults: I. Laboratory and epidemiologic observations. *Rev Infect Dis.* 1983;**5**:35-53.
8. CROWLEY N. Some bacteremias encountered in hospital practice. *J Clin Pathol.* 1970;**23**:166-71.
9. SETIA U, GROSS PA. Bacteremia in a community hospital: spectrum and mortality. *Arch Intern Med.* 1977;**137**:1698-701.
10. BEAMAN KD, KASTEN BL, GAVEN TL. Rate of detection of bacteremia. *Cleve Clin Q.* 1977;**44**:129-36.
11. ROBERTS FJ. A review of positive blood cultures: identification and source of microorganisms and patterns of sensitivity to antibiotics. *Rev Infect Dis.* 1980;**2**:329-39.
12. ISENBERG HD, WASHINGTON JA II, BALOWS A, SONNENWIRTH AC. Collection, handling and processing of specimens. In: LENNETTE EH, BALOWS A, HAUSER WJ JR, SHADOMY HJ, eds. *Manual of Clinical Microbiology.* 4th ed. Washington, D.C.: American Society for Microbiology; 1985:73-98.
13. BENNETT IL, BEESON PB. Bacteremia: a consideration of some experimental bacteremias. *Yale J Biol Med.* 1954;**226**:241-62.
14. EVERETT ED, HIRSCHMANN JV. Transient bacteremia and endocarditis prophylaxis: a review. *Medicine (Baltimore).* 1977;**56**:61-77.
15. SOX HC JR. Probability theory in the use of diagnostic tests: an introduction to critical study of the literature. *Ann Intern Med.* 1986;**104**:60-6.
16. MACGREGOR RR, BEATY HN. Evaluation of positive blood cultures: guidelines for early differentiation of contaminated from valid positive cultures. *Arch Intern Med.* 1972;**130**:84-7.
17. FEINSTEIN AR, PRITCHETT JA, SCHIMPFF CR. The epidemiology of cancer therapy: IV. The extraction of data from medical records. *Arch Intern Med.* 1969;**123**:571-90.
18. WASHINGTON JA II. Blood cultures: principles and techniques. *Mayo Clin Proc.* 1975;**50**:91-8.
19. WERNER AS, COBBS CG, KAYE D, HOOK EW. Studies on the bacteremia of bacterial endocarditis. *JAMA.* 1967;**202**:199-203.
20. DUPONT HL, SPINK WW. Infections due to gram-negative organisms: an analysis of 860 patients with bacteremia at the University of Minnesota Medical Center, 1958-1966. *Medicine (Baltimore).* 1969;**48**:307-32.
21. HALL MM, ILSTRUP DM, WASHINGTON JA II. Effect of volume of blood cultured on detection of bacteremia. *J Clin Microbiol.* 1976;**3**:643-5.

22. SCHELD WM, SANDE MA. Endocarditis and intravascular infections. In: MANDELL GL, DOUGLAS RG JR, BENNETT JE, eds. *Principles and Practice of Infectious Diseases.* New York: John Wiley & Sons, Inc.; 1985:505-30.

23. ROBERTS RB. *Streptococcus pneumoniae.* In: MANDELL GL, DOUGLAS RG JR, BENNETT JE, eds. *Principles and Practice of Infectious Diseases.* New York: John Wiley & Sons; 1985:1147-8.

24. AUSTRIAN R, GOLD J. Pneumococcal bacteremia with especial reference to bacteremic pneumococcal pneumonia. *Ann Intern Med.* 1964;**60**:759-76.

25. BEESON PB, BRANNON ES, WARREN JV. Observations on the sites of removal of bacteria from the blood in patients with bacterial endocarditis. *J Exp Med.* 1945;**81**:9-23.

26. BELLI J, WASIBREN BA. The number of blood cultures necessary to diagnose most cases of bacterial endocarditis. *Am J Med Sci.* 1956;**232**:284-8.

27. BARRITT DW, GILESPIE WAS. Subacute bacterial endocarditis. *Br J Med.* 1960;**1**:1235-9.

28. KELSON SR, WHITE PD. Notes on 250 cases of subacute bacterial (streptococcal) endocarditis studied and treated between 1927 and 1939. *Ann Intern Med.* 1945;**22**:40-60.

29. CATES JE, CHRISTIE RV. Subacute bacterial endocarditis: a review of 442 patients treated in 14 centers appointed by the Penicillin Trials Committee of the Medical Research Council. *Q J Med.* 1951;**20**:93-130.

30. VON REYN CF, LEVY BS, ARBEIT RD, FRIEDLAND G, CRUMPACKER CS. Infective endocarditis: an analysis based on strict case definitions. *Ann Intern Med.* 1981;**94**(4 pt 1):505-18.

31. GARVEY GJ, NEU HC. Infective endocarditis—an evolving disease. *Medicine (Baltimore).* 1978;**57**:105-27.

32. PELLETIER LL JR, PETERSDORF RG. Infective endocarditis: a review of 125 cases from the University of Washington Hospitals, 1963-72. *Medicine (Baltimore).* 1977;**56**:287-313.

33. WILSON WR, DANIELSON GK, GUILIANI ER, GERACI JE. Prosthetic valve endocarditis. *Mayo Clin Proc.* 1982;**57**:155-61.

34. VAN SCOY RE. Culture-negative endocarditis. *Mayo Clin Proc.* 1982;**57**:149-54.

35. WILSON WR. Sepsis: definitions, underlying conditions, manifestations. In: WASHINGTON JA II, ed. *The Detection of Septicemia.* West Palm Beach, Florida: CRC Press, Inc.; 1978:1-21.

36. ILSTRUP DM. Sepsis: organisms from blood cultures at the Mayo Clinic: 1968 to 1975. In: WASHINGTON JA II, ed. *The Detection of Septicemia.* West Palm Beach, Florida: CRC Press, Inc.; 1978:23-5.

37. WILSON WR, VAN SCOY RE, WASHINGTON JA II. Incidence of bacteremia in adults without infection. *J Clin Microbiol.* 1975;**2**:94-5.

38. REITH AF, SQUIER TL. Blood cultures of apparently healthy persons. *J Infect Dis.* 1932;**51**:336-43.

39. EORTC INTERNATIONAL ANTIMICROBIAL THERAPY PROJECT GROUP. Three antibiotic regimens in the treatment of infection in febrile granulocytopenic patients with cancer. *J Infect Dis.* 1978;**137**:14-29.

40. MAKI DG, WEISE CE, SARAFIN HW. A semiqualitative culture method for identifying intravenous-catheter-related infections. *N Engl J Med.* 1977;**296**:1305-9.

41. WEISS H, OTTENBERG R. Relation between bacteria and temperature in subacute bacterial endocarditis. *J Infect Dis.* 1932;**50**:61-8.

Syphilis Tests in Diagnostic and Therapeutic Decision Making

GAVIN HART, M.D., M.P.H.

DESPITE ACCESS to highly effective diagnostic tests for syphilis, deficiencies in diagnosis still occur because the tests are not used or are used improperly (1). Widely accepted strategies of proven effectiveness have been developed for many clinical situations (for example, screening to prevent congenital syphilis), but in some clinical situations, firm guidelines are not available (and may be difficult to obtain) and guidelines must be developed on the basis of reasoned estimation in the face of uncertainty. There is uncertainty about the need for cerebrospinal fluid examination in asymptomatic patients with positive treponemal tests; about which patients to screen to balance excessive costs generated from low-yield screening and dissemination of infection by failing to detect persons with infectious disease; and about the precise performance of tests in detecting asymptomatic neurosyphilis. Misleading indications about the performance of diagnostic tests in some clinical situations have been produced by the study design or faulty interpretation of some investigations. This article provides guidelines for use of the available diagnostic tests based on a synthesis of the data currently available.

Diagnostic Tests for Syphilis

Syphilis may be diagnosed by the direct identification of *Treponema pallidum* in specimens taken from the lesions of primary, secondary, or congenital syphilis, or indirectly by the detection of antibodies in the blood or cerebrospinal fluid.

DARKFIELD EXAMINATION

Exudate from suspected lesions is examined with a

▶ This chapter was originally published in *Annals of Internal Medicine.* 1986;**104**:368-76.

compound microscope equipped with a darkfield condenser (2). Exudate is collected on a glass slide, covered, and examined immediately. *Treponema pallidum* are corkscrew-shaped organisms with regular, deep spirals; they are slightly longer than the diameter of an erythrocyte and have characteristic motility.

DIRECT FLUORESCENT ANTIBODY *TREPONEMA PALLIDUM* TEST

The specimen is collected on a glass slide, as for darkfield examination, but is fixed with acetone and sent to the laboratory (3). Alternatively, exudate may be sent to the laboratory in a capillary tube. Fluorescein-labeled anti-*T. pallidum* globulin is incubated with the exudate, and the stained smear is examined by fluorescence microscopy.

SEROLOGIC TESTS

Treponemal tests, which detect antibodies against *T. pallidum* or its components, and nontreponemal tests, which detect antibodies directed against lipoidal antigens, are the two types of serologic tests for syphilis. The main nontreponemal test used in the United States is the Venereal Disease Research Laboratory (VDRL) test, and the standard treponemal tests are the fluorescent treponemal antibody absorption test (FTA-ABS) and microhemagglutination tests for syphilis (for example, MHA-TP).

Some have advocated doing a large battery of serologic tests to provide maximum diagnostic information (4), but interpretation may be complex when test results disagree. Furthermore, many tests are closely related (that is, they lack independence for statistical analysis), and, in reality, additional tests may not provide additional diagnostic information. An alternative approach emphasizes perfecting the technical performance and interpretation of a limited number of tests (5, 6). In the United States, this strategy favors restricting serologic tests for syphilis to the VDRL, FTA-ABS, and MHA-TP tests and their variants.

Venereal Disease Research Laboratory Test: Purified cardiolipin-lecithin-cholesterol antigen is mixed with heated serum on a glass slide that is rotated mechanically (2). Flocculation is read microscopically, and the result is reported as reactive (medium and large clumps), nonreactive (no clumps), or weakly reactive (small clumps).

This test may be quantitated by serial dilution of serum, and the titer is recorded as the greatest serum dilution that produces a fully reactive result. The same test may be done on cerebrospinal fluid (which should not be heated), and the result is reported as reactive or nonreactive.

Simplified variations of the VDRL test (all of which use unheated serum) are the unheated serum reagin test; the rapid plasma reagin card test, in which carbon particles are included in the antigen suspension; and the automated reagin test, which uses autoanalyzer continuous-flow equipment and the antigen suspension for the rapid plasma reagin card test. The performance characteristics of these tests are generally similar, although an occasional significant divergence in reactivity is reported (7). Likewise, most positive sera show a similar titer with these variants (8). However, some sera may show a marked divergence of the titers, so the same test should be used to follow the course of any particular infection in a patient. In the remainder of this article, VDRL will be used generically to refer to all the flocculation tests using purified cardiolipin-lecithin-cholesterol antigen.

Fluorescent Treponemal Antibody Absorption Test: Heated test serum is mixed with sorbent (sonicate of Reiter treponemes or other appropriate material to remove low-grade nonspecific antibody) and incubated on slides containing *T. pallidum* antigen (2). Fluorescein-labeled antihuman globulin (conjugate) is applied to the slides, which are examined by fluorescence microscopy. The test is reported as reactive, nonreactive, or reactive minimal. A reactive minimal report indicates the need for a follow-up specimen to verify the results.

*Microhemagglutination-*Treponema pallidum *Test:* Sensitized (coated with lyzed *T. pallidum*) sheep erythrocytes agglutinate in the presence of antitreponemal antibody in test serum (9). Failure to agglutinate allows the erythrocytes to settle as a smooth ring or as a button of cells, and the result is reported as negative or nonreactive. Complete agglutination produces a uniformly thin, granular deposit covering the entire bottom of the test well. This test was initially described as the *T. pallidum* hemagglutination test (TPHA), but its versatility for use in widespread screening is increased when it is done on a microtechnical basis (MHA-TP), particularly in the automated form (AMHA-TP) (10). A further modification, the hemagglutination treponemal test for syphilis (HATTS), uses sonicated *T. pallidum* coupled to glutaraldehyde-stabilized turkey erythrocytes by the bis-diazotized benzidine procedure (11). In the remainder of this article, MHA-TP will be used generically to refer to all hemagglutination tests that use sensitized erythrocytes to detect antitreponemal antibody.

CEREBROSPINAL FLUID TESTS

Total protein determination and cerebrospinal fluid cell count are the most appropriate indicators of inflammation of the central nervous system (although they are nonspecific for syphilis). Abnormality is indicated by a total protein content in excess of 40 mg/100 mL or a cell count of greater than 5/mm^3 (the cell count should only be done on freshly drawn fluid). The VDRL (2) and FTA test may be done on cerebrospinal fluid, but an acceptable form of the latter test for routine service is not currently available in the United States.

Limitations of Decision-Making Analysis

Despite the abundance of literature on diagnostic tests for syphilis, many findings are not useful for decision analysis because of features of study design. Some studies have relied on a dubious "gold-standard" test to determine the true state of the patient. Not surprisingly, other tests then appear to be less specific and sensitive. Ideally, disease status should be assigned independently of the tests being evaluated.

A major difficulty occurs in defining noninfected persons, because it is practically impossible to show that any person has never been exposed to treponemal infection. Methods for eliciting infection status include history and case review on patients and their sexual contacts, but longitudinal assessment (detecting changes in VDRL titers or other serologic tests, and the development of symptoms in the patient or contacts) is highly desirable if misassignment is to be minimized. In one study, 50% of one group of patients with false-positive results were subsequently considered to have true-positive results on the basis of longitudinal assessment (12).

Data analysis is complicated by the absence of an adequate "gold-standard" test for late latent syphilis. A stable titer or nonreactive VDRL test in association with a positive treponemal test may be regarded as diagnostic of late latent syphilis (13), but these findings may be due to biological or technical false-positive treponemal tests, nonsyphilitic treponemal disease, or adequately treated (either intentionally or unknowingly) syphilis. No studies have adequately assessed the quantitative contribution of these causes to long-term stable results of serologic tests for syphilis, and the quantitative pattern could vary greatly between different environments.

A second fault of study design in many analyses is performance of treponemal tests only on sera producing a positive cardiolipin test. The greater probability of disease after a positive treponemal test (due to increased prevalence in the population tested) is then assumed to indicate a greater specificity of this test. The widely held view that the FTA-ABS test is more specific than the VDRL test (14) is not supported by studies in which both tests were done in parallel on unselected sera (11, 15, 16).

Finally, some studies have compared the results of one test with those of another or a group of other tests without independent assessment of the disease status of the patients tested. This strategy is useful for comparing positive tests (for example, degree of reactivity or titers) but is misleading when applied to both positive and negative tests (17). In other words, comparison with a "gold-standard" test is a prerequisite for measuring the sensitivity or specificity of a test.

These limitations of available data have necessitated some assumptions and generalizations. Predictive value calculations, using Bayes' theorem (18), have been based on sensitivity and specificity findings that cannot automatically be extrapolated to situations differing from those in which they were determined. However, laboratories may measure this variation by participating in national or international proficiency testing programs.

For simplicity, pretest probabilities in the following analysis have been based on single variables, such as sexual contact, individual symptoms, or test results. In clinical practice, multiple variables, often with a quantitative component, are usually considered. For instance, the significance of genital ulceration is influenced by the age and sexual behavior of the patient as well as by the clinical characteristics of the ulceration.

Performance Characteristics of Diagnostic Tests
DIRECT IDENTIFICATION OF TREPONEMES

In general, the darkfield examination is regarded as highly sensitive and specific in primary syphilis (13). In practice, however, insensitivity may occur because excess debris or erythrocytes obscure treponemes, recent local or systemic antibiotic treatment has been applied, or an inadequate sample has been collected. This well-recognized phenomenon is responsible for the general practice of performing three multiple examinations before a negative result is accepted (13).

The direct fluorescent test shows test characteristics similar to those of the darkfield examination, and it has a definite role when the lesion is in an area (for example, the mouth) that normally harbors saprophytic treponemes or when logistical considerations prevent performance of darkfield examination. The delay (usually 1 to 2 days, depending on logistics) in obtaining a result contrasts with a major advantage of the darkfield test, which is diagnosis and immediate treatment when the patient is first seen. There are no adequate data on the sensitivity of the darkfield test. One study (19) has suggested a sensitivity of 73.8%, but the tests were done under suboptimal conditions (for example, some patients had received oral or systemic antibiotics), and some clinicians claim the sensitivity should be at least 95% when the test is done under ideal conditions. The contrasting interpretation of the darkfield examination for these two sensitivities is shown in Table 1, which highlights the desirability of a high level of expertise in performing this test.

SEROLOGIC TESTS

Sensitivity: The VDRL test usually becomes reactive at some time during primary syphilis. The titer rises rapidly and remains at a peak in the first year of infection, after which it falls slowly, reaching low levels in late syphilis and reverting to nonreactive in about 25% of patients (Figure 1). After adequate treatment, the titer falls at a rate that is related to the duration of infection before treatment. Treatment within the first 6 months usually produces seronegativity within 12 months, whereas seroreversal may take 2 years for later infections (20). In late syphilis, the decline may be very slow or nonexistent (21).

Table 1. Post-Test Probabilities of Syphilis After Testing in Groups with Differing Disease Prevalences

Darkfield Result	VDRL*	Probability	
		75% Sensitivity, 98% Specificity	95% Sensitivity, 99% Specificity
		%	%
Prevalence = 50%			
+	. . .	97	99
−	. . .	20	5
−	+	97	88
−	−	6	1
Prevalence = 5%			
+	. . .	66	83
−	. . .	1	0.3
−	+	66	28
−	−	0.3	0.07
Prevalence = 1%			
+	. . .	27	49
+	+	98	99
+	−	9	19
−	. . .	0.3	0.05

* This analysis assumes a sensitivity of 75% and specificity of 99.5% for the VDRL test. The two sets of sensitivities and specificities listed under Probability are for the darkfield test.

The FTA-ABS and MHA-TP tests usually become reactive in primary syphilis and remain reactive for the patient's lifetime, regardless of treatment (very early treatment may prevent seroreactivity, and some reversion of seropositivity does occur in patients treated in the early stages of infection). The FTA-ABS test tends to be the first serologic test to become positive, followed by the MHA-TP (some authors in Europe have reported superior sensitivity of the MHA-TP test in primary syphilis [22]) and the VDRL test marginally later.

The sensitivity of serologic tests for primary syphilis increases with increasing duration of infection. Thus, one study has shown a higher than usual sensitivity of 84% for the VDRL test, possibly because primary lesions had been present for 8 to 14 days in 22% of participants and for more than 14 days in 19% of participants at the time the test was done (23).

The sensitivities of the VDRL, MHA-TP, and FTA-ABS tests for primary syphilis obtained in some studies are shown in Table 2. The relationship of sensitivity to duration of infection has been described in one study

(24). For infections of less than 30 days' duration, of 30 to 40 days', and of over 40 days', the respective sensitivities were 40%, 67.7%, and 95.8% for the VDRL test; 62.8%, 87%, and 100% for the FTA-ABS; and 71.4%, 80%, and 100% for the MHA-TP test.

Cross-reactivity of the three serologic tests in dark-field-positive primary syphilis has been reported in several studies. (7, 25-27). The FTA-ABS test is rarely negative when either the VDRL or MHA-TP test is positive, but it may be positive in about 25% of patients with either a negative VDRL or MHA-TP test and in about 10% of patients with primary syphilis in whom both the VDRL and MHA-TP tests are negative. Up to 16% of patients with primary disease may have a positive VDRL, negative MHA-TP pattern, and about the same proportion may have the reverse pattern.

A sensitivity of 100% is normally recorded for all tests in patients with untreated secondary syphilis (15, 24, 27). In those with symptomatic late syphilis, sensitivity has been reported as 70% to 71% for the VDRL test (15, 25), 93.5% to 100% for the MHA-TP test (15, 27), and 100% for the FTA-ABS test (15, 25, 27).

Specificity: Reactive VDRL tests on sera with negative treponemal tests are known as biological false-positive reactions and have been reported in a wide variety of conditions (28, 29) including leprosy (30), drug addiction (31, 32), aging (33, 34), and infectious mononucleosis (35, 36). However, biological false-positive reactions have become much less common since the introduction of purified cardiolipin-lecithin-cholesterol antigen in place of less refined antigen (35, 36) and the replacement of

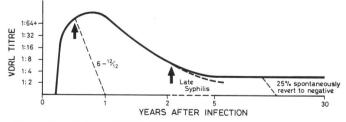

Figure 1. Variation of VDRL (Venereal Disease Research Laboratory test) titer in untreated syphilis. The arrows indicate treatment and the dashed lines show the course after treatment, following infection at time O. Widespread variation from this simplified generalization may occur.

Table 2. Sensitivity of Various Diagnostic Tests for Primary Syphilis

VDRL	MHA-TP	FTA-ABS	Reference*
← —————— % ————— →			
72.5	72.5	98.2	7
75.7	. . .	86.4	25
68.5	82.3	91.5	26
69.7	88.6	97.5	15
74.0	77.0	100.0	27
62.2	83.3	81.1	24

* References 7, 25, 26 and 15 refer to studies done in the United States (all cases darkfield-positive); 27 refers to a study in Poland (diagnostic standard not specified); and 24 refers to a study in Italy (darkfield-positive cases). VDRL = Venereal Disease Research Laboratory test; MHA-TP = microhemagglutination-*Treponema pallidum* test; FTA-ABS = fluorescent treponemal antibody absorption test.

complement fixation tests with flocculation tests (37). There must be serious doubts as to the causative role of pregnancy in biological false-positive reactions, and a positive serologic test detected in a pregnant woman is more likely to be due to syphilis or some other illness (38-40). Some inexperienced technicians tend to overread the VDRL test and report "roughness" (nonreactive) as weakly reactive or reactive, leading to a high proportion of weakly reactive results being false-positive, and a smaller proportion of reactive undiluted results being false-positive.

False-positive FTA-ABS results have been associated with various conditions, including autoimmune or connective tissue diseases, genital herpes, and narcotic addiction. However, underlying illness cannot be implicated in most false-positive FTA-ABS results (41, 42). Similarly, the causes of varying false-positivity rates of the MHA-TP test are usually unclear. Technical factors probably play an important role in the false-positivity rate of the treponemal tests (43), particularly the FTA-ABS test (41, 44, 45).

Many studies on the specificity of serologic tests suggest that both treponemal and nontreponemal tests have high specificity (99.5% to 100%) in healthy persons and decreased specificity (75% to 85%) in sick persons (16, 27, 38, 46-49). The specificities of the VDRL, MHA-TP, and FTA-ABS tests obtained in three of the most conclusive studies are shown in Table 3 (11, 15, 50). These studies involved parallel testing with all tests, well-defined criteria excluding syphilis, a well-documented target population, and control of bias in test interpretation.

CEREBROSPINAL FLUID TESTS

A conclusive evaluation of cerebrospinal fluid tests cannot be done, mainly because of the difficulty in assigning disease status (particularly in asymptomatic patients) with criteria independent of the tests being evaluated. Blood contamination of cerebrospinal fluid, either in the sample collection process or due to disruption of the blood-brain barrier, may produce false findings. Whereas it is most convenient to evaluate tests in patients with proven symptomatic neurosyphilis, the behavior of diagnostic tests may be quite different in those with asymptomatic neurosyphilis.

The traditional hallmarks for the diagnosis of asymptomatic neurosyphilis were the cerebrospinal fluid VDRL test and cerebrospinal fluid cell count. The inadequacy of relying solely on these tests is now recognized, and alternative tests are being investigated (5). Although occasional false-positive results may occur (51), the cerebrospinal fluid VDRL test is a highly specific indicator of neurosyphilis (52). On the other hand, it is insensitive, being positive in only 22% to 69% of patients with active neurosyphilis (based on clinical diagnosis by unspecified criteria) (53-55).

The cerebrospinal fluid FTA test may be more sensitive than the VDRL test (5, 53, 56), but false-positive

Table 3. Specificities of Various Serologic Tests for Syphilis

Source of Sera (Reference)	Sera	VDRL	MHA-TP	FTA-ABS
	n		%	
Healthy volunteers (11)	1048	99.7	99.4	99.2
Sick patients (11)	255	83.9	84.7	77.3
Frozen sera (15)	187	99.5	98.4, 100*	99.5
Fresh sera (15)	379	98.7	99.2, 100*	95.5
Nuns (50)	250	100	. . .	98.8

* Both microhemagglutination-*Treponema pallidum* test (MHA-TP; higher value) and *T. pallidum* hemagglutination test (HATTS; lower value) were done. VDRL = Venereal Disease Research Laboratory test; FTA-ABS = fluorescent treponemal antibody absorption test.

reactions (nonspecificity) can occur (54, 57); thus, diagnosis of neurosyphilis should not be based solely on a positive cerebrospinal fluid FTA test. Because of its lack of specificity and uncertainties about its interpretation, the test is not recommended for use in the United States (13).

The cerebrospinal fluid VDRL titer may persist for an extended period after adequate treatment of neurosyphilis, and the test is unsatisfactory in determining either the extent of inflammatory activity or the response to therapy. Traditionally, this role has been filled by the cell count and by clinical findings in symptomatic patients. The cerebrospinal fluid protein level may also be elevated in patients with neurosyphilis, but it subsides more slowly and is less useful as an indicator of the adequacy of treatment. After adequate treatment, the cell count should return to normal within 6 to 12 weeks, and re-treatment must be considered if significant abnormality persists after 6 months (58). In view of the possible insensitivity of the cell count and total protein level as indicators of neurosyphilitic activity (59, 60), presence of plasma cells and elevated immunoglobulin fractions have been suggested as alternative measures, but these have not been adequately validated (60).

Diagnostic Tests in Specific Clinical Situations

The following section provides guidelines for the use of the available diagnostic tests in specific clinical situations (Table 4). The situations discussed include evaluation of both symptomatic and asymptomatic persons, follow-up after treatment, and cerebrospinal fluid assessment.

SYMPTOMATIC PERSONS

Genital Ulceration (Primary Syphilis): Darkfield microscopy is the test of choice for primary syphilis, because it is sensitive and highly specific and it provides an immediate result. Syphilis should not be overlooked as a cause of oral and anorectal lesions, and sexual history and syphilis testing are important elements of the investigation of lesions at these sites. If available, the direct fluorescent test should be used for testing oral lesions.

The VDRL titer should be used for assessing the adequacy of treatment, the first test being done at the first visit. Although the exact prevalence of syphilis in groups with various symptoms is not known, the presence of

Table 4. Recommendations for the Use of Diagnostic Tests for Syphilis*

Immediate Diagnostic or Therapeutic Action	Further Investigation or Action
Primary syphilis	
Darkfield or direct fluorescent test	VDRL titer for follow-up
Secondary syphilis	
VDRL titer (darkfield for immediate result)	VDRL titer for follow-up
Selected asymptomatic persons†	
VDRL	MHA-TP if VDRL is positive
Adequacy of treatment for early and late syphilis	
VDRL titer 3, 6, and 12 mos after treatment	Re-treat if high titer has not fallen by 12 mos, or if titer has increased after initial fall
Seropositive persons‡	
CSF-VDRL and CSF cell count	Treat for neurosyphilis if CSF-VDRL is positive and cell count is elevated
Follow-up after treatment for asymptomatic neurosyphilis	
CSF cell count 6 wks, 3 mos, and 6 mos after treatment	CSF cell count at 12 mos and 24 mos if normal at 6 mos
Suspected syphilis§	
Treat as for early syphilis	VDRL titer 1, 3, and 6 mos after treatment

* VDRL = Venereal Disease Research Laboratory test; MHA-TP = micro-hemagglutination-*Treponema pallidum* test; CSF = cerebrospinal fluid.

† Includes all pregnant women; proven contacts of persons with infectious disease; and persons in demonstrated high-risk groups.

‡ Includes persons with neurologic abnormalities; persons before treatment with nonpenicillin regimens; and persons before re-treatment after treatment failure.

§ Includes women with newly discovered syphilis seropositivity late in pregnancy; infants of mothers with inadequately treated syphilis; and proven contacts of persons with infectious syphilis.

single, indurated, painless lesions suggests a high probability of syphilis because few other conditions produce this type of lesion. Multiple painful lesions suggest only a moderate probability of disease, whereas shallow, painful, multiple ulcerations suggestive of genital herpes (61) indicate a low probability of syphilis. The relative interpretation of diagnostic tests in these three types of clinical presentation is indicated by Table 1, which indicates post-test probabilities associated with pretest probabilities of 50%, 5%, and 1% arbitrarily taken to represent high, moderate, and low risk of disease.

Sequential probabilities were calculated because sensitivity and specificity values of darkfield microscopy and serologic tests used in combination are not available. Because these tests have a different biological basis, conditional independence of the darkfield and serologic tests was assumed. Because of uncertainty about the performance characteristics of the darkfield test, probabilities were calculated for two sensitivities and specificities of this test. Where two test results are shown on the one line of Table 1, the probability of disease after the darkfield result was used as the disease prevalence for calculating disease probability after a VDRL result.

If one assumes a darkfield sensitivity of 75% and specificity of 98% (that is, performed under adverse conditions) with high disease prevalence, diagnosis is confirmed either by a positive darkfield test or by a positive VDRL test following a negative darkfield result. A negative VDRL test following a negative darkfield test suggests a probability of infection of 6%, which is too high to ignore. Repeated darkfield examinations may be done to confirm the diagnosis, and longitudinal assessment of the VDRL results will resolve any remaining uncertainty. A VDRL test in 1 week will provide prompt evidence of infection if the result is positive; a negative result 1 month later makes the diagnosis of syphilis highly unlikely, and a negative test 3 months later virtually excludes syphilis (62). For a disease prevalence of 5%, diagnosis is suggested (probability of 66%) by a positive darkfield result or by a positive VDRL test following a negative darkfield result, whereas syphilis is unlikely (0.3%) when a negative VDRL test follows a negative darkfield test.

For a pretest probability of 1%, only a single darkfield or VDRL test may be warranted. However, a single positive result alone may not justify the diagnosis. A positive darkfield result gives an infection probability of 27%, and confirmation should be sought before accepting the diagnosis. A positive VDRL test provides confirmation with a probability of infection of 98%. A negative VDRL test following a positive darkfield result suggests an infection probability of 9%, and longitudinal follow-up is required to confirm or exclude the diagnosis.

With a darkfield sensitivity of 95% and specificity of 99% (that is, performed under ideal conditions), positive results substantially increase the probability of disease in populations with prevalences of 5% and 1%, but this increase is insufficient to alter the diagnostic algorithm or therapeutic decisions. A negative darkfield result is stronger evidence for ruling out syphilis, but a VDRL test is still desirable to increase the certainty of diagnosis (either negative or positive) in high-prevalence settings. However, for lower disease prevalence (that is, atypical lesions), a positive VDRL test following a negative dark-field result is not strong evidence of syphilis and further investigation (darkfield and VDRL tests) is warranted. Age of patient, contact with persons with infectious syphilis, recent sexual behavior, and other epidemiologic factors may greatly increase the pretest probability suggested by the clinical lesions discussed (63).

Lesions Suggesting Secondary Syphilis or Early Congenital Syphilis: Secondary syphilis is noted for the array of symptoms it may produce (63). Typical condyloma lata and maculopapular or squamous rash on the palms and soles indicate a reasonably high likelihood of disease. Pruritus, once considered to exclude a diagnosis of secondary syphilis, has been reported in significant numbers of patients (64, 65). However, even for symptoms not highly suggestive of syphilis, serologic tests are recommended to rule out the disease (when negative) because of virtual 100% sensitivity of both treponemal and non-treponemal tests in secondary syphilis. Thus, the VDRL test is highly diagnostic for ruling out disease when the result is negative, regardless of disease prevalence.

Darkfield examination (on exudate from moist or scarified dry lesions) may be performed to provide an immediate result. An initial VDRL titer of less than 1:8 (in association with darkfield-negative lesions) should raise significant doubts about the diagnosis. Further tests 1 week and 1 month later are recommended. A rising titer confirms the diagnosis of secondary syphilis, whereas a stable VDRL titer below 1:8 over the 1-month period virtually precludes the disease. In a patient with a stable, low titer, results of an MHA-TP test will distinguish a false-positive VDRL test from adequately treated syphilis or latent syphilis.

ASYMPTOMATIC PERSONS (SCREENING)

Preferred Test for Screening: Recently, some European authors have recommended the combined use of the VDRL and MHA-TP tests for screening, because of the marginally greater detection rate in primary syphilis and the increased sensitivity of the treponemal test in late syphilis (5, 66, 67). Where a microautomated form of the treponemal test (AMHA-TP) is available at a cost similar to that of the VDRL test (68, 69), an argument can be made for using the MHA-TP alone for screening. However, in the United States, where the VDRL test is cheaper than the treponemal tests and where there is extensive experience with its use, the VDRL test is the preferred serologic test for screening. Positive VDRL results should be confirmed by the MHA-TP test.

Pregnancy: The prevalence of syphilis is usually low in pregnant women, but the costs of congenital syphilis are so high that screening may be cost-beneficial with prevalences as low as 0.005% (70). At this prevalence, however, serologic tests have low predictive value when positive. A positive screening test will indicate a probability of infection of less than 1%, and a positive confirmatory test will increase this probability to 66%, if the two tests are conditionally independent. Consequently, diagnosis is often uncertain in pregnancy. In early pregnancy, this uncertainty is often resolved by longitudinal assessment of the VDRL titer. When uncertainty cannot be resolved, treatment in pregnancy is advocated. Despite a negative screening test early in pregnancy, syphilis may be acquired later in pregnancy and produce a fatal outcome in the infant (71). Consequently, in areas where syphilis is common, women should be screened both early and late in pregnancy.

Congenital Syphilis: The main aim of screening should be prevention of congenital syphilis by detection and treatment of infection in the pregnant mother. Although the significance of positive serologic tests in asymptomatic infants can be assessed by weekly measurement of VDRL titers for 6 weeks, this course is not recommended. If the mother received adequate treatment for syphilis with penicillin, congenital syphilis is very unlikely, and surveillance of the infant with VDRL titers monthly for 3 months is satisfactory. In other cases, the infant should be treated for possible syphilis, rather than awaiting signs or symptoms that will confirm the diagnosis.

Screening on Admission to the Hospital: Screening of all hospitalized patients has been recommended (72) because of reports of unrecognized syphilis producing clinical manifestations responsible for hospitalization (73, 74). However, there is no evidence of a significant prevalence of syphilis in general hospital patients, and the specificity of both nontreponemal and treponemal tests tends to be low in patients with nonsyphilitic disease (11) and in the elderly (33, 34). If the specificity of both the VDRL and MHA-TP tests was 95% (the maximum that could be expected in a hospital population), the post-test probabilities of disease following a positive VDRL test confirmed with a positive MHA-TP test would be 3.9% and 27.9% if the pretest probabilities were 0.01% and 0.1%, respectively. For these reasons, routine syphilis screening preoperatively or on admission to the hospital is difficult to justify.

General Risk Factors: In the United States, homosexual activity causes a high proportion of cases of syphilis. A detailed sexual history is an essential element of the diagnostic process in all patients with oral, genital, or anorectal lesions or in those with symptoms suggesting disseminated infection (for example, lymphadenopathy and fever), even when initial presentation suggests a nonsyphilitic lesion.

The risk of acquiring syphilis from sexual contact varies greatly, depending on the nature of the lesions present in the partner and the type and frequency of sexual activity, but the risk range has been suggested to be 5% to 30% (13). Many contacts may have incubating syphilis, and the sensitivity of both treponemal and nontreponemal tests is low in this stage of disease. Consequently, a negative serologic test is inadequate for ruling out disease. Proven exposure to a person with infectious disease probably warrants immediate treatment to preclude further dissemination of disease.

Routine testing for syphilis in patients with gonorrhea is a time-honored practice, but it may not be universally rewarding (75, 76). The prevalence of 0.1% in female patients in one setting in the United States (76) would lead to a probability of syphilis of only 10%, even if both the VDRL and MHA-TP tests were positive. There are other potential indicators of risk (such as occupation) that vary greatly by time or location. Unless resources are unlimited, it is recommended that the yield from existing screening programs be monitored, and periodic sample screening be conducted on a regional basis to identify new risk factors in a particular locality.

FOLLOW-UP AFTER THERAPY

The major aims of follow-up are to show the effectiveness of therapy and to allow prompt re-treatment when
treatment has failed. A secondary role may be the detection of reinfection in selected groups. A recent analysis
has shown that after treatment of primary or secondary
syphilis, the VDRL titer declined approximately fourfold
at 3 months and eightfold at 6 months (77). The VDRL
titer may fall a little more slowly in patients with early
latent syphilis, but a decline will almost certainly be noted 6 months after treatment. Relapse is highly unlikely if
a satisfactory decline, in the absence of symptoms and
signs of disease, has been maintained for 12 months. For
both late latent and early syphilis, satisfactory serologic
surveillance in the absence of complications involves
quantitative VDRL assessment 3, 6, and 12 months after
treatment.

CEREBROSPINAL FLUID ASSESSMENT

Routine cerebrospinal fluid assessment in patients with
early acquired syphilis is not warranted, because the frequent abnormalities at this stage of disease tend to be
transient (78). Abnormal cerebrospinal fluid findings after the early stage have more serious prognosis, suggesting the need for extensive cerebrospinal fluid testing
(79). However, the yield from screening all patients with
positive serologic findings may be low (80), and the outcome with standard penicillin therapy (using regimens
recommended by the Centers for Disease Control [13])
appears excellent (81), even though penicillin levels in
the cerebrospinal fluid may be negligible after treatment
with some regimens (82). A recent article describing a
decision-analysis model has concluded that lumbar puncture offers little additional benefit and may increase morbidity in patients with asymptomatic late syphilis (83).

The confidence in penicillin therapy cannot be extended to nonpenicillin regimens or to benzathine penicillin in
congenital neurosyphilis, because of limited experience
with these forms of therapy. Patients with syphilis who
have not responded to treatment adequately or who have
neurologic abnormalities clearly have an increased risk of
neurosyphilis and require cerebrospinal fluid assessment.

Cerebrospinal fluid examination therefore should be

restricted to four situations: in patients with syphilis with neurologic abnormalities; before re-treatment of patients who have had relapses after any forms of treatment; as a baseline measure in all patients with syphilis for whom nonpenicillin regimens are prescribed; and in all infants suspected of having congenital syphilis. A positive VDRL test indicates the presence of neurosyphilis, and an elevated cell count indicates active disease. If the cell count is normal, further cerebrospinal fluid testing is not required after uneventful treatment for latent syphilis. If initial examination reveals an elevated cell count, the cerebrospinal fluid examination should be repeated 6 weeks, 3 months, and 6 months after therapy. Re-treatment should be considered for patients with persistent elevated cell counts at 6 months. If the cell count is normal at 6 months, further normal cell counts 12 and 24 months after therapy indicate a high probability of cure.

Data are inadequate to quantify the interpretation of a nonreactive cerebrospinal fluid VDRL test in combination with an elevated cell count and seropositivity. In view of the insensitivity of the cerebrospinal fluid VDRL, this pattern does not exclude asymptomatic neurosyphilis, and standard surveillance after treatment for neurosyphilis is indicated. Investigation for other causes of cerebrospinal disease must be considered, particularly if the cell count does not subside as expected.

References

1. JAFFE HW. The laboratory diagnosis of syphilis: New concepts. *Ann Intern Med.* 1975;**83**:846-50.
2. *Manual of Tests for Syphilis*—Atlanta: Venereal Disease Program, U.S. Communicable Disease Center; 1969. (PHS publication no. 411).
3. *Technique for Direct Immunofluorescent Identification of* Treponema Pallidum *in Body Fluids and Tissue Secretions.* Atlanta: Venereal Disease Research Laboratory, Center for Disease Control; 1971.
4. SHANNON R, BOOTH SD. The pattern of immunological responses at various stages of syphilis. *Br J Vener Dis.* 1977;**53**:281-6.
5. WHO SCIENTIFIC GROUP ON TREPONEMAL INFECTIONS. *Treponemal Infections.* Geneva: World Health Organization; 1982. (WHO technical report series 674).
6. WALLACE AL, NORINS LC. Syphilis serology today. *Prog Clin Pathol.* 1969;**2**:198-215.
7. HUBER TW, STORMS S, YOUNG P, et al. Reactivity of microhemagglutination, fluorescent treponemal antibody absorption, Venereal Disease Research Laboratory, and rapid plasma reagin tests in primary syphilis. *J Clin Microbiol.* 1983;**17**:405-9.

8. PETTIT DE, LARSEN SA, POPE V, PERRYMAN MW, ADAMS MR. Unheated serum reagin test as a quantitative test for syphilis. *J Clin Microbiol.* 1982;**15**:238-42.

9. RATHLEV T. Haemagglutination test utilizing pathogenic *Treponema pallidum* for the sero-diagnosis of syphilis. *Br J Vener Dis.* 1967;**43**:181-5.

10. COX PM, LOGAN LC, NORINS LC. Automated, quantitative microhemagglutination assay for *Treponema pallidum* antibodies. *Appl Microbiol.* 1969;**18**:485-9.

11. WENTWORTH BB, THOMPSON MA, PETER CR, BAWDON RE, WILSON DL. Comparison of a hemagglutination treponemal test for syphilis (HATTS) with other serologic methods for the diagnosis of syphilis. *Sex Transm Dis.* 1978;**5**:103-11.

12. TUFFANELLI DL, WUEPPER KD, BRADFORD LL, WOOD RM. Fluorescent treponemal-antibody absorption tests: studies of false-positive reactions for syphilis. *N Engl J Med.* 1967;**276**:258-62.

13. *Criteria and Techniques for the Diagnosis of Early Syphilis.* Atlanta: Centers for Disease Control; 1979. (DHEW publication no. 98-376).

14. RUDOLPH AH. Syphilis. In: WEHRLE PF, TOP FH, eds. *Communicable and Infectious Diseases.* 9th ed. St. Louis: C.V. Mosby Co.; 1981:621-34.

15. LARSEN SA, HAMBIE EA, PETTIT DE, PERRYMAN MW, KRAUS SJ. Specificity, sensitivity, and reproducibility among the fluorescent treponemal antibody-absorption test, the microhemagglutination assay for *Treponema pallidum* antibodies, and the hemagglutination treponemal test for syphilis. *J Clin Microbiol.* 1981;**14**:441-5.

16. KIRALY K, PRERAU H. Evaluation of the *T. pallidum* haemagglutination (TPHA) test for syphilis on "problem sera." *Acta Derm Venereol (Stockh).* 1974;**54**:303-10.

17. HART G. Screening to control infectious diseases: evaluation of control programs for gonorrhea and syphilis. *Rev Infect Dis.* 1980;**2**:701-12.

18. VECCHIO TJ. Predictive value of a single diagnostic test in unselected populations. *N Engl J Med.* 1966;**274**:1171-3.

19. DANIELS KC, FERNEYHOUGH HS. Specific direct fluorescent antibody detection of *Treponema pallidum. Health Lab Sci.* 1977;**14**:164-71.

20. FIUMARA NJ. Treatment of early latent syphilis of less than a year's duration: an evaluation of 275 cases. *Sex Transm Dis.* 1978;**5**:85-8.

21. FIUMARA NJ. Serologic responses to treatment of 128 patients with late latent syphilis. *Sex Transm Dis.* 1979;**6**:243-6.

22. LUGER A, SPENDLINGWIMMER I. Appraisal of the *Treponema pallidum* haemagglutination test. *Br J Vener Dis.* 1973;**49**:181-2.

23. CHAPEL TA. The variability of syphilitic chancres. *Sex Transm Dis.* 1978;**5**:68-70.

24. ALESSI E, SCIOCCATI L. TPHA test: experience at the Clinic of Dermatology, University of Milan. *Br J Vener Dis.* 1978;**54**:151-4.

25. DEACON WE, LUCAS JB, PRICE EV. Fluorescent treponemal antibody-absorption (FTA-ABS) test for syphilis. *JAMA.* 1966;**198**:624-8.

26. DYCKMAN JD, STORMS S, HUBER TW. Reactivity of microhemagglutination, fluorescent treponemal antibody absorption, and Venereal Disease Research Laboratory tests in primary syphilis. *J Clin Microbiol.* 1980;**12**:629-30.

27. LESINSKI J, KRACH J, KADZIEWICZ E. Specificity, sensitivity, and diagnostic value of the TPHA test. *Br J Vener Dis.* 1974;**50**:334-40.

28. CATTERALL RD. Presidential address to the M.S.S.V.D.: systemic disease and the biological false positive reaction. *Br J Vener Dis.* 1972;**48**:1-12.

29. HARVEY AM, SHULMAN LE. Connective tissue disease and the chronic biologic false-positive test for syphilis (BFP reaction). *Med Clin North Am.* 1966;**50**:1271-9.

30. MURRAY KA. Syphilis in patients with Hansen's disease. *Int J Lepr Other Mycobact Dis.* 1982;**50**:152-8.

31. TUFFANELLI DL. Narcotic addiction with false-positive reaction for syphilis: immunologic studies. *Acta Derm Venereol (Stockh).* 1968;**48**:542-6.
32. KAUFMAN RE, WEISS S, MOORE JD, FALCONE V, WIESNER PJ. Biological false positive serological tests for syphilis among drug addicts. *Br J Vener Dis.* 1974;**50**:350-3.
33. TUFFANELLI DL. Ageing and false positive reactions for syphilis. *Br J Vener Dis.* 1966;**42**:40-1.
34. CARR RD, BECKER SW, CARPENTER CM. The biological false-positive phenomenon in elderly men. *Arch Dermatol.* 1965;**93**:393-5.
35. CABRERA HA, CARLSON J. Biologic false-positive reactions and infectious mononucleosis. *Am J Clin Pathol.* 1968;**50**:643-5.
36. HOAGLAND RJ. False-positive serology in mononucleosis. *JAMA.* 1963;**185**:783-5.
37. BRITISH COOPERATIVE CLINICAL GROUP. Acute and chronic biological false positive reactors to serological tests for syphilis: ABO blood groups and other investigations. *Br J Vener Dis.* 1974;**50**:428-34.
38. MANIKOWSKA-LESINSKA W, LINDA B, ZAJAC W. Specificity of the FTA-ABS and TPHA tests during pregnancy. *Br J Vener Dis.* 1978;**54**:295-8.
39. SALO OP, AHO K, NIEMINEN E, HORMILA P. False-positive serological tests for syphilis in pregnancy. *Acta Derm Venereol (Stockh).* 1969;**49**:332-5.
40. MOORE MB, KNOX JM. Sensitivity and specificity in syphilis serology. *South Med J.* 1965;**58**:963-8.
41. DANS PE, JUDSON FN, LARSEN SA, LANTZ MA. The FTA-ABS test: a diagnostic help or hindrance? *South Med J.* 1977;**70**:312-5.
42. PETER CR, THOMPSON MA, WILSON DL. False-positive reactions in the rapid plasma reagin-card, fluorescent treponemal antibody-absorbed, and hemagglutination treponemal syphilis serology tests. *J Clin Microbiol.* 1979;**9**:369-72.
43. JAFFE HW, LARSEN SA, JONES OG, DANS PE. Hemagglutination tests for syphilis antibody. *Am J Clin Pathol.* 1978;**70**:230-3.
44. GOODHART GL, BROWN ST, ZAIDI AA, POPE V, LARSEN S, BARROW JE. Blinded proficiency testing of FTA-ABS test. *Arch Intern Med.* 1981;**141**:1045-50.
45. BAERTSCHY D, GOLUBJATNIKOV R, STEADMAN M, INHORN SL. Serologic study of specimens with borderline FTA-ABS test reactivity. *Health Lab Sci.* 1977;**14**:177-82.
46. BLUM G, ELLNER PD, MCCARTHY LR, PAPACHRISTOS T. Reliability of the treponemal hemagglutination test for the serodiagnosis of syphilis. *J Infect Dis.* 1973;**127**:321-4.
47. LUGER A, SCHMIDT BL, SPENDLINGWIMMER I, STEYRER K. Specificity of the *Treponema pallidum* haemagglutination test: analysis of results. *Br J Vener Dis.* 1981;**57**:178-80.
48. SEQUEIRA PJL, ELDRIDGE AE. Treponemal haemagglutination test. *Br J Vener Dis.* 1973;**49**:242-8.
49. O'NEILL P, WARNER RW, NICOL CS. *Treponema pallidum* haemagglutination assay in the routine serodiagnosis of treponemal disease. *Br J Vener Dis.* 1973;**49**:427-31.
50. GOLDMAN JN, LANTZ MA. FTA-ABS and VDRL slide test reactivity in a population of nuns. *JAMA.* 1971;**217**:53-5.
51. MADIEDO G, HO KC, WALSH P. False-positive VDRL and FTA in cerebrospinal fluid. *JAMA.* 1980;**244**:688-9.
52. PERDRUP A. *Late Syphilis, with Particular Reference to Clinical Manifestations, Serology and Treatment.* Geneva: World Health Organisation; 1980. (WHO publication no. INT/VDT/80.371.)
53. LECLERC G, GIROUX M, BIRRY A, KASATIYA S. Study of fluorescent treponemal antibody test on cerebrospinal fluid using monospecific anti-immunoglobulin conjugates IgG, IgM, and IgA. *Br J Vener Dis.* 1978;**54**:303-8.

54. ESCOBAR MR, DALTON HP, ALLISON MJ. Fluorescent antibody tests for syphilis using cerebrospinal fluid: clinical correlation in 150 cases. *Am J Clin Pathol.* 1970;**53**:886-90.

55. SCHMIDT BL, LUGER A. *Diagnosis of Neurosyphilis by CSF Examination.* Geneva: World Health Organisation; 1980. (WHO publication no. INT/VDT/80.360.)

56. LUGER A. Diagnosis of syphilis. *Bull WHO.* 1981;**59**:647-54.

57. JAFFE HW, LARSEN SA, PETERS M, JOVE DF, LOPEZ B, SCHROETER AL. Tests for treponemal antibody in CSF. *Arch Intern Med.* 1978;**138**:252-5.

58. DATTNER B, THOMAS EW, DE MELLO L. Criteria for the management of neurosyphilis. *Am J Med.* 1951;**10**:463-7.

59. KOLAR OJ, BURKHART JE. Neurosyphilis. *Br J Vener Dis.* 1977;**53**:221-5.

60. DEWHURST K. The composition of the cerebro-spinal fluid in the neurosyphilitic psychoses. *Acta Neurol Scand.* 1969;**45**:119-23.

61. TRAMONT EC. *Treponema pallidum* (syphilis). In: MANDELL GL, DOUGLAS RG, BENNETT JE, eds. *Principles and Practice of Infectious Diseases.* New York: John Wiley and Sons; 1979:1820-37.

62. BERLIN SI. [Preventive treatment of syphilis]. *Vestn Dermatol Venereol.* 1972;**46**:46-9.

63. *Venereal Disease Epidemiology.* Report 12. Atlanta: Center for Disease Control; 1973. (DHEW publication no. HSM 73-8232).

64. CHAPEL TA. The signs and symptoms of secondary syphilis. *Sex Transm Dis.* 1980;**7**:161-4.

65. COLE GW, AMON RB, RUSSELL PS. Secondary syphilis presenting as a pruritic dermatosis. *Arch Dermatol.* 1977;**113**:489-90.

66. LUGER A, SCHMIDT B, SPENDLINGWIMMER I, HORN F. Recent observations on the serology of syphilis. *Br J Vener Dis.* 1980;**56**:12-6.

67. YOUNG H, HENRICHSEN C, ROBERTSON DHH. *Treponema pallidum* haemagglutination test as a screening procedure for the diagnosis of syphilis. *Br J Vener Dis.* 1974;**50**:341-6.

68. PUCKETT A, PRATT G. Modification of the system of screening for antisyphilis antibodies in a blood transfusion centre, featuring a miniaturisation of the *Treponema pallidum* haemagglutination assay. *J Clin Pathol.* 1982;**35**:1349-52.

69. BARBARA J, SALKER R, LALJI F, DAVIES TD, HARRIS JB. An economical, simplified haemagglutination test for mass syphilis screening. *J Clin Pathol.* 1980;**33**:1216-8.

70. STRAY-PEDERSEN B. Economic evaluation of maternal screening to prevent congenital syphilis. *Sex Transm Dis.* 1983;**10**:167-72.

71. BELLINGHAM FR. Syphilis in pregnancy: transplacental infection. *Med J Aust.* 1973;**2**:647-8.

72. FELMAN Y. How useful are the serologic tests for syphilis? *Int J Dermatol.* 1982;**21**:79-81.

73. DRUSIN LM, HOMAN WP, DINEEN P. The role of surgery in primary syphilis of the anus. *Ann Surg.* 1976;**184**:65-7.

74. DRUSIN LM, SINGER C, VALENTI AJ, ARMSTRONG D. Infectious syphilis mimicking neoplastic disease. *Arch Intern Med.* 1977;**137**:156-60.

75. HART G. Venereal disease in a war environment: incidence and management. *Med J Aust.* 1975;**1**:808-10.

76. JUDSON FN. The importance of coexisting syphilitic, chlamydial, mycoplasmal, and trichomonal infections in the treatment of gonorrhea. *Sex Transm Dis.* 1979;**6**(2 suppl):112-9.

77. BROWN ST, ZAIDI A, LARSEN SA, REYNOLDS GH. Serological response to syphilis treatment: a new analysis of old data. *JAMA.* 1985;**253**:1296-9.

78. MILLS CH. Routine examination of cerebrospinal fluid in syphilis: its value in regard to a more accurate knowledge, prognosis and treatment. *Br Med J.* 1927;**2**:527-32.

79. JAFFE HW, KABINS SA. Examination of cerebrospinal fluid in patients with syphilis. *Rev Infect Dis.* 1982;**4**(suppl):842-7.
80. TRAVIESA DC, PRYSTOWSKY SD, NELSON BJ, JOHNSON KP. Cerebrospinal fluid findings in asymptomatic patients with reactive serum fluorescent treponemal antibody absorption tests. *Ann Neurol.* 1978;**4**:524-30.
81. SHORT DH, KNOX JM, GLICKSMAN J. Neurosyphilis, the search for adequate treatment. *Arch Dermatol.* 1966;**93**:87-91.
82. MOHR JA, GRIFFITHS W, JACKSON R, SAADAH H, BIRD P, RIDDLE J. Neurosyphilis and penicillin levels in cerebrospinal fluid. *JAMA.* 1976;**236**:2208-9.
83. WIESEL J, ROSE DN, SILVER AL, SACKS HS, BERNSTEIN RH. Lumbar puncture in asymptomatic late syphilis: an analysis of the benefits and risks. *Arch Intern Med.* 1985;**145**:465-8.

Throat Cultures and Rapid Tests for Diagnosis of Group A Streptococcal Pharyngitis

ROBERT M. CENTOR, M.D.; FREDERICK A. MEIER, M.D.; and HARRY P. DALTON, Ph.D.

PATIENTS COMMONLY seek medical care for sore throats (1, 2). Although they usually desire symptomatic relief rather than a specific diagnosis, the medical literature has focused on the diagnosis of one etiologic organism, the group A beta-hemolytic streptococcus, and prevention of its nonsuppurative complications. For the last 30 years, throat culture has been the standard technique for diagnosing pharyngitis caused by this organism. However, many physicians now use non-culture-based, antigen-detection techniques to make this diagnosis (3, 4).

Diagnostic test results should not always change management decisions. The tests for group A beta-hemolytic streptococcal pharyngitis are not perfect, and therefore a negative test result should not necessarily change a physician's decision to treat a patient whose clinical presentation strongly suggests streptococcal pharyngitis. In this review, we use the threshold model of decision making, in which a test is done only if the test result can change the probability of disease enough to change the decision to treat (or not treat) (5). The threshold model follows from Bayes' theorem and requires knowledge of the pretest probability of disease, the sensitivity and specificity of the test, and the threshold for treatment. When these values are known, a physician can specify one of three preferred actions—do nothing, test, or treat—for each level of pretest probability. Accordingly, this article focuses on the problem of obtaining accurate estimates of the pretest probability of streptococcal pharyngitis, of the

▶ This chapter was originally published in *Annals of Internal Medicine.* 1986;**105**:892-9.

sensitivity and specificity of tests, and the thresholds for treatment. This review also examines the reasons for establishing the diagnosis of streptococcal pharyngitis; analyzes both the use of throat cultures and the use of the antigen-detection kits; and considers the influence of other possible microbiologic diagnoses on the medical management of pharyngitis.

The Clinical Problem

Denny (6) has enumerated four reasons for diagnosing (and treating) group A streptococcal pharyngitis:

> . . . the illness is shortened with early treatment; the streptococcus is eradicated from the pharynx and thus cannot spread to other individuals; suppurative complications can probably be prevented; and rheumatic fever and possibly acute glomerulonephritis are prevented.

Prompt antibiotic therapy decreases the morbidity from group A streptococcal pharyngitis. In the early 1950s, studies from the Warren Air Force Base showed a consistently favorable effect of antibiotic therapy on the duration of symptoms (7). Brumfitt and Slater (8), in a British general practice population, showed that penicillin decreased the duration of both fever and sore throat by approximately 1 day. Other investigators have reported studies in which early penicillin therapy shortened disease duration by approximately 24 hours (9-11). Krober and colleagues (9) and Merenstein and Rogers (11) randomly assigned patients to receive antibiotics either immediately or after culture results became available. They found significant decreases in morbidity rates among those patients treated soon after symptoms had started. More recently, Randolph and colleagues (12) have reported the largest double-blind, randomized, controlled trial of the effect of antibiotics on the clinical course of streptococcal pharyngitis. The antibiotic-treated groups showed significantly greater clinical improvement after 24 hours, whether judged by physicians, patients, or parents.

Because antibiotic therapy usually eradicates the organism from the pharynx, early treatment reduces the chance of spread to other persons (13).

Bennike and associates' (14) study of penicillin therapy for tonsillitis provided evidence that antibiotics prevent suppurative complications of pharyngitis. Although entry into this study did not require that patients have culture evidence of infection, untreated patients developed suppurative complications more frequently than did penicillin-treated patients. Chamovitz and colleagues (15) also found a decrease in suppurative complications when patients with streptococcal pharyngitis received penicillin. In their study, only 1 of 522 penicillin-treated patients developed such complications, whereas 18 of 391 placebo-treated patients did. The combination of these results and the clinical observation that the incidence of suppurative complications has decreased during the antibiotic era supports the conclusion that antibiotics decrease the probability of suppurative complications.

The classic studies of Denny and colleagues (16) and Wannamaker and colleagues (17) showed the importance of antibiotic therapy in decreasing the incidence of rheumatic fever after group A streptococcal pharyngitis. Rates of rheumatic fever decreased tenfold after penicillin therapy. These outcomes led the American Heart Association (18) to recommend that all patients having streptococcal pharyngitis receive antibiotic treatment. In contrast, prompt antibiotic therapy probably does not prevent the other nonsuppurative complication of streptococcal infections, glomerulonephritis (19).

Current Practice

Despite consensus on the four reasons for identifying and treating group A streptococcal pharyngitis, there are several major areas of variation in the clinical approach to patients with a sore throat. First, physicians vary in whether or not they use any diagnostic tests at all. Furthermore, test results may or may not influence management decisions. To compound the problem, the tests themselves have three sources of variation: some physicians now use antigen-detection tests rather than cultures; laboratories use a variety of culture techniques; and many physicians do testing in their offices rather than sending samples to a laboratory.

Cochi and associates (20) have documented, in a survey of U.S. medical practitioners, the great variation in current practice. Only 25% of primary care physicians (and only 16% of internists) stated that they always obtain cultures for patients with pharyngitis. Another 23% never use cultures (Table 1). Most physicians who obtain cultures start antibiotic treatment before culture results

Table 1. Current Use Among Primary Care Physicians of Throat Culture for Patients with an Acute Sore Throat

	%
Always culture	25
Selectively culture	52
Never culture	23

are available, and only 60% of this group stop antibiotic treatment after receiving a negative culture report.

Technical Description of Tests

All tests for group A streptococcal pharyngitis begin with collection of a specimen from the posterior pharynx. In culture methods, the swab specimen is inoculated onto a blood agar plate, and then the specimen is streaked across the blood agar to isolate individual bacterial colonies.

Laboratory culture techniques vary in two major ways: the atmospheres in which the culture plates are incubated, and the culture media used. Investigators have used three atmospheres of incubation: air, air enriched with 3% to 5% carbon dioxide, and anaerobic conditions. Conflicting studies have found each of these atmospheres to be clearly superior to the other two (21-24). Such contradictory conclusions from large, well-done studies suggest that other variables, in particular the media used, contribute to the differences in isolation rates that these studies reported (25-27).

Similar problems occur in the identification of group A streptococcal isolates. The commonest identification technique relies on selective inhibition of group A isolates by a bacitracin disk (28). Microbiologists designate this identification technique *presumptive* because it disagrees with the reference standard (Lancefield capillary precipitation) in about 22% of isolates (29-32). This technique identifies about 17% of non-group-A organisms as group A and misidentifies about 5% of group A organisms. Pollack and Dahlgren (33) showed that 11% of group G and 13% of group C streptococci were bacitracin sensitive. The other identification (confirmation) tests currently available—fluorescent antibody assays, coagglutination, and latex agglutination—also have error rates of 4% to 16% when compared to the reference standard

(34-37), Lancefield capillary precipitation, which is too tedious and lengthy for routine use in the clinical laboratory. These technical variations must influence the accuracy of "routine" throat cultures.

Many companies now market rapid diagnostic tests for diagnosing group A streptococcal pharyngitis. Rapid tests use either an acid or enzyme extraction procedure to remove the group A carbohydrate from a throat swab (38). These tests use the extract either in a latex agglutination, coagglutination, or enzyme-linked immunosorbent assay procedure to combine antibody identification of the carbohydrate with various mechanisms for detecting group A antigen-antibody complexes (39-44). The time needed to do these tests varies from about 7 to 70 minutes.

Definitions

Another difficulty in evaluating the literature stems from semantic differences. We define four types of streptococcal throat infections:

Definite Streptococcal Pharyngitis: The patient is symptomatic, has a positive culture, and has a host antibody response to the infection (for example, fourfold rise in antistreptolysin O, anti-DNAse B, or other antistreptococcal antibody titers).

Possible Streptococcal Pharyngitis: The patient is symptomatic and has a positive culture, but no antibody information is available.

Streptococcal Carriage: The patient may be symptomatic or asymptomatic, has a positive culture, has no host response, and has persistent positive cultures despite treatment.

Streptococcal Colonization: The patient is asymptomatic but has positive cultures.

Given the current medical practice of not obtaining acute and convalescent serum tests, few studies can identify a population as having definite streptococcal pharyngitis. Even when one collects serologic data, the rate of "definite" infection varies because of the following three factors: antibiotic therapy decreases the percentage of patients who will show a rise in antibody titer, that is, decrease the rate of "definite" infection (45, 46); if one increases the time interval before measuring the second titer, the percentage of patients with a significant rise increases, that is, the rate of "definite" infection increases

(46); and if one increases the number of different types of antibodies (for example, antistreptolysin O, anti-DNAse B, anti-group A antigen) for which one tests, the percentage of patients who have positive cultures and show "definite" infection will increase (47).

Few studies have included complete serologic data, let alone serologic data controlled for the effect of these interventions. The designation possible streptococcal pharyngitis, therefore, describes most patients reported in the literature. Because one cannot know which symptomatic patients have positive cultures yet another cause for their symptoms, we advocate the evaluation of test specificity using the streptococcal colonization rate—that is, test positivity in asymptomatic persons. We thus define the false-positive rate as the colonization rate (note that false-positive rate plus specificity equal one).

Establishing sensitivity provides a challenge in the absence of an agreed-on "gold-standard" test for disease. Determining a "gold-standard" test for streptococcal pharyngitis would require methods that would provide certainty both that the patient had streptococci present in the throat and that those organisms were causing the pharyngitis. Researchers have used multiple swabs and tonsillar cultures as a proxy for sensitivity estimation. These methods only approximate the probability of organism detection and cannot prove causation of pharyngitis. Multiple swab tests are used to estimate the probability that a single throat swab will detect the presence of group A beta-hemolytic streptococci in the throat. Either sampling variation (errors due to the nonhomogeneous presence of streptococci in the throat) or failure of test technique (inability to demonstrate streptococci actually present on one or both swabs) can cause multiple swabs to have different results. The tonsillar culture study measures the probability that a routine throat swab will detect group A beta-hemolytic streptococci growing in surgically removed tonsils (48). No investigators have (or could have) applied this technique as a reference standard in patients with acute pharyngitis.

In the absence of a "gold-standard" test, physicians generally would agree to treat all symptomatic patients having positive cultures. Either multiple swabs or a tonsillar culture provides a standard against which to evaluate one throat swab, because these techniques detect patients whom all physicians would treat.

Test Performance

LABORATORY THROAT CULTURE

Specificity: As presented in the definitions section, the specificity of throat culture depends on the colonization rate in a population. In adults, we have data from two studies. Laatsch (49) performed 958 throat cultures from asymptomatic medical technology students, and only 8 of these cultures (0.84%) grew group A beta-hemolytic streptococci. In a study done in our emergency room (50), we found only 4 positive cultures for 329 control patients (1.22%). According to these studies, the specificity of throat culture approximates 99% in adults. Because of low colonization, neither study documents seasonal variation. However, children generally have a higher colonization rate (and thus a lower specificity) (51) and also exhibit seasonal variations (52).

Sensitivity: Double swab studies provide data for estimating the sensitivity of a single throat culture. When investigators have obtained and cultured two swabs from a single patient, they have noted a 9% to 12% discordance for positive cultures (53). These data indicate that one swab has about a 90% probability of detecting group A streptococci in the throat. A study in 1944 among Army personnel showed a lesser sensitivity for a single culture (54). In that study, the investigators obtained throat cultures on 3 consecutive days, and of patients having at least one of the three cultures positive, only 76% grew group A beta-hemolytic streptococci on the initial culture.

When Saslaw and colleagues (48) compared 174 throat swabs taken before tonsillectomy with cultures from minced tonsillar homogenates, 34 of the tonsillar specimens grew group A beta-hemolytic streptococci but only 28 of the corresponding throat swabs yielded positive cultures. In no instance did a patient with a negative tonsillar culture have a positive throat swab. This study suggests a sensitivity of 82% for throat swabs when judged against a tonsillar culture standard.

Although these sensitivity estimates range between 76% and 90%, in accord with previous medical-decision analyses, we will accept the high sensitivity of 90% for our baseline analysis (55). This convention equates the probability of detecting group A streptococci in the throat with sensitivity, without addressing the question of whether the streptococci cause the patient's sore throat.

OFFICE CULTURES

Mondzac (56), in 1967, warned that office cultures showed variable results when compared with simultaneously obtained cultures submitted to a state bacteriology laboratory. In six offices, the probability of a positive office culture, given a positive culture at the state laboratory, ranged from 29% to 60%; and the probability of a negative office culture, when the state laboratory had a negative culture, ranged from 76% to 99%. As a result of this report, investigators in several subsequent studies calculated sensitivity and specificity using microbiology laboratory cultures as a reference standard. These studies only address the ability of an office laboratory to grow and identify group A streptococci from throat swabs (microbiologic sensitivity and specificity), and not the sensitivity and specificity of office cultures for diagnosing group A streptococcal pharyngitis (clinical sensitivity and specificity).

Using this convention, Rosenstein and coworkers (57) found that physicians' laboratories had a microbiologic sensitivity of 81% and a microbiologic specificity of 99%. Battle and Glasgow (58) found a sensitivity of 96% and a specificity of 90%. More recently, Morris (59), using a commercial bacitracin disk culture technique, reported a sensitivity of only 40% and a specificity of 92%. Office-based cultures thus have variable agreement with cultures from microbiology laboratories. Although some office laboratories perform very well, one should not assume good performance unless the office provides quality-control data (60).

RAPID TESTS

Specificity: In the one study that performed rapid antigen testing on asymptomatic persons (49), only 2 of 329 adults had positive rapid tests. Thus, specificity was greater than 99% for rapid antigen tests.

Sensitivity: Using one throat culture as a reference standard, several studies have addressed the sensitivity of rapid antigen testing. Various authors have reported sensitivities between 80% and 95% (4). McCusker and colleagues (61) noted a discrepancy between adult and pediatric samples in a laboratory-based study. Gerber and coworkers (62) found a sensitivity of 84% in their pediatric practice. In a study of adult patients, Centor and colleagues (50) observed a sensitivity of 96%. Studying a subset of the same population as Centor and colleagues, Graham and coworkers (27) compared a rapid test with three culture methods (two sheep blood agar plates and one selective agar plate). They defined their reference standard as a positive result in any of the three cultures. The probability of a positive result on the rapid test (95%) exceeded that on the sheep blood agar plates, regardless of whether the plates were incubated in air (86%), carbon dioxide (86%), or anaerobically (94%).

We will assume that the sensitivity of rapid tests approaches 95% in adults. This estimate derives from our studies that used experienced technicians to do the tests. No study has reported data on these tests done in a routine practice setting (using untrained office personnel), although several authors have questioned how these tests will perform in such settings (63, 64). As with office cultures, quality control remains a critical consideration to clinicians considering the adoption of this new technology.

Pretest Probabilities

Before a threshold analysis can be done, the pretest probability of streptococcal pharyngitis must be estimated. The prevalence of positive throat cultures could be used as an estimate of pretest probability, but such an analysis would disregard clinical information. Several studies have shown that patients with differing clinical presentations have different pretest probabilities.

We have developed a simple model that combines prevalence with information from the clinical examination to estimate pretest probabilities. Rather than relying on subjective pretest probability estimates, we used logistic regression to develop a method for estimating the probability of a positive culture given prevalence and the presence or absence of selected signs and symptoms. Emergency room physicians recorded data for 286 adult patients from whom throat cultures were obtained. The resulting model gives one point to each of four signs or symptoms: tonsillar exudates; swollen, tender, anterior cervical nodes; history of fever; and lack of cough (65). For example, if a patient presents with no cough, a history of a fever, normal cervical nodes, and tonsillar exudates, that patient would get three points. Table 2 shows the corresponding probabilities of a positive culture given

Table 2. Effect of Prevalence of Group A Streptococcal Pharyngitis on Probability Estimates

Symptom Score*	Prevalence		
	5.00%	10.00%	20.00%
	←———————— % ————————→		
0	0.64	1.34	2.96
1	1.71	3.55	7.65
2	4.53	9.10	18.38
3	11.42	21.39	37.97
4	25.95	42.52	62.47

* A patient is assigned a score according to the total number of signs and symptoms present. Each of the following signs is worth 1 point: tonsillar exudates; swollen, tender, anterior cervical nodes; history of fever; and lack of cough.

different assumptions about the prevalence of group A streptococcal pharyngitis in a population. Note that the probability of a positive culture for any patient depends on the prevalence of streptococcal pharyngitis in that population.

Other investigators have examined models for estimating pretest probabilities. Walsh and coworkers (66) described an algorithm for classifying adults with sore throats. Similarly, Komaroff and associates (67) have reported a nomogram derived from a discriminant score. Wigton and coworkers (68) have prospectively validated our model in an emergency room population in Nebraska. Recently, Poses and colleagues (69) have prospectively evaluated several scores. In that study, our model, after being adjusted for the different prevalence, performed similarly in a university student health center as it had in our emergency room.

Post-Test Probabilities

A positive culture or antigen test increases the probability that a patient actually has streptococcal pharyngitis, whereas a negative result decreases this probability. As we noted in the introduction, positive tests do not establish the diagnosis of streptococcal pharyngitis, nor do negative tests exclude it. Test results allow the physician to generate a higher or lower revised probability of disease. Post-test probabilities depend on the variables that we have considered thus far: pretest probability of disease and the sensitivity and specificity of the test. Sox

Table 3. Post-test Probability Estimates for Various Pretest Probabilities

Test	Sensitivity	Specificity	Post-test Probability	
			After a Positive Test	After a Negative Test
			%	
Pretest probability = 4.5%				
Rapid test	95	99	82	1
Throat culture	90	99	80	1
Pretest probability = 38%				
Rapid test	95	99	98	3
Throat culture	90	99	98	6
Pretest probability = 50%				
Rapid test	95	99	99	5
Throat culture	90	99	99	9

(70), in the introductory article of this series, presented Bayes' theorem and discussed its implications. Table 3 shows the results of applying Bayes' theorem using the estimates that we have developed in this review. We have used a sensitivity of 95% and a specificity of 99% for rapid tests, and a sensitivity of 90% and a specificity of 99% for routine throat culture.

Threshold Analysis

Physicians manage patients who have sore throat with one of three options: reassurance without testing or treatment; testing, with treatment based on the test results; or treatment based on clinical presentation without laboratory testing. Several aspects of group A streptococcal pharyngitis and its treatment influence the management choice for an individual patient. A patient's risk/benefit ratio will vary according to the pretest probability, because the likelihood of benefit depends on the probability of disease. The risks of treating patients include allergic reactions (especially to penicillin) and undesirable side effects (for example, nausea from erythromycin). Earlier in this review, we enumerated the benefits of treating streptococcal pharyngitis. Several authors have formally analyzed this problem (71-73). However, these analyses have not included the effect of penicillin on the duration of symptoms. Moreover, these analyses used society's viewpoint rather than that of the individual patient.

Hillner and coworkers (74) recently analyzed this problem from the patient's viewpoint. Their analysis used the patient utilities developed by Hermann (75) (Table 4). Hermann used a time-tradeoff method for defining various conditions (for example, acute rheumatic fever, mild penicillin allergy, and death) in terms of sick-days due to pharyngitis. The probabilities of adverse outcomes, shown in Table 5, came from various literature sources.

The baseline analysis found a threshold below which a physician would neither treat nor test the patient of only 0.2% and a threshold above which a physician would treat the patient without testing of 11% (assuming a 1-day turnaround time for test results). Thus, this analysis recommends treating patients who have a pretest probability of greater than 11% and testing essentially all other patients. If one could get rapid (< 2 hours) results, however, the threshold below which one would test increases to 49%. Two variables have major opposing influences on the threshold between testing and treating: quicker symptomatic relief in patients treated immediately (which encourages treatment at a lower pretest probability), and avoidance of allergic reactions in patients not having streptococcal infections (which discourages treatment and thus raises the threshold).

Table 4. Utility Assumptions Used in the Threshold Analysis

	Sick-Day Equivalents
Untreated pharyngitis	5
Treated streptococcal pharyngitis	4
Mild penicillin reaction	15
Severe penicillin reaction	180
Peritonsillar abscess	100
Uncomplicated rheumatic fever	1000
Complicated rheumatic fever	10 000
Death (due to penicillin allergy or acute rheumatic fever)	20 000

Table 5. Probability Assumptions for Threshold Analysis

Condition	Probability
	%
Penicillin reaction (allergy)	0.5
Acute rheumatic fever after untreated streptococcal pharyngitis	0.05
Complicated course for acute rheumatic fever	10
Death from acute rheumatic fever	1
Suppurative complication (peritonsillar abscess) after untreated streptococcal pharyngitis	2
Severe reaction in patient having penicillin reaction	0.5
Fatal reaction in patient having penicillin reaction	0.05

Other Infectious Causes of Pharyngitis

Investigators have suggested various other nonviral causes of pharyngitis. Streptococci other than group A beta-hemolytic organisms can cause both epidemic and endemic pharyngitis. Komaroff and colleagues (76) have published data on the possible role of chlamydiae in endemic pharyngitis. Several authors have listed mycoplasma as an etiologic agent. Additionally, *Neisseria gonorrhoeae*, is often listed as a cause of sore throats in adults.

The evidence supporting non-group-A streptococci as a cause of pharyngitis includes several documented epidemics (77-80). Investigators have also noted rises in antibody titers in patients having non-group-A streptococcal infections (81). Recently, we have presented case-control data supporting group C streptococci as a cause of adult endemic pharyngitis (82).

The non-group-A streptococci can cause pharyngitis, but we cannot, at this time, ascertain the importance or need for treating patients with these infections. Most current culture techniques do not identify these organisms; the rapid tests identify only group A antigens. If patients would benefit from having non-group-A streptococcal infections treated, then neither most culture protocols nor rapid testing specific for group A streptococci would suffice for diagnosis.

Komaroff and colleagues (76), using only serologic testing, estimated that chlamydia cause approximately 20% of adult pharyngitis and mycoplasma cause 10% of these infections. Although both serologic and culture studies have documented mycoplasmas as a probable cause of pharyngitis (83), investigators have not yet supported the serologic findings of chlamydia with culture substantiation (84). The positive serologic results may be due to immunologic cross-reaction of *Chlamydia trachomatis* with other organisms. Alternatively, the serologic assays may have detected chlamydial strains that standard culture techniques cannot isolate. The TWAR agent, a *C. psittaci* requiring special isolation techniques, has recently been detected in patients with upper respiratory tract symptoms (85). Detection of this agent may resolve the discrepancy between serologic evidence of chlamydial pharyngitis and failure to isolate *C. trachomatis* from patients with sore throats.

Several reports have verified oropharyngeal gonorrhea infection due to *N. gonorrhoeae*. Whether these organisms cause symptomatic pharyngitis remains unclear. Weisner and colleagues' (86) studies in a venereal disease clinic failed to show a significant difference in the rate of gonococcal pharyngeal infection between patients having sore throats and those who had no pharyngeal symptoms. Komaroff and associates (87), in a study of adult pharyngitis, found a prevalence of positive gonorrhea cultures of only 1%. On the basis of these studies, physicians need not routinely obtain cultures for this organism from patients with sore throats.

Other organisms probably can cause pharyngitis (for example, *Legionella* species, *Haemophilus influenzae*, and nonhemolytic streptococci). As research expands our knowledge of etiology, we must always ask the relevant clinical question: Does treating patients with this newly described infection decrease morbidity? A recent randomized controlled study has examined the effect of treating patients who have pharyngitis with erythromycin (88). This study excluded all patients having culture documentation of group A streptococcal infection. The study failed to show a clinical effect, leading us to conclude that, in 1986, the management of pharyngitis still revolves around the diagnosis and treatment of group A streptococcal pharyngitis.

Recommendations

We recommend that all patients having clinical signs and symptoms predicting a high probability (> 47%) of streptococcal pharyngitis should be treated without testing. If a clinician has rapid tests (with known quality-control data) available, then we recommend using these tests in most other patients, treating patients who have positive tests, and not treating patients who have negative results. If rapid tests are not available, we recommend immediately treating those patients who have a pretest probability of disease of greater than 11%. We would do cultures for all remaining patients and predicate eventual treatment on the culture result. This last recommendation assumes that the physician can achieve perfect follow-up of all culture-positive patients from whom therapy has been withheld pending culture results (89). In many medical settings, this assumption is unrealistic (Table 6).

Our recommendations follow from Hillner and co-workers' (74) decision analysis. The clinical model in Table 2 can be used to estimate the clinical probability of disease. The decrease in disease duration due to immediate treatment has the most influence on decreasing the treatment threshold. Medication side effects represent the second most important factor in the analysis. If one assumes either an increased rate of allergic reactions or an increased severity of these reactions, then the testing thresholds would rise, that is, a physician would require a higher clinical probability of group A streptococcal pharyngitis before prescribing immediate antibiotic treatment. These recommendations pertain only to adult patients, as most of the data derive from studies of adults.

Table 6. Recommendations for the Diagnosis and Treatment of Group A Streptococcal Pharyngitis

1. Treat all adult patients having clinical signs and symptoms predicting a high probability (> 47%) of streptococcal pharyngitis without further diagnostic efforts.

2. If rapid tests with known quality-control data are available, test all adult patients with a pretest probability of < 47%, and treat only those having positive results on rapid tests.

3. If rapid test are not available and follow-up is possible, treat all adult patients with a pretest probability of > 11%. Cultures should be done for patients having pretest probabilities of < 11%, and only those having a positive culture should be treated.

ACKNOWLEDGMENTS: The authors thank Dr. Harold Sox for his invaluable assistance. Dr. Centor is a Teaching and Research Scholar of the American College of Physicians.

References

1. KOMAROFF AL. A management strategy for sore throat. *JAMA.* 1978;**239**:1429-32.
2. O'MALLEY MS, FREY JJ, HOOLE AJ. The clinical management of sore throat: a comparison of three ambulatory settings. *NC Med J.* 1984;**45**:291-5.
3. Rapid office diagnostic tests for streptococcal pharyngitis. *Med Lett Drugs Ther.* 1985;**27**:49-51.
4. RADETSKY M, WHEELER RC, ROE MH, TODD JK. Comparative evaluation of kits for rapid diagnosis of group A streptococcal disease. *Pediatr Infect Dis.* 1985;**4**:274-81.
5. PAUKER SG, KASSIRER JP. The threshold approach to clinical decision making. *N Engl J Med.* 1980;**302**:1110-6.
6. DENNY FW. Effect of treatment on streptococcal pharyngitis: is the issue really settled? *Pediatr Infect Dis.* 1985;**4**:352-4.
7. BRINK WR, RAMMELKAMP CH, DENNY FW, et al. Effect of penicillin and aureomycin on the natural course of streptococcal tonsillitis and pharyngitis. *Am J Med.* 1951;**10**:300-8.
8. BRUMFITT W, SLATER JDM. Treatment of acute sore throat with penicillin. *Lancet.* 1957;**1**:8-11.
9. KROBER MS, BASS JW, MICHELS GN. Streptococcal pharyngitis: placebo-controlled double-blind evaluation of clinical response to penicillin therapy. *JAMA.* 1985;**253**:1271-4.
10. NELSON JD. The effect of penicillin therapy on the symptoms and signs of streptococcal pharyngitis. *Pediatr Infect Dis.* 1984;**3**:10-3.
11. MERENSTEIN JH, ROGERS KD. Streptococcal pharyngitis: early treatment and management by nurse practitioners. *JAMA.* 1974;**227**:1278-82.
12. RANDOLPH MF, GERBER MA, DEMEO KK, WRIGHT L. Effect of antibiotic therapy on the clinical course of streptococcal pharyngitis. *J Pediatr.* 1985;**106**:870-5.
13. POSKANZER DC, FELDMAN HA, BEADENKOPF WG, KURODA K, DRISLANE A, DIAMOND EL. Epidemiology of civilian streptococcal outbreaks before and after penicillin prophylaxis. *Am J Public Health.* 1956;**46**:1513-24.
14. BENNIKE T, BROCHNER-MORTENSEN K, KJAER E, SKADHANGE K, TROLLE E. Penicillin therapy in acute tonsillitis, phlegmonous tonsillitis and ulcerative tonsillitis. *Acta Med Scand.* 1951;**139**:253-74.
15. CHAMOVITZ R, RAMMELKAMP CH, WANNAMAKER LW, DENNY FW. The effect of tonsillectomy on the incidence of streptococcal respiratory disease and its complications. *Pediatrics.* 1960;**26**:355-67.
16. DENNY FW, WANNAMAKER LW, BRINK WR, et al. Prevention of rheumatic fever: treatment of preceding streptococcic infection. *JAMA.* 1950;**143**:151-3.
17. WANNAMAKER LW, RAMMELKAMP CH, DENNY FW, et al. Prophylaxis of acute rheumatic fever. *Am J Med.* 1951;**10**:673-95.
18. SHULMAN ST, AMREN DP, BISNO AL, et al. Prevention of rheumatic fever: a statement for health professionals by the Committee on Rheumatic Fever and Infective Endocarditis of the Council on Cardiovascular Disease in the Young. *Circulation.* 1984;**70**:1118A-22A.
19. WEINSTEIN L, LE FROCK J. Does antimicrobial therapy of streptococcal pharyngitis or pyoderma alter the risk of glomerulonephritis? *J Infect Dis.* 1971;**124**:229-31.
20. COCHI SL, FRASER DW, HIGHTOWER AW, FACKLAM RR, BROOME CV. Diagnosis and treatment of streptococcal pharyngitis: survey of U.S. medical practitioners. In: SHULMAN ST, ed. *Pharyngitis—Manage-*

ment in an Era of Declining Rheumatic Fever. New York: Praeger Press; 1984:73-94.

21. LIBERTIN CR, WOLD AD, WASHINGTON JA II. Effects of trimethoprim-sulfamethoxazole and incubation atmosphere on isolation of group A streptococci. *J Clin Microbiol.* 1983;**18**:680-2.

22. MURRAY PR, WOLD AD, SCHRECK CA, WASHINGTON JA II. Effects of selective media and atmosphere of incubation on the isolation of group A streptococci. *J Clin Microbiol.* 1976;**4**:54-6.

23. KUNZ LJ, MOELLERING RC. Streptococcal infections. In: BALOWS A, HAUSLER WJ, eds. *Diagnostic Procedures for Bacterial, Mycotic and Parasitic Infections.* 6th ed. Washington, D.C.: American Public Health Association; 1981:603-60.

24. LAUER BA, RELLER LB, MIRRETT S. Effect of atmosphere and duration of incubation on primary isolation of group A streptococci from throat cultures. *J Clin Microbiol.* 1983;**17**:338-40.

25. KURZYNSKI TA, VAN HOLTEN CM. Evaluation of techniques for isolation of group A streptococci from throat cultures. *J Clin Microbiol.* 1981;**13**:891-4.

26. CARLSON JR, MERZ WG, HANSEN BE, RUTH S, MOORE DG. Improved recovery of group A beta-hemolytic streptococci with a new selective medium. *J Clin Microbiol.* 1985;**21**:307-9.

27. GRAHAM L, MEIER FA, CENTOR RM, GARNER BK, DALTON HP. The effect of media and conditions of cultivation on comparisons between latex agglutinations and culture detection of group A streptococci. *J Clin Microbiol.* 1986;**24**:644-6.

28. Results of the throat culture questionnaire. *Clin Microbiol Newslett.* 1980;**2**(13):1-5.

29. EDERER GM, HERRMANN MM, BRUCE R, MATSEN JM, CHAPMAN SS. Rapid extraction method with pronase B for grouping beta-hemolytic streptococci. *Appl Microbiol.* 1972;**23**:285-8.

30. LEVINSON MC, FRANK PF. Differentiation of group A from other beta-hemolytic streptococci with bacitracin. *J Bacteriol.* 1955;**69**:284-7.

31. GUNN BA. SXT and Taxo A disks for presumptive identification of group A and B streptococci in throat cultures. *J Clin Microbiol.* 1976;**4**:192-3.

32. FACKLAM RR, PODULA JF, THACKER LG, WORTHAM EC, SCONYERS BJ. Presumptive identification of group A, B, and D streptococci. *Appl Microbiol.* 1974;**27**:107-13.

33. POLLACK HM, DAHLGREN BJ. Distribution of streptococcal groups in clinical specimens with evaluation of bacitracin screening. *Appl Microbiol.* 1974;**27**:141-3.

34. WELLSTOOD S. Evaluation of Phadebact and Streptex kits for rapid grouping of streptococci directly from blood cultures. *J Clin Microbiol.* 1982;**15**:226-30.

35. TAYLOR N, MEIER FA, BECK JR, HILL HR. Latex agglutination is more accurate and less expensive than fluorescent antibody in identifying group A streptococci from culture [Abstract]. In: *Abstracts of the 85th Annual Meeting of American Society for Microbiology.* Washington, D.C.: American Society for Microbiology; 1985:C60.

36. BIXLER-FORELL E, MOODY M, MARTIN W. Evaluation of slide agglutination methods for identification of beta-hemolytic streptococci [Abstract]. In: *Abstracts of the 83rd Annual Meeting of the American Society for Microbiology.* Washington, D.C.: American Society for Microbiology; 1983:C392.

37. LESHER RJ, CASIANO-COLON AE. Comparison of fluorescent antibody, bacitracin susceptibility, latex agglutination, coagglutination, and API20S for identifying group A streptococci [Abstract]. In: *Abstracts of the 83rd Annual Meeting of the American Society for Microbiology.* Washington, D.C.: American Society for Microbiology; 1983:C389.

38. GERBER MA. Culturing of throat swabs: end of an era [Editorial]? *J Pediatr.* 1985;**107**:85-8.

39. EL KHOLY A, WANNAMAKER LW, KRAUSE RM. Simplified extraction procedure for serological grouping of beta-hemolytic streptococci. *Appl Microbiol.* 1974;**28**:836-9.

40. SLIFKIN M, GIL GM. Serogrouping of beta-hemolytic streptococci from throat swabs with nitrous acid extraction and the Phadebact streptococcus test. *J Clin Microbiol.* 1982;**15**:187-9.

41. GERBER MA. Micronitrous acid extraction-coagglutination test for rapid diagnosis of streptococcal pharyngitis. *J Clin Microbiol.* 1983;**17**:170-1.

42. EDWARDS EA, PHILLIPS IA, SUTTER WC. Diagnosis of group A streptococcal infections directly from throat secretions. *J Clin Microbiol.* 1982;**15**:481-3.

43. OTERO JR, REYES S, NORIEGA AR. Rapid diagnosis of group A streptococcal antigen extracted directly from swabs by an enzymatic procedure and used to detect pharyngitis. *J Clin Microbiol.* 1983;**18**:318-20.

44. KNIGGE KM, BABB JL, FIRCA JR, ANCELL K, BLOOMSTER TG, MARCHLEWICZ BA. Enzyme immunoassay for the detection of group A streptococcal antigen. *J Clin Microbiol.* 1984;**20**:735-41.

45. WEINSTEIN L, TSAO CCL. Effect of types of treatment in the development of antistreptolysin in patients with scarlet fever. *Proc Soc Exp Biol Med.* 1946;**63**:449-50.

46. DENNY FW, PERRY WD, WANNAMAKER LW. Type-specific streptococcal antibody. *J Clin Invest.* 1957;**36**:1092-100.

47. KAPLAN EL, TOP FH JR, DUDDING BA, WANNAMAKER LW. Diagnosis of streptococcal pharyngitis: differentiation of active infection from the carrier state in the symptomatic child. *J Infect Dis.* 1971;**123**:490-501.

48. SASLAW MS, JABLON JM, JENKS SA, BRANCH CC. Beta-hemolytic streptococci in tonsillar tissue. *Am J Dis Child.* 1962;**103**:51-8.

49. LAATSCH LJ. Pharyngeal carriage of beta-hemolytic streptococci and the effect of laboratory exposure in medical technology students. *J Med Technol.* 1985;**2**:106-10.

50. CENTOR RM, DALTON HP, CAMPBELL MS, et al. Rapid diagnosis of streptococcal pharyngitis in adult emergency room patients. *J Gen Intern Med.* 1986;**1**:248-51.

51. KAPLAN EL. The group A streptococcal upper respiratory tract carrier state: an enigma. *J Pediatr.* 1980;**97**:337-45.

52. MARKOWITZ M. Cultures of the respiratory tract in pediatric practice. *Am J Dis Child.* 1963;**105**:46-52.

53. HALFON ST, DAVIES AM, KAPLAN O, LAZAROV E, BERGNER-RABINOWITZ S. Primary prevention of rheumatic fever in Jerusalem schoolchildren: II. Identification of beta-hemolytic streptococci. *Isr J Med Sci.* 1968;**4**:809-14.

54. DINGLE JH, et al. Endemic exudative pharyngitis and tonsillitis. *JAMA.* 1944;**125**:1163-9.

55. TOMPKINS RK, BURNES DC, CABLE WE. An analysis of the cost-effectiveness of pharyngitis management and acute rheumatic fever prevention. *Ann Intern Med.* 1977;**86**:481-92.

56. MONDZAC AM. Throat culture processing in the office—a warning [Letter]. *JAMA.* 1967;**200**:1132-3.

57. ROSENSTEIN BJ, MARKOWITZ M, GORDIS L. Accuracy of throat cultures processed in physician's offices. *J Pediatr.* 1970;**76**:606-9.

58. BATTLE CU, GLASGOW LA. Reliability of bacteriologic identification of beta-hemolytic streptococci in private offices. *Am J Dis Child.* 1971;**122**:134-6.

59. MORRIS SD. Reliability of office-based diagnostic tools in streptococcal pharyngitis. *W Va Med J.* 1984;**80**:89-94.

60. PETER G, SMITH AL. Group A streptococcal infections of the skin and pharynx. *N Engl J Med.* 1977;**297**:311-7, 365-70.

61. MCCUSKER JJ, MCCOY EL, YOUNG CL, ALAMARES R, HIRSCH LS. Comparison of Directigen Group A Strep Test with a traditional culture

technique for detection of group A beta-hemolytic streptococci. *J Clin Microbiol.* 1984;**20**:824-5.

62. GERBER MA, SPADACCINI LJ, WRIGHT LL, DEUTSCH L. Latex agglutination tests for rapid identification of group A streptococci directly from throat swabs. *J Pediatr.* 1984;**105**:702-5.

63. Rapid detection of beta haemolytic streptococci [Editorial]. *Lancet.* 1986;**1**:247-8.

64. GERBER MA. Diagnosis of group A beta-hemolytic streptococcal pharyngitis: use of antigen detection tests. *Diagn Microbiol Infect Dis.* 1986;**4**(3 suppl):5S-15S.

65. CENTOR RM, WITHERSPOON JM, DALTON HP, BRODY CE, LINK K. The diagnosis of strep throat in adults in the emergency room. *Med Decis Making.* 1981;**1**:239-46.

66. WALSH BT, BOOKHEIM WW, JOHNSON RC, TOMPKINS RK. Recognition of streptococcal pharyngitis in adults. *Arch Intern Med.* 1975;**135**:1493-7.

67. KOMAROFF AL, PASS TM, ARONSON MD, et al. The prediction of streptococcal pharyngitis in adults. *J Gen Intern Med.* 1986;**1**:1-7.

68. WIGTON RS, CONNOR JL, CENTOR RM. Transportability of a decision rule for the diagnosis of streptococcal pharyngitis. *Arch Intern Med.* 1986;**146**:81-3.

69. POSES RM, CEBUL RD, COLLINS M, FAGER SS. The importance of disease prevalence in transporting clinical prediction rules: the case of streptococcal pharyngitis. *Ann Intern Med.* 1986;**105**:586-91.

70. SOX HC. Probability theory in the use of diagnostic tests: an introduction to critical study of the literature. *Ann Intern Med.* 1986;**104**:60-6.

71. GIAUQUE WC, PEEBLES TC. Application of multidimensional utility theory in determining optimal test-treatment strategies for streptococcal sore throat and rheumatic fever. *Oper Res.* 1976;**24**:933-50.

72. KOMAROFF AL, PASS TM, PAPPIUS EL. A cost-effectiveness analysis of alternative strategies for management of sore throat [Abstract]. *Clin Res.* 1983;**31**:299A.

73. SMITH DL, BRAUER WA. Comparative costs of diagnosis and treatment in acute pharyngitis. *South Med J.* 1981;**74**:332-4.

74. HILLNER BE, CENTOR RM, CLANCY CM. What a difference a day makes: the importance of turnaround time of diagnostic tests in sore throats. *Med Decis Making.* 1985;**5**:363.

75. HERMANN JM. Patients' willingness to take risks in the management of pharyngitis. *J Fam Pract.* 1984;**6**:767-72.

76. KOMAROFF AL, ARONSON MD, PASS TM, ERVIN CT, BRANCH WT JR, SCHACHTER J. Serologic evidence of chlamydial and mycoplasmal pharyngitis in adults. *Science.* 1983;**222**:927-9.

77. STRYKER WS, FRASER DW, FACKLAM RR. Foodborne outbreak of group G streptococcal pharyngitis. *Am J Epidemiol.* 1982;**116**:533-40.

78. BENJAMIN JT, PERRIELLO VA JR. Pharyngitis due to group C hemolytic streptococci in children. *J Pediatr.* 1976;**89**:254-6.

79. HILL HR, CALDWELL GG, WILSON E, HAGER D, ZIMMERMAN RA. Epidemic of pharyngitis due to streptococci of Lancefield group G. *Lancet.* 1969;**2**:371-4.

80. MCCUE JD. Group G streptococcal pharyngitis: an analysis of an outbreak at a college. *JAMA.* 1982;**248**:1333-6.

81. BAUMGARTEN A, VON GRAEVENITZ A, GRECO T. Serological evidence for a causative role of non-group A hemolytic streptococci in pharyngitis. *Zentralbl Backeriol Mikrobiol Hyg [A].* 1981;**249**:460-5.

82. MEIER FA, CENTOR RM, GRAHAM L, DALTON HP. Group C streptococci in endemic pharyngitis in young adults [Abstract]. In: *Proceedings of the 26th Interscience Conference on Antimicrobial Agents and Chemotherapy.* Washington, D.C.: American Society for Microbiology; 1986:1005.

83. GLEZEN WP, CLYDE WA JR, SENIOR RJ, SHEAFFER CI, DENNY FW. Group A streptococci, mycoplasmas, and viruses associated with acute pharyngitis. *JAMA.* 1967;**202**:455-60.

84. HUSS H, JUNGKIND D, AMADIO P, RUBENFELD I. Frequency of *Chlamydia trachomatis* as the cause of pharyngitis. *J Clin Microbiol.* 1985;**22:**858-60.

85. GRAYSTON JT, KUO CC, WANG SP, ALTMAN J. A new *Chlamydia psittaci* strain, TWAR, isolated in acute respiratory tract infections. *N Engl J Med.* 1986;**315:**161-8.

86. WIESNER PJ, TRONCA E, BONIN P, PEDERSEN AH, HOLMES KK. Clinical spectrum of pharyngeal gonococcal infection. *N Engl J Med.* 1973;**288:**181-5.

87. KOMAROFF AL, ARONSON MD, PASS TM, ERVIN CT. Prevalence of pharyngeal gonorrhea in general medical patients with sore throats. *Sex Transm Dis.* 1980;**7:**116-9.

88. MCDONALD CJ, TIERNEY WM, HUI SL, FRENCH ML, LELAND DS, JONES RB. A controlled trial of erythromycin in adults with nonstreptococcal pharyngitis. *J Infect Dis.* 1985;**152:**1093-4.

89. CENTOR RM, WITHERSPOON JM. Treating sore throats in the emergency room: the importance of follow-up in decision making. *Med Decis Making.* 1982;**2:**463-9.

Urinalysis and Urine Culture in Women with Dysuria

ANTHONY L. KOMAROFF, M.D.

ONE OF THE COMMONEST reasons for ordering a urinalysis and urine culture is to evaluate the possibility of a urinary tract infection in a woman having acute dysuria. In this article, I consider what is known about the value of these tests in aiding the diagnosis and treatment of such symptomatic patients and also patients suspected of having asymptomatic bacteriuria. Topics not considered include the role of urinalysis or urine culture in evaluating possible urinary tract infection in pregnant women, children of either sex, adult men, or patients with indwelling urinary catheters; and the value of urinalysis in the diagnosis of noninfectious disorders of the urinary tract or in various systemic diseases.

Recent research indicates that the urinalysis has an even more important role in the diagnosis of symptomatic urinary tract infection than previously had been believed. Whereas until recently the urine culture had been regarded as the "gold-standard" for determining the presence of a real and treatable urinary tract infection in symptomatic patients, it now appears that this is not the case (1). Indeed, there is no single "gold-standard" test of urinary infection, because there are several types of urinary tract and vaginal infection that produce dysuria. The reason for the growing importance of urinalysis is the recognition that the presence of pyuria, in the symptomatic patient, is a useful indicator of a potentially treatable urinary tract infection.

Test Description

URINALYSIS

The urinalysis includes a description of the urine color,

▶ This chapter was originally published in *Annals of Internal Medicine.* 1986;**104**:212-8.

measurement of the specific gravity, and an estimate of the pH and concentrations of glucose, protein, ketones, blood, and bilirubin, determined in most laboratories by a rapid "dipstick" method. Examination of the urine sediment typically is done by centrifuging the urine at 2000 rev/min for 5 minutes, pouring off all the supernatant, mixing the sediment pellet with the residual 0.5 to 1 mL of supernatant, and examining the resulting suspension under the "high-power" field (that is, magnification of approximately $450\times$). The sediment is examined for leukocytes, erythrocytes, epithelial cells, crystals, casts, and bacteria. The quantity of cells typically is reported as the average number (after viewing at least five separate areas of the slide) per high-power field.

The most important variable in the prediction of infection is pyuria. The assessment of pyuria is imperfect. The leukocyte count on urinalysis, like the colony count on urine culture, can be affected by factors that alter the concentration of the urine. Furthermore, error may be introduced by variation in the amount of supernatant in which the sediment pellet is resuspended and by variation in the volume of urine placed under the cover slip (2). A leukocyte counting chamber controls some of these variables (3-8) but has not been used widely in primary care settings.

Despite these limitations, the assessment of pyuria can be of great value. This conclusion has been established primarily by Stamm and colleagues (9), who measured pyuria by examining uncentrifuged urine samples with a hemocytometer. They defined pyuria as eight or more leukocytes per cubic millimetre, which corresponds to approximately two to five leukocytes per high-power field in centrifuged urine sediment (10). The predictive value of pyuria, defined in this manner, is discussed subsequently.

Because neutrophils contain several unique esterases not present in serum, urine, or kidney tissue, it has been proposed that a rapid dipstick method to detect this esterase activity in urine would provide a reliable semiquantitative means of detecting pyuria (11). Indeed, use of the dipstick containing the leukocyte esterase assay is growing. The specificity of this test in predicting pyuria appears to be high, ranging from 94% to 98% (that is, false-positive rates of 2% to 6%) (11-14). Reports of the sensitivity of the test have varied, with sensitivity rates ranging from 74% to 96% (false-negative rates of 4% to 26%) (11-14). Substitution of this rapid assay for microscopic examination may prove cost effective, but information is sacrificed by forgoing examination of the urine sediment in favor of a dipstick: Hematuria and bacteriuria are more crudely estimated, and the presence of casts cannot be determined. How often this loss of information would prove detrimental is not yet clear.

URINE CULTURE

Specimen Collection and Handling: In most practices, a clean-voided, midstream urine specimen is obtained for culture (and urinalysis). The nonmenstruating woman should be instructed to clean the labia with gauze moistened with sterile water or saline or with green soap. The use of antiseptic agents to clean the perineum, although widely practiced, should be discouraged, because small amounts of antiseptic agent in the collected urine can artifactually reduce the colony count (15). The urine must be planted on culture media within 20 minutes to avoid erroneously high colony counts due to bacterial growth in urine left at room temperature. If the urine cannot be planted on culture media within 20 minutes, then the urine should be promptly refrigerated until it can be cultured.

Colony counts can be greatly affected by circumstances that alter the concentration of bladder urine. For example, colony counts can be much greater in concentrated, first-voided morning urines than in urines obtained from the same patient later that day (15).

Methods for Performing Culture: Culture media that encourage the growth of gram-negative coliforms (such as eosin-methylene blue or MacConkey agar) and media that encourage the growth of gram-positive cocci (such as sheep blood agar) should be used. The traditional pour-plate method for quantitatively culturing the urine is the most accurate, but also the most cumbersome. Typically, 0.1 mL of urine is added to 10 mL of a diluent broth or buffer solution, and shaken to achieve even dispersion. Then 0.1 mL of this mixture, along with 10 mL of molten agar, are poured into a petri dish. One colony on the plate represents 1000 organisms in the original urine specimen.

The simpler streak-plate method employs a flamed,

sterile bacteriologic loop that delivers a relatively constant amount of urine (typically 0.001 mL) to an agar plate. Because a much smaller amount of urine is sampled, when compared with that of the pour-plate method, low colony counts (for example, 100 to 100 000 bacteria/mL of urine) will be less reliably detected with the loop method than with the pour-plate method.

Several simpler methods are now common and are particularly useful for the physician's office. The most widely used is the "dip-slide," in which a glass slide, like that used for microscopic analysis, is coated with an agar medium on each side (16). The slide is kept in a sterile container, then dipped in freshly voided urine, and returned to the sterile container. The dip-slide may be incubated or even left at room temperature (17). The density of colonies on the slide is compared with a series of pictures that comes with the kit and that gives an approximation of the number of bacteria per millilitre of urine. Because a larger sample of urine is used than with the pour-plate or loop methods, sampling error is less likely. However, the colony count is a semiquantitative estimate, susceptible to observer error.

Interpretation of Colony Count: The meaning of quantitative urine cultures has recently been reviewed in detail by Stamm (18) and Platt (19) and is discussed only briefly here. The definition of an abnormal urine culture result depends on the way the urine specimen was obtained and the clinical circumstances. Any growth generally is regarded as indicative of real infection if the specimen has been obtained by suprapubic aspiration or catheterization. Catheterization clearly introduces a few organisms into the bladder urine (increasing the chance of a false-positive result) (20-22). Some believe that suprapubic aspiration also may sometimes produce a false-positive result by provoking a contraction of the perineal musculature and causing retrograde movement of urethral organisms into the otherwise sterile bladder urine. Most observers believe this is uncommon, but the question has not been well studied.

Traditionally, the urine culture has been thought to have two putative virtues: First, quantitating the colony count was held to have diagnostic value in separating true infection from contamination. Second, testing for antibacterial sensitivities guided the choice of therapeutic agent.

The value of quantitating bacteriuria is questionable in a woman with acute dysuria. There is now strong evidence that the traditional definition of a "positive" urine culture (100 000 bacteria/mL) will fail to diagnose many women with bacterial infection of the lower urinary tract who could benefit from treatment. In one study, Stamm and colleagues (23) have shown that up to 50% of acutely dysuric women who really had a gram-negative coliform infection of the urinary tract (as determined by suprapubic aspiration or catheterization) did not have greater than 100 000 bacteria/mL of urine on culture of simultaneously voided urine. Furthermore, the urine culture cannot identify chlamydial, gonococcal, or other forms of urethritis, nor the presence of vaginal infection.

Also, the value of antibacterial sensitivity testing is uncertain in patients with acute dysuria. Most organisms will be sensitive to the antibacterial agents commonly used, except in patients with persistent or relapsing infection with the same organism. Even organisms that are labeled as "resistant" on Kirby-Bauer disk testing often are sensitive to the high concentrations of antibacterial present in the urine (24-26). Therefore, sensitivity testing can be misleading. Fortunately, an increasing number of laboratories are reporting minimal inhibitory concentrations as well as levels of each antibacterial that usually are achieved in the blood and urine. This method is clearly more useful, but its cost effectiveness remains to be shown.

Clinical Applications

The patient with acute dysuria may have any of seven clinical conditions, each diagnosed and managed differently (1). The roles of urinalysis and urine culture are different in each of these conditions and are different still in asymptomatic patients suspected of having bacteriuria. I briefly describe each of these clinical conditions and the role of urinalysis and culture in them (Table 1).

ACUTE PYELONEPHRITIS

Dysuria, frequency, and urgency (although these symptoms sometimes may be absent) in association with fever, flank pain, nausea and vomiting, rigors, costovertebral angle tenderness, and other findings suggest acute pyelonephritis. Urinalysis and urine culture are mandatory in any patient suspected clinically of having this disorder.

Urinalysis: Almost always, urinalysis in these patients reveals marked pyuria and bacteriuria (20). Hematuria and proteinuria also may be present during the first several days of symptoms. Furthermore, Gram stain of uncentrifuged urine or sediment is valuable, primarily in identifying possible enterococcal infection (for which ampicillin but not aminoglycoside therapy would be chosen); microscopic examination of unstained sediment, though sufficient for recognizing bacteriuria with motile gram-negative rods, is less reliable in demonstrating gram-positive cocci (27). In my judgment, a Gram stain should always be done in patients with acute pyelonephritis, although it is not usually necessary in patients with other causes of dysuria.

Urine Culture: The urine culture is mandatory in patients with acute pyelonephritis, primarily because sensitivity testing can be of great value in the patient who does not respond to initial therapy. Also, isolation of the responsible organisms and the pattern of antibacterial sensitivities (the "antibiogram") are useful in subsequently identifying relapsing infection with the same organism.

The colony count is less useful. In most patients with acute pyelonephritis, the colony count is greater than 100 000 bacteria/mL of urine, although it may be lower than 100 000/mL in 5% to 10% of women with this disease (20). A "negative" colony count should not automatically cause the clinician to reconsider the clinical diagnosis of acute pyelonephritis.

A colony count of less than 100 000 bacteria/mL in a patient with the clinical findings of acute pyelonephritis (and no other obvious explanation such as the recent use of antibacterials) suggests urinary tract obstruction or perinephric abscess. "Test-of-cure" cultures 2 to 3 days after completion of therapy are fully justified in patients with acute pyelonephritis, because upper urinary tract infection is generally regarded as harder to eradicate than lower tract infection.

SUBCLINICAL PYELONEPHRITIS

Evidence over the past 10 to 15 years indicates that a surprising number of patients (up to 30% in most primary care settings and up to 80% in emergency rooms serving indigent populations [25]) who have the clinical

Table 1. Recommended Use of Urinalysis and Urine Culture (and Other Tests) in Women with Different Suspected Causes of Acute Dysuria

Suspected Cause and Clinical Findings	Diagnostic Tests and Expected Results
Acute pyelonephritis 　Fever, rigors, nausea, vomiting, flank pain, costovertebral angle tenderness	Urinalysis 　Pyuria and bacteriuria Urine culture 　> 100 000 bacteria/mL Urine Gram stain 　Gram-negative bacilli or gram-positive cocci
Subclinical pyelonephritis 　Underlying urinary tract disease 　Diabetes mellitus 　Immunocompromised state 　Urinary infections before age 12 　Symptoms for 7 to 10 d before seeking care 　Documented relapsing infection with same organism at any time in the past 　Three or more urinary infections in past year 　Acute pyelonephritis in past year	Urinalysis 　Pyuria and bacteriuria Urine culture 　> 100 000 bacteria/mL
Chlamydial urethritis 　Sexual partner with recent urethritis 　New sexual partner 　Stuttering onset of symptoms 　Absence of hematuria 　Mucopurulent cervical discharge with edematous exocervix	Urinalysis 　Pyuria without bacteriuria
Gonococcal urethritis 　Sexual partner with recent urethritis 　Recent history of documented gonorrhea in patient or sexual partner	Urinalysis 　Pyuria without bacteriuria Gram stain of purulent discharge from urethral or cervical os 　Gram-negative intracellular diplococci Culture on Thayer-Martin or New York City media 　*Neisseria gonorrhoeae*

Table 1 (Continued)

Vaginitis
  Symptoms of vaginal discharge, itch, or irritation (always ask about such symptoms; patients may not volunteer them)
	Vaginal examination
	  Abnormal discharge
	  Microscopic examination of abnormal discharge
	    Budding yeast and pseudohyphae, trichomonads, "clue cells"

Lower urinary tract bacterial infection
    None of the above clinical indicators, but presence of pyuria
	Urinalysis
	  Pyuria and bacteriuria

No apparent infectious pathogen
    None of the above clinical indicators and absence of pyuria
	Urinalysis
	  No pyuria, no bacteriuria

picture of lower urinary tract infection or "cystitis" (dysuria, frequency, and urgency without fever or other symptoms or signs of acute pyelonephritis) nevertheless have upper urinary tract infection. This finding has been shown in studies that used bilateral ureteral catheterization (28), the bladder wash-out technique (29, 30), and the antibody-coated bacteria assay (31-33).

These patients with "subclinical pyelonephritis" (1) are initially indistinguishable from patients with true lower tract bacterial infection. They may have minimal symptoms that smolder for long periods of time and that are difficult to eradicate. Several clinical risk factors seem to increase the likelihood of subclinical pyelonephritis and therefore justify obtaining urine studies: known underlying urinary tract disease; diabetes mellitus or other conditions or therapies producing an immunocompromised state; a history of urinary tract infections in childhood; a history of documented relapsing infection with the same bacterium; symptoms for 7 to 10 days before seeking care; acute pyelonephritis in the past year; and residence in a poor, inner-city neighborhood.

There are no studies comparing antibacterial with placebo therapy for subclinical pyelonephritis. However, the prompt clinical response and the evidence that longer courses of therapy (beyond 10 to 14 days) may be required in some patients (31) suggest that proper diagnosis and treatment improve patient outcome. Although the optimum therapeutic regimen is unknown, some patients may require prolonged therapy (for example, 6 weeks of full-dose therapy) to achieve eradication of a persistent renal focus of infection.

Urinalysis: When subclinical pyelonephritis is suspected, a urinalysis should be obtained. At the initial visit, the urinalysis typically shows pyuria and bacteriuria; hematuria and proteinuria may also be present transiently.

Urine Culture: In subacute pyelonephritis, urine culture and colony count almost always reveal more than 100 000 bacteria/mL of urine (9). A culture should be obtained from any patient in whom the disease is suspected, both before and after completion of treatment ("test-of-cure" culture). First, treatment failure is more likely; in patients with subclinical pyelonephritis, the organism may be more likely to be resistant to the first-line benign antibacterial agents used. Second, the consequences of treatment failure may be more serious; because the patient has an uneradicated upper tract infection, with tissue invasion, recurrent symptoms may be more likely to develop suddenly and to take the form of significant pain, bacteremia, and clinical sepsis. I know of no data to support this fear, and clinical experience suggests that it is an unusual event, except perhaps in the elderly or immunocompromised patient. However, given current knowledge, it seems prudent to obtain cultures before and after treatment when subclinical pyelonephritis is suspected.

LOWER URINARY TRACT BACTERIAL INFECTION

Over the past 15 years, it has become apparent that many women with symptoms of lower urinary tract infection (and associated pyuria) have what has been called a "negative" culture: fewer than 100 000 bacteria/mL of urine (34-36). Until recently, it had been conventional to say that patients with a "positive" culture (> 100 000 bacteria/mL) had "cystitis," whereas patients with "low-count" bacteriuria had infection limited to the urethra, the "acute urethral syndrome" (34). Thus, the degree of bacteriuria had been thought to define two groups with different pathologic conditions: one group, with putative "cystitis," clearly benefiting from antibacterial therapy, and the other group, with putative acute urethral syndrome, not clearly benefiting from therapy.

It now appears that this widely held hypothesis is unjustified. First, the presence of hematuria, proteinuria, and suprapubic pain in many patients with low-count bacteriuria suggests inflammation of the bladder as well as the urethra. Second, as argued earlier, there now is strong evidence that symptomatic women with low-count bacteriuria, as shown on culture of clean-voided urine, have infection of the bladder, as determined by culture of urine collected by suprapubic aspiration or catheterization (1). Third, treatment of symptomatic patients having low-count bacteriuria results in prompt clinical and bacteriologic cure, as compared with placebo therapy (37).

Therefore, the terms "cystitis" and "acute urethral syndrome" falsely suggest distinct clinical conditions and should be abandoned. Instead, the symptomatic woman with pyuria on urinalysis and a colony count of greater than only 100 bacteria/mL of urine on a clean-voided specimen should be regarded as having a single clinical entity—lower urinary tract bacterial infection—infection of both the bladder and urethra, with low-count bacteriuria (1, 23).

In fact, most patients with lower tract bacterial infection have greater than 100 000 bacteria/mL of urine. But a large minority do not; in the symptomatic woman who also has pyuria, low-count bacteriuria (100 to 100 000 bacteria/mL) in clean-voided specimens does not usually reflect contamination (23). This argument can be made most strongly for infections with pure cultures of *Escherichia coli* and *Staphylococcus saprophyticus* (18, 38), the two most frequent urinary pathogens in women with lower urinary tract infection or subclinical pyelonephritis.

Urinalysis: In the patient suspected of having lower urinary tract infection (because the clinical features suggesting other causes of acute dysuria are absent), urinalysis is indicated. The presence of pyuria justifies giving immediate therapy, whereas the absence of pyuria justifies withholding therapy (1, 39). This is because pyuria is found in 90% to 95% of patients with lower tract infection and colony counts of greater than 100 000 bacteria/mL of urine, in over 70% of patients with lower tract infection and colony counts of 100 to 100 000 bacteria/mL, and in only 1% of asymptomatic, nonbacteriuric patients (18). If the patient has pyuria without bacteriuria (as determined by examination of unstained sediment), chlamydial urethritis, gonococcal urethritis, or urinary infection with gram-positive cocci may be more likely.

Urine Culture: The value of urine culture is much less in lower urinary tract bacterial infection than in upper tract infection. A recent cost-effectiveness analysis has indicated that the small added benefits (a reduction in duration of symptoms by 10%) were not worth the considerable added costs (an increase of 40%) required to treat the episode of dysuria (40). For reasons mentioned earlier, the colony count is not very helpful. More important, oral therapy with any of several benign antibacterials is highly effective; sensitivity testing proves valuable very infrequently. Indeed, single-dose therapy may be as effective as 7 to 10 days of therapy and is associated with far fewer adverse drug reactions (32). I do not obtain urine cultures routinely when I suspect the patient has lower tract bacterial infection.

"Test-of-cure" cultures following treatment are of little usefulness when lower tract bacterial infection is suspected. Most recurrent infections will be reinfections of the lower tract, and virtually all such recurrent infections will declare themselves by producing symptoms (41); repeat cultures in asymptomatic patients have a very low yield. Indeed, it has recently been reported that selected women with a history of recurrent infection can reliably recognize early symptoms of recurrent infection and successfully achieve clinical and bacteriologic cure by treating themselves with a single dose of trimethoprim-sulfamethoxazole (four regular-strength tablets of 80 mg-400 mg each, or two double-strength tablets) (42). This drug probably is the most effective of several widely used single-dose regimens (43).

CHLAMYDIAL URETHRITIS

Urethral infection with *Chlamydia trachomatis* accounts for some cases of acute dysuria in women (9). Chlamydial urethritis should be suspected when the patient has a stuttering and prolonged onset of dysuria (and frequency or urgency), has a partner with symptoms of urethritis, or has a new sexual partner. Chlamydial urethritis also should be suspected when mucopurulent endocervical secretions are noted on speculum examination, a finding that is further confirmed by seeing 10 or more polymorphonuclear leukocytes per 1000-power microscopic field in samples of the endocervical secretions (44). Treatment with tetracycline hydrochloride or erythromycin for at least 7 days is effective (37).

Urinalysis: Urinalysis may be of help in estimating the likelihood of chlamydial urethritis, because the finding of pyuria without microscopic bacteriuria is suggestive of chlamydial urethritis. Hematuria is very unusual, as is proteinuria.

Urine Culture: Because *C. trachomatis,* an obligate intracellular parasite, grows only in cell culture and not on nutrient agar media, culture is of no value (45). Methods for isolating *C. trachomatis* do not provide results for several days, are not readily available in many places, are probably insensitive, and are expensive. However, recently developed rapid assays for chlamydial antigens using monoclonal antibodies appear to be highly sensitive and specific, and may become an effective means for diagnosing this entity accurately at the time the patient first presents with acute dysuria (46).

OTHER URETHRAL INFECTIONS

Occasionally urethritis may be caused by *Neisseria gonorrhoeae* or herpes simplex virus. In my experience, *Trichomonas vaginalis* or *Candida albicans* may occasionally cause urethritis without symptoms of vaginitis (although abnormal vaginal discharge and cervicitis are seen on a pelvic examination). Standard treatment regimens are effective.

Urinalysis: All of these forms of urethritis except candidal urethritis typically produce pyuria (47). Urinalysis may be of some utility in suggesting these entities: Pyuria without microscopic bacteriuria suggests urethritis, and the finding of budding yeast forms or motile trichomonads may also be helpful.

Urine Culture: When the usual culture media are used, urine culture is of no value in establishing the diagnosis. If *N. gonorrhoeae* is suspected, culture on appropriate media of samples from the urethral os and cervical os are valuable. Rapid antigen detection techniques are not yet sufficiently sensitive in women to replace the culture (48). Future improvements in test sensitivity may allow this rapid and simple technique to provide the clinician and patient with accurate and immediate information.

NO RECOGNIZED PATHOGEN

Many women with dysuria have no recognized pathogen, do not have pyuria, and do not respond to antimicrobial treatment (9, 37). The absence of pyuria in these patients is useful because it indicates that antimicrobial treatment is probably unnecessary. The cause of the dysuria may be an urethral inflammation from physical or chemical agents or from trauma.

VAGINITIS

Patients with vaginitis may present with a chief complaint of dysuria (plus frequency and urgency) and not vaginal discharge or irritation, although these latter symptoms can be elicited by the clinician (36, 47, 49). We have found that in college-aged women vaginal infections actually are more frequent causes of the presenting complaint of dysuria than are urinary infections (36). Typically, pyuria is absent except when a trichomonal infection involves the urethra as well as the vagina (36, 47).

When patients describe symptoms of vaginitis, a vaginal examination is mandatory, but urinalysis and urine culture are not. The one exception to this case is when the woman describes dysuria as an "internal," visceral, and dull sensation (which indicates inflammation of the urinary tract) rather than as an "external," somatic, and sharp pain felt as the jet of urine streams past the inflamed vaginal labia (36, 50). "Internal" dysuria in a woman with vaginal discharge suggests coexisting urinary and vaginal infections (36).

A Recapitulation: The Dysuria-Pyuria Syndrome

In the woman with dysuria and without symptoms and signs of acute pyelonephritis or vaginitis, the presence of pyuria strongly suggests the presence of any of several treatable entities: subclinical pyelonephritis, lower urinary tract bacterial infection, chlamydial urethritis, and other forms of urethritis. Conversely, pyuria is almost always absent in patients in whom no recognized pathogen can be found; these patients also do not respond to antibacterial treatment (37). The utility of pyuria in predicting the presence or absence of treatable infection is greater when urine specimens are handled carefully as part of a formal study, than when urine specimens are handled in a normal manner in the "real world" of clinical practice (51, 52). These observations only stress the importance of promptly examining freshly voided urine.

In brief, patients with acute dysuria and pyuria have a syndrome, the dysuria-pyuria syndrome (39), that almost always can benefit from immediate antibacterial treatment, whereas patients without pyuria do not. Thus, the finding of pyuria not only is more readily available than the result of a urine culture, but also appears to be a better predictor of treatable infection. The finding of pyuria does not help determine which of the several treatable clinical conditions is present, however; only the aforementioned clinical findings can do that.

Besides the assessment of pyuria, the urinalysis provides other useful information. The presence of hematuria is helpful in ruling out chlamydial and other forms of urethritis, as well as vaginitis; probably the same is true of proteinuria. When seen, leukocyte casts clearly indicate upper urinary tract infection. Urine pH may on occasion be useful (when it is greater than 7) in suggesting infection with urea-splitting organisms and possibly-associated struvite stones. Urine glucose levels have value in suggesting previously unrecognized diabetes mellitus, which in turn raises the possibility of papillary necrosis and (possibly) perinephric abscess, in the patient with symptoms and signs of acute pyelonephritis. We speculate that diabetes also increases the likelihood of subclinical pyelonephritis.

Other elements of the urinalysis do not have established value in caring for the woman with acute dysuria. Patients with acute pyelonephritis lose the ability to concentrate the urine, as reflected in the specific gravity. However, specific gravity may also be low in patients with lower urinary tract infection who drink hypoosmolar fluids to reduce their symptoms or to replace perceived fluid loss. Also, specific gravity may be higher than expected in patients with acute pyelonephritis because of fever-induced insensible losses or vomiting. Other elements of the urinalysis that have no known value in caring for women with acute dysuria include urine color, urinary ketone concentrations, urinary bilirubin concentrations, sedimentary crystals, and epithelial cells.

In summary, in the woman with acute dysuria and without symptoms and signs of acute pyelonephritis, a urinalysis is almost always of some value, but a urine culture is of value primarily in patients with suspected subclinical pyelonephritis. It could be argued that a urine culture, when sterile, increases the likelihood of chlamydial or gonococcal urethritis, but using the urine culture for that purpose seems less cost effective than attempting to make the diagnosis directly with appropriate diagnostic tests.

Asymptomatic Women

The value of identifying asymptomatic bacteriuria in the asymptomatic, nonpregnant woman, is controversial. Asymptomatic bacteriuria (> 100 000 bacteria/mL of urine), especially when there is also pyuria (18), does correlate with definable urinary tract abnormalities (such as renal scars on intravenous pyelogram), but there is little evidence that further scars (or renal dysfunction) are prevented by treatment. Asymptomatic bacteriuria also appears to be correlated with increased mortality in the elderly (53, 54), but there is no evidence that treatment of asymptomatic bacteriuria alters the mortality rate. The one group that appears to benefit from treatment of asymptomatic bacteriuria is pregnant women; randomized, double-blind trials indicate that treatment reduces the occurrence of acute pyelonephritis and possibly low-birth-weight babies (55-59). Therefore, I recommend regular urinalyses in the prenatal period, with urine cultures if pyuria is noted.

Unresolved Issues

Among women with acute dysuria coming to a primary care practice setting, the following two unanswered questions about *urinalysis* seem most important to address with further investigation. First, in each of the different classes of patients with acute dysuria described above, what is the frequency with which findings seen only on examination of the urine sediment (for example, casts, microscopic hematuria, microscopic bacteriuria) provide information essential to diagnosis and treatment? If this information, which the counting chamber and leukocyte esterase techniques cannot provide, is found to influence patient management frequently, then it will be harder to abandon the examination of the sediment. Second, how would patient outcome (clinical and microbiologic cure) differ in patients treated according to three different strategies: basing a decision to treat (and possibly to obtain a urine culture) on the urine sediment findings; basing the decision(s) on the counting chamber findings; and basing the decision(s) on the leukocyte esterase test?

Among many unanswered questions about *urine culture,* the following seem most important to address through further investigation: What is the frequency with which organisms reported to be "resistant" to benign antibacterials on Kirby-Bauer disk testing are really sensitive to the concentrations of these antibacterials found in the urine? In those (presumably unusual) cases of organisms truly resistant to urinary concentrations of all "benign" antibacterials, how often are these organisms also truly resistant to urinary concentrations of the commonly used second-step aminoglycosides?

Recommendations

Table 1 summarizes the recommendations for when to obtain urinalysis, urine culture, and several other commonly used tests in the woman with acute dysuria. The urinalysis and urine culture should not be routinely used to screen for asymptomatic bacteriuria, except in pregnant women.

ACKNOWLEDGMENTS: The author thanks Harold Sox, Richard Platt, and the two anonymous manuscript reviewers for the *Annals* for making many helpful suggestions regarding this manuscript.

Grant support: in part by grants HS 02063 and HS 04066 from the National Center for Health Services Research.

References

1. KOMAROFF AL. Acute dysuria in women. *N Engl J Med.* 1984;**310**:368-75.
2. GADEHOLT H. Quantitative estimation of urinary sediment, with special regard to sources of error. *Br Med J.* 1964;**1**:1547-9.
3. LITTLE PJ. A comparison of the urinary white cell concentration with the white cell excretion rate. *Br J Urol.* 1964;**36**:360-3.
4. MABECK CE. Studies in urinary tract infections: IV. Urinary leucocyte excretion in bacteriuria. *Acta Med Scand.* 1969;**186**:193-8.
5. GADEHOLT H. Quantitative estimation of cells in urine: an evaluation of the Addis count. *Acta Med Scand.* 1968;**183**:369-74.
6. BRUMFITT W. Urinary cell counts and their value. *J Clin Pathol.* 1965;**18**:550-5.
7. MUSHER DM, THORSTEINSSON SB, AIROLA VM. Quantitative urinalysis: diagnosing urinary tract infection in men. *JAMA.* 1976;**236**:2069-72.
8. FAIRLEY K, BARRACLOUGH M. Leucocyte-excretion rate as a screening test for bacteriuria. *Lancet.* 1967;**1**:420-1.

9. STAMM WE, WAGNER KF, AMSEL R, et al. Causes of the acute urethral syndrome in women. *N Engl J Med.* 1980;**303**:409-15.

10. STANSFELD JM. The measurement and meaning of pyuria. *Arch Dis Child.* 1962;**37**:257-62.

11. KUSUMI RK, GROVER PJ, KUNIN CM. Rapid detection of pyuria by leukocyte esterase activity. *JAMA.* 1981;**245**:1653-5.

12. PERRY JL, MATTHEWS JS, WEESNER DE. Evaluation of leukocyte esterase activity as a rapid screening technique for bacteriuria. *J Clin Microbiol.* 1982;**15**:852-4.

13. GELBART SM, CHEN WT, REID R. Clinical trial of leukocyte test strips in routine use. *Clin Chem.* 1983;**29**:997-9.

14. CHERNOW B, ZALOGA GP, SOLDANO S, et al. Measurement of urinary leukocyte esterase activity: a screening test for urinary tract infections. *Ann Emerg Med.* 1984;**13**:150-4.

15. ROBERTS AP, ROBINSON RE, BEARD RW. Some factors affecting bacterial colony counts in urinary infection. *Br Med J.* 1967;**1**:400-3.

16. COHEN SN, KASS EH. A simple method for quantitative urine culture. *N Engl J Med.* 1967;**277**:176-80.

17. ARNEIL GC, McALLISTER TA, KAY P. Detection of bacteriuria at room-temperature. *Lancet.* 1970;**1**:119-21.

18. STAMM WE. Measurement of pyuria and its relation to bacteriuria. *Am J Med.* 1983;**75**(1B):53-8.

19. PLATT R. Quantitative definition of bacteriuria. *Am J Med.* 1983;**75**(1B):44-52.

20. KASS EH. Asymptomatic infections of the urinary tract. *Trans Assoc Am Physicians.* 1956;**69**:56-63.

21. SANFORD JP, FAVOUR CB, MAO FH, HARRISON JH. Evaluation of the positive urine culture: an approach to positive differentiation of significant bacteria from contaminants. *Am J Med.* 1956;**20**:88-93.

22. GUZE LB, BEESON PB. Observations on the reliability and safety of bladder catheterization for bacteriologic study of the urine. *N Engl J Med.* 1956;**255**:474-5.

23. STAMM WE, COUNTS GW, RUNNING KR, FIHN S, TURCK M, HOLMES KK. Diagnosis of coliform infection in acutely dysuric women. *N Engl J Med.* 1982;**307**:463-8.

24. DEAN R, HERLIHY E, McGUIRE EJ. The accuracy of antimicrobial disk sensitivity testing in urinary tract infections. *J Urol.* 1978;**120**:80-1.

25. SAVARD-FENTON M, FENTON BW, RELLER LB, LAUER BA, BYYNY RL. Single-dose amoxicillin therapy with follow-up urine culture. *Am J Med.* 1982;**73**:808-13.

26. FAIR WR, FAIR WR III. Clinical value of sensitivity determinations in treating urinary tract infections. *Urology.* 1982;**19**:565-9.

27. KUNIN C. The quantitative significance of bacteria visualized in the unstained urinary sediment. *N Engl J Med.* 1961;**265**:589-90.

28. STAMEY TA, GOVAN DE, PALMER JM. The localization and treatment of urinary tract infections: the role of bactericidal urine levels as opposed to serum levels. *Medicine (Baltimore).* 1965;**44**:1-36.

29. FAIRLEY KF, BOND AG, BROWN RB, HABERSBERGER P. Simple test to determine the site of urinary-tract infection. *Lancet.* 1967;**2**:427-8.

30. RONALD AR, BOUTROS P, MOURTADA H. Bacteriuria localization and response to single-dose therapy in women. *JAMA.* 1976;**235**:1854-6.

31. FANG LST, TOLKOFF-RUBIN NE, RUBIN RH. Efficacy of single-dose and conventional amoxicillin therapy in urinary-tract infection localized by the antibody-coated bacteria technic. *N Engl J Med.* 1978;**298**:413-6.

32. RUBIN RH, FANG LST, JONES SR, et al. Single-dose amoxicillin therapy for urinary tract infection: multicenter trial using antibody-coated bacteria localization. *JAMA.* 1980;**244**:561-4.

33. BUCKWOLD FJ, LUDWIG P, HARDING GKM, et al. Therapy for acute cystitis in adult women: randomized comparison of single-dose sulfisoxazole vs trimethoprim-sulfamethoxazole. *JAMA.* 1982;**247**:1839-42.

34. GALLAGHER DJA, MONTGOMERIE JZ, NORTH JDK. Acute infections in the urinary tract and the urethral syndrome in general practice. *Br Med J.* 1965;**1**:622-6.

35. FAIRLEY KF, CARSON NE, GUTCH RC, et al. Site of infection in acute urinary-tract infection in general practice. *Lancet.* 1971;**2**:615-8.

36. KOMAROFF AL, PASS TM, MCCUE JD, COHEN AB, HENDRICKS TM, FRIEDLAND G. Management strategies for urinary and vaginal infections. *Arch Intern Med.* 1978;**138**:1069-73.

37. STAMM WE, RUNNING K, MCKEVITT M, COUNTS GW, TURCK M, HOLMES KK. Treatment of the acute urethral syndrome. *N Engl J Med.* 1981;**304**:956-8.

38. LATHAM RH, RUNNING K, STAMM WE. Urinary tract infections in young adult women caused by *Staphylococcus saprophyticus. JAMA.* 1983;**250**:3063-6.

39. KOMAROFF AL, FRIEDLAND G. The dysuria-pyuria syndrome [Editorial]. *N Engl J Med.* 1980;**303**:452-4.

40. CARLSON KJ, MULLEY AG. Management of acute dysuria: a decision-analysis model of alternative strategies. *Ann Intern Med.* 1985;**102**:244-9.

41. KRAFT JK, STAMEY TA. The natural history of symptomatic recurrent bacteriuria in women. *Medicine (Baltimore).* 1977;**56**:55-60.

42. WONG ES, MCKEVITT M, RUNNING K, COUNTS GW, TURCK M, STAMM WE. Management of recurrent urinary tract infections with patient-administered single-dose therapy. *Ann Intern Med.* 1985;**102**:302-7.

43. HOOTON TM, RUNNING K, STAMM WE. Single-dose therapy for cystitis in women: a comparison of trimethoprim-sulfamethoxazole, amoxicillin, and cyclacillin. *JAMA.* 1985;**253**:387-90.

44. BRUNHAM RC, PAAVONEN J, STEVENS CE, et al. Mucopurulent cervicitis—the ignored counterpart in women of urethritis in men. *N Engl J Med.* 1984;**311**:1-6.

45. SCHACHTER J. Chlamydial infections. *N Engl J Med.* 1978;**298**:428-34.

46. TAM MR, STAMM WE, HANDSFIELD HH, et al. Culture-independent diagnosis of *Chlamydia trachomatis* using monoclonal antibodies. *N Engl J Med.* 1984;**310**:1146-50.

47. DEMETRIOU E, EMANS SJ, MASLAND RP JR. Dysuria in adolescent girls: urinary tract infection or vaginitis? *Pediatrics.* 1982;**70**:299-301.

48. DEMETRIOU E, SACKETT R, WELCH DF, KAPLAN DW. Evaluation of an enzyme immunoassay for detection of *Neisseria gonorrhoeae* in an adolescent population. *JAMA.* 1984;**252**:247-50.

49. DANS PE, KLAUS B. Dysuria in women. *John Hopkins Med J.* 1976;**138**:13-8.

50. BERG AO, HEIDRICH FE, FIHN SD, et al. Establishing the cause of genitourinary symptoms in women in a family practice: a comparison of clinical examination and comprehensive microbiology. *JAMA.* 1984;**251**:620-5.

51. SCHULTZ HJ, MCCAFFREY LA, KEYS TF, NOBREGA FT. Acute cystitis: a prospective study of laboratory tests and duration of therapy. *Mayo Clin Proc.* 1984;**59**:391-7.

52. LATHAM RH, WONG ES, LARSON A, COYLE M, STAMM WE. Laboratory diagnosis of urinary tract infection in ambulatory women. *JAMA.* 1985;**254**:3333-6.

53. EVANS DA, KASS EH, HENNEKENS CH, et al. Bacteriuria and subsequent mortality in women. *Lancet.* 1982;**1**:156-8.

54. PLATT R, POLK BF, MURDOCK B, ROSNER B. Mortality associated with nosocomial urinary-tract infection. *N Engl J Med.* 1982;**307**:637-42.

55. KINCAID-SMITH P, BULLEN M. Bacteriuria in pregnancy. *Lancet.* 1965;**1**:395-9.

56. LITTLE PJ. The incidence of urinary infection in 5000 pregnant women. *Lancet.* 1966;**2**:925-8.

57. SAVAGE WE, HAJJ SN, KASS EH. Demographic and prognostic characteristics of bacteriuria in pregnancy. *Medicine* *(Baltimore)*. 1967;**46**:385-407.

58. BAILEY RR. Urinary infection in pregnancy. *NZ Med J.* 1970;**71**:216-20.

59. ELDER HA, SANTAMARINA BAG, SMITH S, KASS EH. The natural history of asymptomatic bacteriuria during pregnancy: the effect of tetracycline on the clinical course and the outcome of pregnancy. *Am J Obstet Gynecol.* 1971;**111**:441-62.

Carcinoembryonic Antigen

ROBERT H. FLETCHER, M.D., M.Sc.

Cᴀʀᴄɪɴᴏᴇᴍʙʀʏᴏɴɪᴄ ᴀɴᴛɪɢᴇɴ (CEA) is one of a class of oncofetal antigens that are normally present during fetal life, occur at low concentrations in adults, and circulate in high concentrations in patients with certain malignancies, particularly epithelial tumors. Since the first description of CEA in 1965 (1), it was recognized that the concentration of the antigen in body fluids, particularly blood, might serve as a useful guide in the care of patients with cancer. This article reviews the evidence that CEA levels can contribute in clinically important ways to four aspects of patient care: screening for cancer in asymptomatic persons, diagnosing cancer when it is suspected, assigning a prognosis at the time of diagnosis, and monitoring the effects of treatment.

History and Current Use

Since its discovery, CEA has engendered great interest in the medical community. Several thousand journal articles and several excellent reviews have been published (1-4), describing both its basic chemistry and biology and its value in the care of patients. Information about the clinical usefulness of CEA has also been summarized in two major conferences, held in 1977 and 1980 (5-7). Although over a thousand journal articles about the antigen have been published since 1980, the new information has not questioned the basic conclusions of these conferences.

Initially, it was hoped that the CEA level would be both a sensitive and specific marker for the presence of cancer, particularly that of the gastrointestinal tract. As information has accumulated, these hopes have largely

▶ This chapter was originally published in *Annals of Internal Medicine.* 1986;**104**:66-73.

been dispelled and it has become apparent that the antigen circulates in small quantities in normal persons, that its levels are increased in the presence of various benign diseases, and that levels are commonly not elevated in the presence of cancer.

Despite these disappointments, the CEA assay has taken a modest place in the management of patients with cancer. Its proper use is limited to specific clinical situations, and the information it conveys is generally not definitive. Because of the many articles about CEA and the consistency of their findings, experts have had relatively little difficulty agreeing on the situations in which this test is useful.

Although guidelines for prudent use of CEA assays have been reported, physicians in practice apparently have greater belief in the practical value of these levels than do experts. In one study in 1979, over 50% of physicians believed that a CEA assay was worthwhile for initial detection of colonic cancer and that elevated levels in a nonsmoking person without symptoms should prompt an aggressive search for colonic cancer—both beliefs that experts by that time had rejected (8).

Assays

Carcinoembryonic antigen is not a single entity, but rather a family of related glycoproteins (2). These antigens are measured by various methods in research laboratories, and efforts are ongoing to increase the specificity of the assays (9).

Most reports of clinical research and patient care involving measurement of CEA levels by assays have used one of three commercially available kits (10). The Roche assay (Hoffman LaRoche, Inc., Nutley, New Jersey), a radioimmunoassay procedure, was approved for use in the United States in 1973. Specimens are first measured by an "indirect" method; if the CEA concentration is greater than 20 ng/mL, the manufacturer recommends that the specimen be reassayed by a "direct" method. The direct method has been shown to give a higher value than the indirect assay of the same specimen (11, 12). The disparity between the two methods was 31 ± 11 ng/ mL in one study (11), a difference that is clinically important. Two other commercial assays, produced by Abbott Laboratories (Chicago, Illinois), were approved in

1980. One is a solid-phase radioimmunoassay, and the other is an enzyme immunoassay.

In one study (13), the log correlation coefficient between the Roche indirect and the Abbott enzyme immunoassay methods was 0.948. However, there were clinically important differences in the results of the two methods for some patients; for example, in some patients the CEA level measured was as low as 7 ng/mL by one method and 50 ng/mL by the other. One reason for the lack of concordance, other than technical error, may be heterogeneity of the CEA molecules; the different methods may measure different antigens (13).

There is good evidence that CEA measurements should not be used interchangeably from laboratory to laboratory or from method to method. The Centers for Disease Control studied the performance of 125 laboratories throughout the United States in 1976. Although many laboratories performed satisfactorily, almost a quarter of the results were placed in the wrong nominal groups, as defined by generally agreed on ranges (*see* below) (12). Another study has shown systematic error in 4 of 5 laboratories examined (14).

To minimize the effects of these potential sources of error, various guidelines have been recommended for the clinical use of CEA (10, 12): Measurements by different assay methods should not be used interchangeably. Laboratories should establish their own "range of normal," and possibly also the sensitivity and specificity of the test for local patients. Results from different laboratories, even when using the same assay method, should be interpreted with caution. Results of direct and indirect assays by the Roche method should not be regarded as comparable. Assays of serum and plasma levels by the two Abbott methods should not be regarded as comparable.

These cautions are particularly important when serial specimens from the same patient are compared. Disregard for these recommendations could result in clinically important misinterpretation of the information provided by these assays.

The charge to the patient for a single CEA determination varies with time, place, and method. Charges reported in the medical literature are $56.00 (15) and $65.00 (8). The current charge at the teaching hospital of the University of North Carolina at Chapel Hill is $38.00;

the charge is similar at a nearby private laboratory. The cost of the test to the hospital is presumably lower.

Normal Values

Most normal persons have detectable concentrations of circulating CEA. Levels for healthy persons have been described for various unselected populations, and the distributions are similar. The distribution is not Gaussian but is skewed to the right, approximating a log-normal distribution. Levels of 2.5 and 5.0 ng/nL are commonly used cutoff points for distinguishing normal from abnormal levels. In two large surveys of apparently normal persons, 84% to 87% had antigen levels of less than 2.5 ng/mL, 95% to 98% had levels of less than 5 ng/mL, and almost no one had levels of greater than 10 ng/mL (16, 17).

Carcinoembryonic antigen concentrations are, on average, somewhat higher in smokers than in nonsmokers (18). Levels may be higher in men than in women (19), but this finding does not simply reflect the greater prevalence of smoking among men (20). Concentrations also tend to be slightly higher in older persons, and this finding is apparently not explained by the greater prevalence of benign diseases associated with elevated CEA values in the elderly (21, 22). Racial differences in serum levels of CEA have been suggested (20) but not established.

Extreme elevations of CEA levels are unusual in apparently healthy persons. Most "elevations" are in the 2.5- to 10.0-ng/mL range. Relatively high levels in some persons can be attributed to various nonneoplastic diseases associated with CEA elevations. For a few, an undetected malignancy is possible. For most, an explanation is not apparent, at least by cursory examination.

Screening

Screening in medical practice is the process of searching for a disease in persons without symptoms attributable to that disease. The value of screening rests on evidence that early detection can lead to more effective treatment than would be possible if the disease were detected in the ordinary course of events. For a diagnostic test to be useful in screening, several conditions should be satisfied (23): The disease causes substantial suffering; a sensitive, specific, and feasible screening procedure must be available; and earlier treatment after detection by screening should be acceptable to patients and must be efficacious.

Shortly after the discovery of CEA, it was hoped that the test for this antigen would be useful in the early detection of colorectal cancer. This cancer is relatively common, results in high morbidity and mortality, and is more curable at early stages. Screening tests (for example, occult blood in stool or colonoscopy) are available but not well accepted by patients and physicians, so a better screening test would be welcome (24). Moreover, CEA levels are a better indicator for colorectal cancers than for other cancers.

The performance of CEA assays as a screening test for colorectal cancer can be described by the sensitivity and specificity of the test among persons without symptoms suggestive of the cancer. Cancers should be at Dukes stages A and B at detection, because later stages are not "early" and are unlikely to be much more treatable than usual if detected by screening. Also, for any screening test there is a trade-off between sensitivity and specificity depending on where the cutoff point between normal and abnormal is placed, and it is necessary to examine CEA assays for this effect.

The sensitivity and specificity, at various cutoff points between normal and abnormal, of CEA levels used to detect colorectal cancer are shown in Figure 1; Dukes stages A through D are presented separately. The data are from reports of the sensitivity of CEA measurements in detecting colorectal cancer at various stages (25) and the specificity of the assays in normal persons (16). Data are presented for three cutoff points between normal and abnormal: 2.5, 5.0, and 10.0 ng/mL. The curves could be extrapolated for levels below 2.5 ng/mL, but the test would not be used in this range because of unacceptably low specificity.

Figure 2 shows that the earlier the stage of colorectal cancer, the less likely a CEA assay is to detect it. Measurement of antigen levels is a relatively insensitive way of detecting Dukes stage A and B tumors; at the usual upper limit of normal of 2.5 ng/mL, this method has a sensitivity of 36% and a specificity of 87% for these stages. Efforts to increase the sensitivity to clinically useful levels by lowering the cut-off point between normal and abnormal would decrease the specificity unacceptably. Measurement of CEA levels is more sensitive in

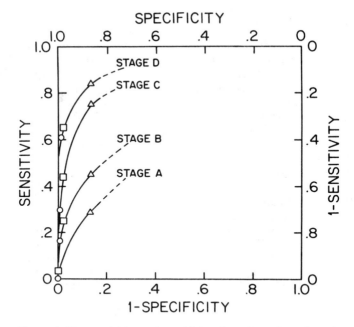

Figure 1. The sensitivity and specificity of carcinoembryonic antigen for detection of colorectal cancer at various Dukes stages (16, 25). Triangles indicate a cutoff point of 2.5 ng/mL; squares, 5.0 ng/mL; and circles, 10.0 ng/mL.

detecting advanced colorectal cancer of Dukes stages C and D. The sensitivity at levels of 2.5 ng/mL is 74% for stage C disease and 83% for stage D disease. However, colorectal cancer is considerably less curable at these stages.

The likelihood that a positive test represents colorectal cancer depends on the prevalence (prior probability) of colorectal cancer among persons tested as well as the sensitivity and specificity of the test. The prevalence of undetected colorectal cancer is low in unselected populations, about 0.4 to 7/1000, depending on the population studied (26, 27). At this prevalence and at usual levels of sensitivity and specificity, the probability of cancer if the serum CEA is abnormal is unacceptably low (Figure 2). For example, at a prevalence of 1/1000, a sensitivity of 40%, and a specificity of 90% (all for stage A and B cancers), there would be 250 false-positive tests for every

1 patient with cancer. Also, 60% of cancers would be missed.

Carcinoembryonic antigen assays perform no better in screening for other cancers commonly associated with elevated CEA levels. Bowel cancers other than colorectal (for example, stomach or pancreas) are not known to be more treatable at eaɪly stages. Breast cancer already has well-established screening tests, mammography and manual examination. In any case, the sensitivity and specificity of CEA assays for detecting these tumors are no better than for detecting colorectal cancer, and the prevalence of these tumors is not higher.

Therefore, measurement of CEA levels is not a useful test for detecting early, potentially curable cancer. The test's relatively low sensitivity and specificity, along with the low prevalence of cancer in asymptomatic populations, lead to too many false-positive and false-negative results. This conclusion is supported by data from a large, population-based cohort study, the Framingham study, in which serum samples from patients with newly detected cancer were examined for CEA levels (28). The conclusion is also in agreement with the recommendations of the National Institutes of Health Consensus Development Conference in 1979 (6).

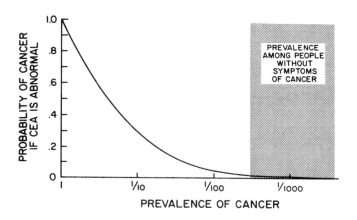

Figure 2. The probability of early colorectal cancer (stages A and B) if serum carcinoembryonic antigen (*CEA*) level is abnormal, according to the prevalence of disease (sensitivity = 40%, specificity = 90%).

Diagnosis

A diagnostic test for cancer is one that confirms or rules out the presence of cancer among patients who are suspected of having that disease. The performance of CEA assays as a diagnostic test is judged by similar criteria as for screening. Although several of these criteria are quantitatively different, the conclusion is the same: Measurement of CEA levels has limited value as the sole diagnostic test for cancer.

The sensitivity of CEA levels for detecting colorectal cancer—that is, the proportion of patients with colorectal cancer who have a positive test result—is similar, for a given stage of disease, to that described for screening. At a cutoff point of 2.5 ng/mL, sensitivity ranges from 30% to 85% depending on the stage of the cancer. However, in general, sensitivity in symptomatic patients is likely to be higher than that in asymptomatic patients, because symptomatic patients are more likely to have advanced disease. The sensitivity is similar for some other gastrointestinal cancers (stomach, pancreas, and liver) and somewhat less (60% to 70%) for cancers of the lung, breast, prostate, and bladder as well as various gynecologic malignancies (29).

The specificity of CEA levels for cancer—that is the likelihood of a negative test result in a patient without cancer—depends on the clinical situation in which the test is used. Various benign conditions are associated with elevated CEA levels (Table 1). Foremost among these is liver disease (30); over 90% of patients with chronic liver disease and 50% of those with acute liver disease have raised plasma CEA levels (31). Beyond the conditions listed in Table 1, there are case reports of CEA elevations for hundreds of conditions. Often the benign conditions associated with elevated levels are the very conditions that must be distinguished from cancer. For example, liver disease may either mimic or be a manifestation of cancer. However, benign conditions are rarely a cause of extreme elevations, or even levels above 10 ng/mL.

Because of its relatively low sensitivity and specificity, CEA is not useful as the sole diagnostic test for a previously undetected cancer. The sensitivity is not high enough, because in our society it is unacceptable for a cancer to be suspected, investigated, and not found. Simi-

Table 1. Some Conditions Associated with Elevated Plasma Levels of Carcinoembryonic Antigen Other Than Cancer

Liver diseases
   Alcoholic
   Chronic active
   Primary biliary
   Cryptogenic
   Obstructive jaundice
Bowel diseases
   Peptic ulcer
   Pancreatitis
   Diverticulitis
   Inflammatory bowel disease
Other*
   Smoking
   Renal failure
   Fibrocystic breast disease

*There are hundreds of case reports of elevations in various other, less common diseases.

larly, the specificity is not high enough, because clinicians must almost never conclude cancer is present when it is not; most treatments, particularly radiotherapy and chemotherapy, are too dangerous to justify false-positive diagnoses. Carcinoembryonic antigen cannot substitute for current methods of diagnosing colorectal cancer if that disease is suspected. Barium enema, sigmoidoscopy, and colonoscopy, with biopsy of abnormal-appearing lesions, are more accurate and must, in any case, be done to stage the disease and direct the surgeon.

It is generally believed that adenomatous colonic polyps can be precursors of invasive cancer. Colonic polyps are usually not associated with elevated CEA levels, and CEA levels are not useful for distinguishing locally invasive polyps from benign ones. This finding is consistent with the poor performance of the antigen in detecting early invasive colorectal cancer (Figure 1).

Although CEA levels are not definitive enough when used alone, they can contribute to the diagnostic process when combined with other tests. Thus, if several tests for cancer (including measurement of CEA levels) are positive, this pattern of results may increase the physician's certainty that cancer is present to where biopsy seems justified. Conversely, if several such tests are negative, the clinician might become sufficiently confident that cancer is not present to curtail further aggressive (invasive) diagnostic procedures.

Prognosis

The plasma CEA concentration, measured at the time of diagnosis, is known to be related to prognosis for many cancers. The higher the level, the more likely the tumor is to recur. This finding has been shown for cancers of the colon and rectum (32-34), breast (35), stomach (36), lung (37,38), and other organs.

It is also apparent that the blood CEA concentration is related to stage of disease: the more advanced the clinical stage, the higher the CEA level at the time of diagnosis. This relationship for colorectal cancer is shown in Table 2. A similar association has been found for breast cancer in one study (35); elevated CEA levels (> 4 ng/mL) were found in 15% of women with stage I tumors and in 73% of women with stage IV tumors. Some reports have suggested an association between CEA level and stage for many other cancers, so this finding appears to be a general phenomenon.

For most cancers, clinical staging is ordinarily done at the time of diagnosis whether or not a CEA measurement is available. The question then arises, does the CEA level convey prognostic information over and above what is available after staging? That is, does the CEA level add information or only duplicate information already in hand? Most studies of CEA levels and prognosis have not been analyzed in a way that would answer this question. However, for colorectal cancer the evidence appears to be

Table 2. Plasma Carcinoembryonic Antigen (CEA) Concentration According to Stage of Colorectal Carcinoma*

	Dukes Stage			
	A	B	C	D
Patients, *n*	58	51	63	31
CEA concentration, %				
0-2.5 ng/mL	72	55	25	16
2.6-5.0 ng/mL	25	20	30	19
5.1-10.0 ng/mL	3	10	14	3
10.1-20.0 ng/mL	0	15	13	19
> 20.0 ng/mL	0	0	18	43

* Data from Wanebo and colleagues (25), adapted by Ladenson and McDonald (4).

sufficient to consider the CEA antigen level a marker of prognosis that is partly independent of clinical stage (33, 34, 39). The same is true for breast cancer (35). There is not enough reported experience to decide just how much new information CEA levels convey after taking stage into account, but apparently its contribution is small. The independence of CEA levels to stage for other tumors has not been sufficiently examined.

When patients are found to have cancer, they are generally offered the most efficacious treatment available, whatever their CEA level. It could be argued that predicting the course of disease with greater precision, without improving the clinician's ability to alter that course, is not useful. Worse, knowledge of a bad prognosis might do more harm than good by removing hope of cure earlier than that would ordinarily occur. However, informing patients of the expected course of their disease has been a traditional responsibility of physicians. If used wisely, knowledge of CEA levels might result in more good than harm.

In summary, determining the circulating CEA concentration at the time of diagnosis provides information about prognosis for many cancers. For colorectal and breast cancer, and perhaps for others, this information may be in addition to that available through staging. Although this information may not lead directly to decreased morbidity and mortality, assigning a prognosis more precisely can, by itself, be helpful in the care of patients.

Monitoring

A rise in the blood CEA concentration in a patient after apparently successful treatment for cancer has been shown repeatedly to signal a recurrence of the tumor. This finding has been shown for a variety of tumors.

The best evidence is for colorectal cancer. After apparently complete surgical resection of colorectal cancer, the blood CEA concentration, if elevated before surgery, falls to normal levels in nearly all patients (40). The fall usually occurs within 1 month but sometimes takes up to 4 months (41). If levels do not fall to the normal range, an incomplete resection is likely. In one series, only 6 of 90 patients (7%) with colorectal cancer and elevated CEA levels did not have a fall in antigen level to below 20 ng/mL after surgery, and all 6 patients subsequently had a recurrence of tumor (40).

After the initial fall, it is not uncommon for transient, small elevations in CEA levels to occur in the absence of recurrent tumor. However, a sustained and progressive rise in levels is strong evidence for recurrence. This rise has been variously defined as any elevation above a certain level (for example, 10 ng/mL) (42), a number of consecutive measurements above a level, or the slope of the rise (for example, > 5% per month) (43). By such criteria, CEA monitoring apparently identifies recurrence of tumor with a sensitivity of about 80%; sensitivity has been reported to be as high as 89% and as low as 17%. Specificity of CEA levels for recurrence is apparently about 70%, with a range in various reports of 34% to 91%. It is uncertain why these ranges for sensitivity and specificity are so broad, but apparently the differences are related to different definitions of rise, initial stage of disease, and duration of follow-up. The higher values seem more valid. The lead time between detection of recurrent tumor by CEA assay and discovery by ordinary clinical means is commonly several months, but there are reports of lead times in individual patients of as long as 1 to 2 years.

When monitoring patients with colorectal surgery, the usual interval between CEA determinations is 3 months. The relative utility of various intervals has not been studied. Presumably, the choice of 3 months reflects a trade-off between the potential value of early detection of recurrence and the inefficiency of too-frequent monitoring.

Of what value to patients is early detection of recurrent cancer? Ordinarily, we do not consider recurrent cancer of the colon, breast, or lung any more curable when discovered early than when found late. Moreover, treatment need not be instituted early for palliation if the patient does not yet have symptoms.

For colorectal cancer, it has been hypothesized that early detection of recurrence by means of CEA monitoring might lead to cure in some patients. This hypothesis has been tested in several large clinical trials (44). After apparently complete resection, patients were monitored at approximately 3-month intervals; if the CEA level rose, second-look surgery was done in hopes that if a recurrence were found it would be resectable and that the second resection would result in cure. None of these trials included a control group not monitored for the antigen.

Short-term results have been reported for several of these trials, but long-term results are not yet available. However, sufficient information is available to place some limits on what can be accomplished by second-look surgery for colorectal cancer prompted by CEA monitoring (Figure 3). Although a rising CEA level usually marks recurrence of tumor, about half of second-look operations do not disclose resectable tumor, and in the best case only 3% of all patients monitored might be cured by the protocol. The potential for saving lives must be weighed against the possibilities for harm when patients without symptoms are told earlier that their disease has recurred but there is no effective treatment. The financial cost per resectable tumor is estimated to be $24 779 (45).

The poor performance of CEA monitoring in detecting resectable cancer recurrences may result in part from the test's poor performance in purely local disease. In one

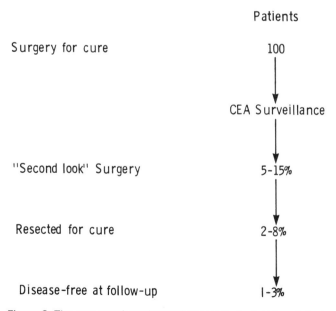

Figure 3. The cure rate for colorectal cancer that might be attributed to postoperative monitoring of carcinoembryonic antigen (*CEA*) levels and second-look surgery (25, 32, 44). Although often not specified, the median follow-up appears to be a few years in most series.

study, "sensitivity of the carcinoembryonic antigen test was good for metastatic recurrent disease, fairly good for residual neoplastic disease, but insufficient for local recurrence" (46).

There was no significant difference in disease-free interval or survival between the two treatment groups (47). Therefore, the value of using serial CEA determinations to monitor patients with colorectal cancer after apparently complete resection, and then responding to elevations in levels by second-look surgery or chemotherapy is currently uncertain. This management strategy should be considered experimental, and not ordinary, patient care.

Early chemotherapy prompted by CEA monitoring has been tried. A randomized controlled trial has compared chemotherapy, with fluorouracil and semustine, begun after relatively early detection of recurrence of colonic cancer by CEA measurement to treatment with the same drug regimen begun only when there were clinical indications.

The CEA level has been used as a marker of response to treatment and of recurrence for other cancers. Serial measurements of antigen levels have been shown to rise and fall with extent of disease for breast (48) and lung cancers (49). However, there is no evidence that this information leads to effective treatment of these tumors if they recur. Carcinoembryonic antigen has not been found useful in monitoring for various other tumors, including hepatocellular, urothelial, and gynecologic cancers.

Monitoring CEA levels may be useful as an adjunct to the management of patients with gastrointestinal, breast, and lung tumors that are known to be metastatic and that are being managed by chemotherapy or radiotherapy. If cancer can be evaluated by other means—for example, metastases to the skin or lung—there is no need for a less accurate measure like CEA. However, not uncommonly, response to treatment cannot be measured directly. Under these circumstances, CEA levels may be the only way of estimating the extent of disease. Knowing the presence or absence of response in individual patients may be useful because it can lead to more precise tailoring of therapy and hence better results.

Summary

Carcinoembryonic antigen, which is often found in abnormally high concentrations in the plasma of patients with cancer, has been suggested to be of practical value in detecting cancer among persons without complaints, in diagnosing cancer when it is suspected, in assigning a more precise prognosis at the time of diagnosis, and in monitoring the effects of treatment. Now, almost 20 years after this antigen was first described, there is sufficient evidence to weigh these assertions. The recommended uses based on these considerations are summarized in Table 3 .

Carcinoembryonic antigen is not useful for detecting cancer when the disease is not suspected, mainly because the sensitivity and specificity of CEA levels are not high enough, particularly for the detection of early cancer, and because the prevalence of undetected cancer is low in unselected populations. As a result, many cancers would

Table 3. Clinical Usefulness of Carcinoembryonic Antigen in the Management of Colorectal Cancer

Potential Use	Usefulness	Rationale
Screening	Not useful	Sensitivity and specificity are not high enough and are lowest in early stages of disease.
Diagnosis	Limited value	Serum levels alone cannot establish the diagnosis. They may be useful, in conjunction with findings of other noninvasive tests, in deciding how actively to pursue a diagnostic work-up for colorectal cancer.
Prognosis	Limited value	Serum levels predict recurrence of colorectal cancer independently of stage, but this information cannot be used to improve prognosis.
Monitoring after surgery	Limited value	Serum levels can detect recurrence of colorectal cancer after surgery earlier than other methods, but this information does not increase the opportunity for effective therapeutic interventions in most patients.

not be detected by CEA assays and many abnormal test results would turn out not to represent cancer after more careful diagnostic evaluation.

The antigen is also not useful, when used alone, for definitively diagnosing or ruling out cancer. The reasons are similar to those for detecting unsuspected cancer. Also, the requirements for accuracy of diagnostic tests for cancer when used alone are much more stringent than for screening. However, CEA assays may make a useful contribution to the diagnostic process, prior to a definitive conclusion, when used in conjunction with other tests.

Levels of CEA at the time of diagnosis are clearly related to prognosis. For the most part, this is because the level is related to the extent of disease, which would ordinarily be assessed in any case. However, some of the information contributed by CEA monitoring is in addition to that of clinical stage. The value of assigning a more precise prognosis by means of CEA assay depends on whether a more effective treatment can be selected; in most cases one cannot. The value also depends on whether information about a bad prognosis is used humanely.

Finally, the CEA level is a relatively accurate marker of the extent of cancer, and so it can be used to monitor patients for response to treatment or for recurrence. When the cancer is not otherwise evaluable, CEA assay may be the only available test for this purpose. Monitoring CEA levels is justified only if selection of therapy is contingent on this information, as it may be with some chemotherapy regimens.

References

1. GOLD P, FREEDMAN SO. Demonstration of tumor-specific antigens in human colonic carcinomata by immunological tolerance and absorption techniques. *J Exp Med.* 1965;**121**:439-62.
2. BEATTY JD, TERZ JJ. Value of carcinoembryonic antigen in clinical medicine. *Prog Clin Cancer.* 1982;**8**:9-29.
3. COOPER EH, O'QUIGLEY J. Colorectal cancer: biochemical markers. *Recent Results Cancer Res.* 1982;**83**:67-76.
4. LADENSON JH, McDONALD JM, LANDT M, SCHWARTZ MK. Colorectal carcinoma and carcinoembryonic antigen (CEA). *Clinc Chem.* 1980;**26**:1213-20.
5. Proceedings of the First International Conference on the Clinical Use of Carcinoembryonic Antigen, June 1-3, 1977, Lexington, Kentucky. *Cancer.* 1978;**42**(suppl):1397-659.

6. GOLDENBERG DM. Carcinoembryonic antigen: its role as a marker in the management of cancer: A National Institutes of Health Consensus Development Conference. *Ann Intern Med.* 1981;**94**:407-9.

7. NEVILLE AM. Carcinoembryonic antigen: its role as a marker in the management of cancer: summary of an NIH consensus statement. *Br Med J [Clin Res].* 1981;**282**:373-5.

8. VEST SL, ROCHE JK. Carcinoembryonic antigen: physician attitudes, patterns of use, and impact upon patient care. *Dig Dis Sci.* 1982;**27**:289-96.

9. SHUSTER J, FREEDMAN SO, GOLD P. Oncofetal antigens: increasing the specificity of the CEA radioimmunoassay. *Am J Clin Pathol.* 1977;**68**(5 suppl):679-87.

10. DIERKSHEIDE WC. Precautions in testing for carcinoembryonic antigen [Letter]. *JAMA.* 1981;**246**:1547.

11. LOEWENSTEIN MS, KUPCHIK HZ, ZAMCHECK N. Disparity between CEA-Roche "indirect" and "direct" carcinoembryonic antigen values: clinical relevance [Letter]. *N Engl J Med.* 1976;**294**:1123.

12. TAYLOR RN, FULFORD KM, HUONG AY. Results of a nationwide proficiency test for carcinoembryonic antigen. *J Clin Microbiol.* 1977;**5**:433-8.

13. FLEISHER M, NISSELBAUM JS, LOFTIN L, SMITH C, SCHWARTZ MK. Roche RIA and Abbott EIA carcinoembryonic antigen assays compared. *Clin Chem.* 1984;**30**:200-5.

14. LAVIN PT, ZAMCHECK N, HOLYOKE ED. A carcinoembryonic antigen standardization experiment for the conduct of multi-institutional clinical trials: Gastrointestinal Tumor Study Group. *Cancer Treat Rep.* 1979;**63**:2031-3.

15. MEEKER WR JR. The use and abuse of CEA test in clinical practice. *Cancer.* 1978;**41**:854-62.

16. HERBETH B, BAGREL A. A study of factors influencing plasma CEA levels in an unselected population. *Oncodev Biol Med.* 1980;**1**:191-8.

17. TABOR E, GERETY RJ, NEEDY CF, ELISBERG BL, COLON AR, JONES R. Carcinoembryonic antigen levels in asymptomatic adolescents. *Eur J Cancer.* 1981;**17**:257-8.

18. CLARKE C, HINE KR, DYKES PW, WHITEHEAD TP, WHITFIELD AGW. Carcinoembryonic antigen and smoking. *J R Coll Physicians Lond.* 1980;**14**:227-8.

19. BEAUDONNET A, GOUNON G, PICHOT J, REVENANT MC. Sex- and age-related influences on carcinoembryonic antigen in blood [Letter]. *Clin Chem.* 1981;**27**:771.

20. HAINES AP, LEVIN AG, FRITSCHE HA. Ethnic-group differences in serum levels of carcinoembryonic antigen [Letter]. *Lancet.* 1979;**2**:969.

21. BERARDI RS, RUIZ R, BECKNELL WE JR, KEONIN Y. Does advanced age limit the usefulness of CEA assays? *Geriatrics.* 1977;**32**:86-8.

22. TOUITOU Y, PROUST J, KLINGER E, NAKACHE JP, HUARD D, SACHET A. Cumulative effects of age and pathology on plasma carcinoembryonic antigen in an unselected elderly population. *Eur J Cancer Clin Oncol.* 1984;**20**:369-74.

23. CANADIAN TASK FORCE ON THE PERIODIC HEALTH EXAMINATION. The periodic health examination. *Can Med Assoc J.* 1979;**121**:1193-254.

24. FLETCHER SW, DAUPHINEE WD. Should colorectal carcinoma be sought in periodic health examinations? An approach to the evidence. *Clin Invest Med.* 1981;**4**:23-31.

25. WANEBO HJ, RAO B, PINSKY CM, et al. Preoperative carcinoembryonic antigen level as a prognostic indicator in colorectal cancer. *N Engl J Med.* 1978;**299**:448-51.

26. MOLOFSKY LC, HAYASHI SJ. Proctosigmoidoscopy as a routine part of a multiphasic program. *Am J Med Sci.* 1958;**235**:628-31.

27. GREEGOR DH. Detection of silent colon cancer in routine examination. *CA.* 1969;**19**:330-7.

28. WILLIAMS RR, MCINTIRE KR, WALDMANN TA, et al. Tumor-associated antigen levels (carcinoembryonic antigen, human chorionic gonad-

otropin and alpha-fetoprotein) antedating the diagnosis of cancer in the Framingham study. *J Natl Cancer Inst.* 1977;**58**:1547-51.

29. COOPER MJ, MACKIE CR, SKINNER DB, MOOSSA AR. A reappraisal of the value of carcinoembryonic antigen in the management of patients with various neoplasms. *Br J Surg.* 1979;**66**:120-3.
30. LOEWENSTEIN MS, ZAMCHECK N. Carcinoembryonic antigen and the liver. *Gastroenterology.* 1977;**72**:161-6.
31. BULLEN AW, LOSOWSKY MS, CARTER S, PATEL S, NEVILLE AM. Diagnostic usefulness of plasma carcinoembryonic antigen levels in acute and chronic liver disease. *Gastroenterology.* 1977;**73**(4 pt 1):673-8.
32. STEELE G JR, ELLENBERG S, RAMMING K, et al. CEA monitoring among patients in multi-institutional adjuvant G.I. therapy protocols. *Ann Surg.* 1982;**196**:162-9.
33. KOHLER JP, SIMONOWITZ D, PALOYAN D. Preoperative CEA level: a prognostic test in patients with colorectal carcinoma. *Am Surg.* 1980;**46**:449-52.
34. LAVIN PT, DAY J, HOLYOKE ED, MITTELMAN A, CHU TM. A statistical evaluation of baseline and follow-up carcinoembryonic antigen in patients with resectable colorectal carcinoma. *Cancer.* 1981;**47**:823-6.
35. MYERS RE, SUTHERLAND DJA, MEAKIN JW, MALKIN DG, KELLEN JA, MALKIN A. Prognostic value of postoperative blood levels of carcinoembryonic antigen (CEA) in breast cancer. *Recent Results Cancer Res.* 1979;**67**:26-32.
36. STAAB HJ, ANDERER FA, BRÜMMENDORF T, HORNUNG A, FISCHER R. Prognostic value of preoperative serum CEA level compared to clinical staging: II. Stomach cancer. *Br J Cancer.* 1982;**45**:718-27.
37. STOKES TC, STEVENS JFS, LONG P, LOCKEY E, MILLER AL. Preoperative carcinoembryonic antigen and survival after resection of lung cancer. *Br J Dis Chest.* 1980;**74**:390-4.
38. CONCANNON JP, DALBOW MH, HODGSON SE, et al. Prognostic value of preoperative carcinoembryonic antigen (CEA) plasma levels in patients with bronchogenic carcinoma. *Cancer.* 1978;**42**(3 suppl):1477-83.
39. WOLMARK N, FISHER B, WIEAND HS, et al. The prognostic significance of preoperative carcinoembryonic antigen levels in colorectal cancer: results from NSABP (National Surgical Adjuvant Breast and Bowel Project) clinical trials. *Ann Surg.* 1984;**199**:375-82.
40. ARNAUD JP, KOEHL C, ADLOFF M. Carcinoembryonic antigen (CEA) in diagnosis and prognosis of colorectal carcinoma. *Dis Colon Rectum.* 1980;**23**:141-4.
41. MACH JP, VIENNY H, JAEGER P, HALDEMANN B, EGELY R, PETTAVEL J. Long-term follow-up of colorectal carcinoma patients by repeated CEA radioimmunoassay. *Cancer.* 1978;**42**(3 suppl):1439-47.
42. KOCH M, WASHER G, GAEDKE H, MCPHERSON TA. Carcinoembryonic antigen: usefulness as a postsurgical method in the detection of recurrence in Dukes stages B2 and C colorectal cancers. *JNCI.* 1982;**69**:813-5.
43. BOEY J, CHEUNG HC, LAI CK, WONG J. A prospective evaluation of serum carcinoembryonic antigen (CEA) levels in the management of colorectal carcinoma. *World J Surg.* 1984;**8**:279-86.
44. MARTIN EW JR, COOPERMAN M, CAREY LC, MINTON JP. Sixty second-look procedures indicated primarily by rise in serial carcinoembryonic antigen. *J Surg Res.* 1980;**28**:389-94.
45. SANDLER RS, FREUND DA, HERBST CA JR, SANDLER DP. Cost effectiveness of postoperative carcinoembryonic antigen monitoring in colorectal cancer. *Cancer.* 1984;**53**:193-8.
46. FUCINI C, TOMMASI MS, CARDONA G, MALATANTIS G, PANICHI S, BETTINI U. Limitations of CEA monitoring as a guide to second-look surgery in colorectal cancer follow-up. *Tumori.* 1983;**69**:359-64.
47. HINE KR, DYKES PW. Prospective randomised trial of early cytotoxic therapy for recurrent colorectal carcinoma detected by serum CEA. *Gut.* 1984;**25**:682-8.

48. LAMERZ R. Serial carcinoembryonic antigen (CEA) determinations in the management of metastic breast cancer. *Oncodev Bio Med.* 1980;**1:**123-35.
49. GOSLIN RH, SKARIN AT, ZAMCHECK N. Carcinoembryonic antigen: a useful monitor of therapy of small cell lung cancer. *JAMA.* 1981;**246:**2173-6.

Biochemical Profiles

Applications in Ambulatory Screening and Preadmission Testing of Adults

RANDALL D. CEBUL, M.D.; and J. ROBERT BECK, M.D.

Convenience and the promise of more information at lower cost have led to the wide and routine use of biochemical profiles. Socioeconomic and political forces, however, have made these profiles the subject of considerable debate during the past 2 decades. In this article, we review the evidence and provide recommendations about the routine use of biochemical profiles for adult patients in the settings of ambulatory care screening and preadmission testing. By biochemical profile, we mean a general battery of 12 or more biochemical tests measured on large-volume, automated instruments. We do not address panel testing directed primarily at individual organ systems, such as batteries related to liver or immunologic status. By screening, we mean efforts to detect disease in unselected populations of asymptomatic persons; case-finding (efforts to detect disease in patients seen for unrelated symptoms or diseases [1]) is addressed only tangentially. Finally, routine refers to a policy, of an institution or individual physician, of performing biochemical profiles without regard to the clinical evidence in an individual patient; that is, routine testing is done on all patients in the given setting (ambulatory or preadmission).

A Brief Historical Perspective

Policies and practice with regard to biochemical pro-

► This chapter was originally published in *Annals of Internal Medicine*. 1987; **106**:403-13.

files have been inextricably linked to sociologic, medical, and technologic changes over the past few decades. The roots of testing with biochemical profiles are found in the origins of "multiphasic screening" as a means of detecting disease before symptoms occur (2). First applied to a health survey among industrial employees in San Jose, California, in 1949, multiphasic screening was endorsed early by proponents of health maintenance organizations and quickly became politicized (2). During the 1960s, the incorporation of the biochemical profile as part of multiphasic screening was influenced by the general affluence of American society, social changes that viewed medical care as a right, and the advent of widely available computer technology. In 1966 Collen (3) noted: "The advent of automation and computers may introduce a new era of preventive medicine." And in 1970 Garfield (4) wrote: "Although no long-term evidence exists that the course of disease is influenced by multiphasic health testing, this is largely irrelevant. Such programs are essential for other very important reasons. The . . . concept of medical care as a right . . . is creating a demand for periodic health checkups and health appraisals."

Social and economic changes in American society during the mid- and late 1970s were accompanied by equally strident reappraisals of biochemical profiles and multiphasic screening. The yield of biochemical profiles, in terms of disease detection that materially improved patient health, was found to be very low in various testing situations. Blame for the development and promulgation of these profiles was variably placed on the dehumanizing influence of computers, the for-profit firms that assembled the packages without regard to their medical justification, and the clinical chemists who were said to have "remarkable professional myopia [for having] failed to accept responsibility for evaluating whether the programs in which they are engaged are of benefit to patients" (5, 6).

Social and economic forces have been complex during the past decade. Favoring the use of biochemical profiles have been the patients' rights and consumers' groups, with their high expectations of the health care system. Many authors have claimed that the malpractice crisis of the mid-1970s further increased the use of diagnostic tests for "defensive" purposes (7, 8). Finally, recent changes in health care reimbursement have stimulated increased use of office-based laboratory testing (the effects of which are largely unstudied) and an intense interest in examining the "true costs" and consequences of such practices as multiphasic screening, including the use of biochemical profiles. The inclusion of the "induced costs" of pursuing falsely abnormal test results, for example, makes the use of biochemical profiles far more costly than one might assume at first glance (9, 10). Reimbursement of office-based testing has raised issues of substandard quality control and possible overuse of diagnostic tests because of financial incentives to the practitioner (11). It is in this evolving milieu that the physician must decide when to order a biochemical profile and how to act on its results.

A Sample Profile and Associated Conditions

Several biochemical profiles exist, from a relatively simple 6-test combination to batteries of 20 or more component tests. Commonly used profiles incorporate 12 or 20 tests. Table 1 identifies a sample 12-test battery to be considered in detail for the purposes of this paper. Table 1 also identifies some medical conditions associated with abnormal findings of the component tests. The list of associated conditions, although not all-inclusive, illustrates the breadth of pathophysiologic states that might be considered by the clinician when confronted with abnormalities in one or more biochemical tests. However, most of the listed conditions are uncommon; they are seldom found in patients without clinical signs and symptoms; and with few exceptions, their presence is only weakly indicated by abnormalities of the associated biochemical marker. For example, although an elevated serum level of lactate dehydrogenase is associated with several conditions, these conditions are seldom seen in a person presumed to be free of disease after a careful history and physical examination, and asymptomatic increases in the lactate dehydrogenase level are only weakly predictive of specific underlying disease.

Although specificity of prediction is a desirable feature of a diagnostic test, a test's sensitivity, or detection rate, probably is more important in screening. By this measure, some tests of the sample profile are better than others. For example, the total serum protein level is not very

Table 1. A Sample Twelve-Factor Biochemical Profile and Illustrative Associated Conditions

Test and Abnormal Values	Illustrative Associated Conditions
Calcium	
Increased	Metabolic disease (for example, hyperparathyroidism), malignancy, sarcoidosis, other bone disease (for example, Paget's disease)
Decreased	Hypoparathyroidism, malabsorption, renal failure, osteomalacia, pancreatitis
Glucose	
Increased	Diabetes mellitus, glucagonoma, mineralocorticoid excess (many causes), hyperthyroidism
Blood urea nitrogen	
Increased	Primary renal disease (for example, medullary cystic kidney, hereditary nephritis), secondary renal disease (for example, infectious, immunologic, vascular, metabolic, obstructive), prerenal azotemia
Sodium	
Increased	Mineralocorticoid excess (many causes), heat stroke, diabetes insipidus, cerebral tumor or thromboembolism
Decreased	Volume depletion (many causes), mineralocorticoid deficiency (many causes), antidiuretic hormone excess (many causes)
Potassium	
Increased	Renal failure, metabolic acidosis (many causes), mineralocorticoid deficiency or renal unresponsive states (several causes)
Decreased	Mineralocorticoid excess (many causes)
Uric acid	
Increased	Gout, renal failure (many causes), myeloproliferative disorders, leukemia
Total protein	
Increased	Systemic infection (for example, tuberculosis), systemic inflammation (for example, collagen vascular disease), malignancy (for example, lymphoma, myeloma), liver disease (many causes in addition to those above)
Albumin	
Decreased	Malnutrition, nephrotic syndrome (many causes), protein-losing enteropathies (many causes), severe liver disease (many causes)

Table 1. (Continued)

Test and Abnormal Values	Illustrative Associated Conditions
Cholesterol	
Increased	Primary (for example, familial) and secondary hypercholesterolemia (for example, hypothyroidism, nephrotic syndrome, hepatitis)
Decreased	Hyperthyroidism, malabsorption, liver disease (many causes)
AST*	
Increased	Hepatocellular inflammation (many causes), cardiac inflammation (for example, infarction, myocarditis, pericarditis), skeletal muscle inflammation (for example, virus infection, polymyositis)
LDH*	
Increased	Hemolysis, thromboembolism, systemic infection or inflammation, malignancy
Alkaline phosphatase	
Increased	Liver disease (many causes), bone disease (many causes)

* AST = aspartate aminotransferase; LDH = lactate dehydrogenase.

sensitive for any of the conditions with which it is associated, but increased levels of serum cholesterol or glucose are virtually always detected in the presence of familial hypercholesterolemia or diabetes millitus, respectively.

Current Technology

Biochemical profiles most commonly are measured on large-volume, automated instruments that perform an entire repertoire of tests. By this approach, the labor involved in sample preparation is not duplicated. Typically, the six commonest clinical chemistry tests represent half of a laboratory's workload, and the addition of 14 more tests makes up another 40%. Recent technologic development has focused on the specialized automated instruments for routine chemistry testing that provide results with accuracies similar to benchmark procedures (12).

Continuous flow instruments were the first machines devoted to automated biochemical screening. These instruments pump bulk reagent continuously through tubing to form a stream, and they pump serum samples continuously into that stream. The samples are segmented by air bubbles to minimize carryover between specimens, and sample and reagent proportions are controlled by flow rates. For some analytes (component tests) to be measurable in these systems, modifications of standard chemical procedures have been necessary, leading to the belief that continuous flow procedures are less accurate than manual methods.

Contemporary automated chemistry instruments compartmentalize each sample in its own cuvette. Aliquots are taken from the sample chamber for analysis. The most sophisticated of these machines permit a specific menu of tests to be run on each sample, so as to minimize reagent and sample consumption. Such instruments permit kinetic enzymatic assays and bichromatic measurements (that is, two wavelengths), features found more commonly in manual reference methods. As a result, the precision of discrete analyzers approaches that of reference methods for many analytes (12).

By convention, laboratory precision is expressed as the coefficient of variation for a particular method of analyzing a biochemical. In essence, this coefficient measures the amount of variability in results on repeated determinations for a given aliquot, with lower values indicating higher precision. It is calculated by dividing the standard deviation of values by the average value for a given aliquot. Although this standard of comparison has been challenged (13), it remains the accepted means by which different analytic methods and laboratories are evaluated.

A SAMPLE TWELVE-TEST PANEL

Each test in the sample 12-test biochemical profile is reviewed briefly here, in terms of methods for automated analysis and corresponding within-laboratory precision. Coefficients of variation were obtained from a current reference textbook (14).

Calcium is measured in discrete-sample analyzers by spectrophotometry of Ca^{2+} complexes, commonly with *o*-cresolphthalein. The coefficient of variation is 50% greater than with manual atomic absorption methods at low serum calcium levels (78 mg/L) but comparable at high levels.

Glucose is measured either spectrophotometrically through nicotinamide adenine dinucleotide phosphate (NADP) reduction after hexokinase treatment, or after oxidation with glucose oxidase followed by a peroxidase indicator reaction. Both methods are easily automated, and their results agree closely with proposed reference standards.

Urea nitrogen is detected through a coupled urease-glutamate dehydrogenase reaction, which is automated relatively easily. Flow machines use a standard colorimetric procedure with diacetyl monoxime. Coefficients of variation are equivalent.

Sodium and potassium, univalent cations, are measured manually by flame atomic emission spectroscopy. Sensitive indirect methods use ion-selective electrodes; these are available on automated instruments and have the same coefficients of variation as flame methods.

Uric acid can be measured by phosphotungstic acid reduction or by an enzymatic method using uricase. Both can be adapted to discrete-sample automated analyzers, and both have the same performance characteristics.

Albumin is measured colorimetrically with bromocresol green or bromocresol purple dyes. The coefficient of variation of 2.2% is equivalent to that of reference methods. A biuret reagent method for measuring total protein, used most commonly in automated instruments, forms the basis for a proposed standard.

Cholesterol determinations have been adapted to automated biochemical analyzers through use of a one-step enzymatic endpoint method and an indicator dye such as 4-aminophenanzone. This accurate method achieves a coefficient of variation of 6%, similar to that of the classic reference method of Abell.

The activity of aspartate aminotransferase (AST, formerly serum glutamic-oxaloacetic transaminase or SGOT) is measured through the enzymatic reaction itself: aspartic acid and alpha-ketoglutarate are converted to glutamic acid and oxaloacetate. The oxaloacetate moiety then is either coupled to a dye or treated enzymatically with malate dehydrogenase to form a stable chromophore. All of these procedures can be automated and are essentially equivalent in precision.

Lactate dehydrogenase is measured by its typical reaction: the kinetic reversible conversion of pyruvate to lactate. This reference method also is readily automated and has a coefficient of variation of 3%.

Alkaline phosphatase can be measured by five automated methods that use fluorescent or spectrophotometric assays. Their coefficients of variation average around 5%. The best reference method has a coefficient of 2% for alkaline phosphatase values in the normal range.

CONCLUSION

Thus, the precision of modern discrete-sample analyzers is virtually indistinguishable from the precision of reference methods. On the other hand, automated methods tend to be more susceptible to errors from interfering substances and to technical effects such as carryover (trace amounts of a previous sample remaining in the instrument at the next sample analysis). Nevertheless, in 1986, a result from an automated biochemical profile is likely to be the same as the result for an analyte measured manually.

Biochemical Profiles in Two Settings: Previous Recommendations and Unresolved Issues

AMBULATORY CARE SCREENING

Three premises underlie the development of periodic screening procedures: that asymptomatic adults can harbor organic disease; that periodic screening can detect such disease at an early stage; and that early discovery of disease can lead to its arrest, reversal, or cure and thereby reduce morbidity and mortality (15). General criteria for the evaluation of screening procedures are identified in Table 2. Criteria similar to these have been applied to the relevant medical literature by two panels of experts to formulate screening recommendations (1, 16). The Canadian Task Force on the Periodic Health Examination (1) considered three sets of criteria in evaluating specific screening procedures: the risks and benefits; the sensitivity, specificity, and predictive value; and the safety, simplicity, cost, and acceptability to the patient. Of 128 potentially preventable conditions that were identified, 78 were considered for more detailed study by the Task Force. The impact of the particular condition on the individual person, and on society, was analyzed in determining the "current burden of suffering" of each condition. By this process, rare, untreatable, or self-limited conditions were eliminated from consideration. Similar factors were considered by the Medical Practice Committee of

Table 2. Criteria for Evaluating the Usefulness of Diagnostic Screening Tests

Will the tests detect disease that would otherwise remain undetected until later in time?
  What are the tests' risks, sensitivity, specificity, cost, and patient acceptability?
  How does the tests' diagnostic value compare with unaided clinical judgment?
Will earlier disease detection have a favorable impact on patient status?
  What is the risk, cost, efficacy, and effectiveness of therapy at an earlier stage of disease?
  How will earlier diagnosis affect the patient's psychological well-being?
What are the costs of testing that results from diagnostic misclassification?
  What are the induced costs and risks of further diagnostic evaluation?
  What are the induced costs and risks of mistreatment?
  What are the nonmedical consequences of diagnostic "labeling"?
Do the potential benefits of testing outweigh the costs and risks?
  What is the current societal "burden of suffering" related to the targeted diseases?
  What is the potential impact of testing on the individual person?

the American College of Physicians (16) in its recommendations and by Frame and Carlson (17) in their critical review of periodic screening practices.

Neither the Canadian (1) nor the American commission (16) recommended the use of biochemical profiles for screening purposes. Of the individual components of the profile that might prove useful, only the serum cholesterol test was recommended by both commissions. Lest this conclusion be interpreted as an unqualified indictment of biochemical profiles, it should be noted that the commissions' purpose was not to analyze the specific profiles or their component tests. Furthermore, because the commissions' evaluations began by identifying specific diseases, which did not include all conditions potentially detectable by components of the biochemical profile, the resulting recommendations may have understated the potential value of profile testing. Evidence that bears more specifically on the yield and consequences of profile testing are described later (*see* Biochemical Profiles: Evidence and Recommendations).

PREADMISSION TESTING

Defined as the scheduling of certain diagnostic tests before elective admission to the hospital, preadmission testing may be done routinely or selectively. Selective testing refers to the selection and ordering of particular tests for particular patients or groups of patients (for example, all patients admitted to surgical or medical services). The primary rationale for preadmission testing has been its potential ability to minimize the hospital stay of these patients by completing "all or nearly all of the diagnostic aspects of the patient's care prior to admission" (18). In focusing on enhanced hospital efficiency and reduced length of stay, preadmission testing programs undoubtedly will undergo increased scrutiny in the current era of prospective reimbursement for hospitalization.

As one part of a preadmission testing program, use of biochemical profiles already has been subjected to extensive study in North America and elsewhere (*see* Biochemical Profiles: Evidence and Recommendations). To date, however, no guidelines or recommendations have been published about the use of biochemical profiles in preadmission testing. Recommendations from the Medical Necessity Project of the American College of Physicians and Blue Cross-Blue Shield (19) state that "no diagnostic tests, including . . . biochemical blood screen[ing] . . . should be required as routine procedures for patients admitted to a hospital." The rationale for this position was that diagnostic testing should complement, not replace, a careful history taking and physical examination and that the injudicious use of the diagnostic laboratory greatly affects the cost of medical care. "The burden of proof " of the need for routine preadmission testing, the recommendation states, "rests on the physician who orders it."

Testing on admission to the hospital shares some of the features of ambulatory care screening but also has some distinct features. Specifically, assessment of biochemical profiles in the preadmission setting raises five considerations: the prevalence of unsuspected illness in those patients admitted to the hospital (as compared with the prevalence among asymptomatic persons seeking medical attention in the ambulatory care setting); the yield of unanticipated diagnoses that materially alter patient management at the hospital; the impact of altered patient management on patient health among different patient groups (for example, surgical or medical patients); the effect of preadmission testing on use of in-hospital diagnostic services; and the effect of preadmission testing on overall length of hospital stay and hospital costs. The first three factors take a clinical perspective, focusing on conditions in which early detection would benefit the patient, whereas the last two focus on the effect of preadmission testing on efficient resource utilization in the hospital.

Statistical Principles of Biochemical Profile Interpretation
"NORMAL" RESULTS AND MULTIPLE TESTS

"Normal" results for biochemical tests commonly are defined as the mean value for the test in a population of presumably nondiseased persons, plus or minus 2 SD. Although it has been argued that this definition (6) is a misapplication of statistical sampling theory (6), its practical consequence is to mislabel 5% of results from normal persons as abnormal, by definition; that is, if we accept this definition of "normal," the specificity of each test in a biochemical profile can be no greater than 95%.

The implication of this definition for the results of multiple tests done simultaneously is dramatic. If we assume that each test in the battery is independent of the others, then the probability that a completely normal person will have normal results on all n tests is $(0.95)^n$. Thus, as the number of laboratory tests in the biochemical profile increases, the likelihood that a healthy person will be classified as normal rapidly diminishes (Table 3). For the healthy person subjected to a profile with 12 tests, the

Table 3. The Probability That a Healthy Person Will Have Normal Results on All Tests in a Biochemical Profile

Number of Tests	Probability That All Tests Will Be Normal
	%
1	95
6	74
12	54
20	36
100	0.6

probability that all 12 results will be "normal" is only 54%.

Thus, sources of error in diagnostic classification include analytical imprecision (*see* Current Technology) as well as statistical assumptions in defining the "normal range," the latter source of error being magnified in direct proportion to the number of tests being done. Biologic variability further complicates the problem of accurate diagnosis. Biologic sources of variability include within-person and between-person differences in demographics, diet, drugs, posture (for example, serum iron level), and coexisting illnesses (20, 21). These factors differentially influence the results of the different component tests in a biochemical profile, making the interpretation of an unexpectedly abnormal test result especially problematic.

INTRA-INDIVIDUAL BIOLOGIC VARIABILITY: REGRESSION TO THE MEAN

An important biologic phenomenon known as regression to the mean suggests that because of biologic variation of physiologic processes, extreme values of a parameter are likely to become less extreme on repeated measurement. Thus, an abnormal test result from a presumably normal person is likely to be normal, or at least less abnormal, when measured a second time (6). Although this phenomenon is observed in many biologic measurements, it is largely ignored or explained by other, usually causal, mechanisms. With regard to biochemical profile results, the conflicting values generally are ascribed to laboratory error (6).

The implications of this phenomenon for the interpretation of test profiles are clear. In general, unexpectedly abnormal results will "regress toward the mean" on repeated measurement. The premature initiation of further evaluation generally will lead to a diagnostic "blind alley," in addition to generating unnecessary cost and risk to the patient. If therapy is begun hastily after the initial abnormality, the clinician may derive false assurance that appropriate treatment was begun when subsequent tests reveal more "normal" values.

EFFECT OF DISEASE PREVALENCE ON THE POST-TEST PROBABILITY OF DISEASE

The probability of a disease after an abnormal test result depends highly on test sensitivity, test specificity, and

Table 4. Post-test Probability of Disease Given a Positive Test Result in a Test with 95% Sensitivity and Specificity at Different Disease Prevalences

Prevalence of Disease	Post-test Probability of Disease with a Positive Test
%	%
0.001	0
0.01	0
0.1	2
1	16
2	28
5	50
50	95

the pretest probability of the disease being considered. In screening situations, pretest probability simply can be equated with overall disease prevalence among asymptomatic adults. For diseases detectable by the component tests of a biochemical profile, this prevalence generally is very low, on the order of 0.001% to 1%. In the preadmission setting, the prevalence of clinically inapparent disease is more difficult to estimate because of problems in identifying the appropriate cohort of persons with whom to compare the person being tested. In general, however, prevalence of unsuspected disease will be higher in patients admitted to the hospital than in persons undergoing screening. For example, we can assume that there is a fivefold increase in disease prevalence in the preadmission setting, which results in pretest probability estimates of 0.005% to 5%.

The impact of disease prevalence on the probability of disease after an abnormal test result is shown in Table 4, where the component tests are assumed to have a sensitivity and specificity of 95%. The assumption of 95% test specificity is based on the arbitrary definitions of test "normality" described earlier. In contrast, the assumption of 95% test sensitivity is optimistic in relation to disease-test relations for most component tests of a biochemical profile. Given these assumptions, however, the probability of a disease after an abnormal screening test is very low. For example, if we assume a 1% disease prevalence, the probability of disease after an abnormal test result is only 16%; that is, there remains an 84% likelihood that the person with this test abnormality is free of the disease in question. The yield of abnormal results in preadmission testing is better, although still not impressive (Table 4).

OTHER FACTORS

Biochemical test results are not intrinsically binary (abnormal or normal) but instead are measured and reported in continuous values (for example, milligrams per deciliter). Thus, extreme values of a test result are more predictive of disease than are minimally abnormal results; by similar analyses, however, it also can be shown that such extreme values are less likely to occur in a population presumed to be free of disease. A complete quantitative analysis of the yield of biochemical profile testing would need to include the following additional considerations: the discriminating properties of each test result at each possible level of test abnormality, for all associated diseases; the probability that each level of test abnormality would occur in each testing setting; the probability of different diseases coexisting in the same person; and the degree of correlation among the component tests.

Biochemical Profiles: Evidence and Recommendations

AMBULATORY CARE SCREENING

The statistical principles of testing described above would lead one to expect the following conclusions: the proportion of abnormal results will increase exponentially with the number of component tests in the profile; the probability of any given test being abnormal will be approximately 2% to 5% in a population that is *known* to be free of disease, and only slightly higher in a screening population; the probability of disease if a screening test result is abnormal generally will be low, on the order of 0% to 15%; confirmatory tests performed after initially abnormal results most often will be normal; and the probability of a disease if a test result is abnormal will be greater for some tests than for others. One would also expect that new medical management would be initiated in direct proportion to the probability of disease if an individual test result is abnormal. What have the data actually shown?

Friedman and coworkers (22) studied the relation of

the number of component tests in a profile to the proportion of abnormal results obtained. Test results were documented for a population of 8651 randomly selected patients who were tested as part of a multiphasic health checkup at the San Francisco or Oakland, California, Kaiser Health Plans. When 8 tests were done, 74.1% of these patients had normal results for all component tests in the profile. When 20 tests were done, only 45.1% of these same patients had completely normal results, and 54.9% had 1 or more test abnormalities. These results, obtained from a very large sample of patients attending a routine health evaluation program, strongly support the statistical expectations described in the preceding paragraph. Furthermore, except for serum sodium level, which was reported to be either high or low in 16.6% of all patients, the frequency of individual test abnormalities (of the tests in Table 1) ranged from 1.5% (albumin) to 5.9% (glucose), and abnormal results were confirmed on repeated testing in less than 30% of the patients. Finally, and also in agreement with statistical expectations, among patients with specific test abnormalities, new diagnoses were made in 0% to 16.7% and new therapies were initiated in 0% to 14.1%.

In a similar study, Bates and Yellen (23) obtained follow-up data on 417 physicians who performed biochemical profiles on patients as part of a multiphasic screening program of the Rochester Regional Medical Program in 1969 to 1970. The seven biochemical tests (glucose, cholesterol, calcium, potassium, uric acid, alkaline phosphatase, and aspartate aminotransferase) were selected, in part, because of "reasonable expectation of [new] diagnosis and management"; that is, tests were preselected to include those most likely to yield useful results. The proportion of these presumed healthy patients with completely normal profiles was not reported in the study. The frequency of abnormal results on individual tests ranged from 4% to 10%. At the high end of this range, 9.9% of patients had serum cholesterol values above 260 mg/dL, and 8.4% had serum glucose values above 199 mg/dL 1 hour after ingesting a standard glucose load. Physicians reported that most of these abnormalities were not previously known or clinically apparent. Nevertheless, except for patients with elevated serum glucose values, confirmatory testing was done for less than 30% of those with test abnormalities. New medical management related to specific test abnormalities was initiated in a small and variable proportion of patients. Abnormal serum glucose values resulted in new management in 4.5% of all patients; cholesterol, 2.85%; calcium, 0.25%; potassium, 1.5%; uric acid, 1.15%; and alkaline phosphatase, 0.45%. These results are similar to those of Friedman and colleagues (22) and further identify serum glucose and cholesterol as measures of potentially highest diagnostic and therapeutic yield in the screening setting.

In a retrospective cohort study of ambulatory patients undergoing periodic health screening at the Kaiser-Permanente Medical Care Program in California, Rubenstein and colleagues (10) examined abnormal alkaline phosphatase results uncovered during biochemical profile testing. The probability of active diseases usually associated with abnormal alkaline phosphatase values was about 5% among patients who were not pregnant and who had no prior diagnosis of cancer or liver or bone disease (22 of 471 patients). Of the patients with new diagnoses made during 2 years' follow-up, "clinically useful" findings were made in slightly more than half (13 of 22), or 2.8% of those tested. A comprehensive summary of follow-up investigations done as a result of the initial abnormality was not reported, although 94% of the patients studied had repeated alkaline phosphatase results recorded during the follow-up. The authors of this study proposed a simple follow-up algorithm to minimize these induced costs of biochemical screening, although no evaluation of the proposed protocol has been done.

In summary, the empirical evidence appears to support statistical expectations about the use of biochemical profiles among persons who are seeking medical attention but who have no clinical evidence of disease associated with abnormal biochemical test results. Using larger batteries of tests increases the frequency of abnormal results and decreases the tests' diagnostic yield. The discovery of abnormal results leads to additional testing, increasing both diagnostic yield and the costs of evaluation, although the frequency of follow-up testing is extremely variable for different tests and test results. The yield of new diagnoses is small but greater than zero for most tests, and some tests (notably, glucose and cholesterol measurements) have greater yields than others, both in terms of new diagnoses and changes in patient management.

RECOMMENDATIONS FOR AMBULATORY SCREENING

1. Although it is difficult to place a quantitative value on the utility of biochemical profile testing in the screening situation, the available data suggest that the benefits of screening are not worth their aggregate cost and risk (including the induced costs and risks of repeated and follow-up testing). On the basis of these studies, it is our opinion that the performance of biochemical profiles for screening asymptomatic adults is not warranted.

2. Despite the preceding recommendation, selected components of the usual profiles probably are warranted in screening asymptomatic adults. The serum glucose value may be abnormally elevated in 5% to 8% of such adults. Confirmed abnormalities of the blood glucose level, measured during fasting or after an oral glucose challenge, operationally define the disease diabetes mellitus (24). This finding has important prognostic and therapeutic implications if it is confirmed in a patient. The value of patient education and diet therapy in this setting cannot be overstated (24). These efforts are inexpensive, without risk, and will probably improve the patient's long-term health status (24).

3. Likewise, the serum cholesterol value may be abnormally elevated in many asymptomatic adults in Western society (22, 23, 25-27). Confirmed abnormal values for this test operationally define the disease hypercholesterolemia, which is a known risk factor for atherosclerosis. The Lipid Research Clinics Coronary Primary Prevention Trial showed that lowering serum cholesterol values can reduce the incidence of cardiovascular morbidity and mortality (28); overall, these data support a 2% reduction in symptomatic coronary heart disease rates for each 1% reduction in serum cholesterol values. Other population-based data are consistent with this association and show continuous gradation of risk with increasing cholesterol levels (29, 30). Whereas the benefit/risk ratio for using currently available drugs to reduce cholesterol values is unclear, the effects of simple diet therapy are well known and probably without cost or risk to the patient. Thus, a recent consensus conference of the National Institutes of Health has recommended that per-

sons with hypercholesterolemia be identified and treated (26). The conference has recommended that persons with moderate cholesterol levels (75th to 90th percentile) be treated mainly by dietary means and that drug therapy be reserved for persons in the high-risk category (> 90th percentile) who are insufficiently responsive to dietary changes. Unsettled at this point is whether to include fractionation methods to differentiate high-density from low-density cholesterol in screening. These are not now included in the usual biochemical profiles.

4. With modest enthusiasm, we also recommend screening for renal dysfunction with the serum creatinine test with or without the blood urea nitrogen test. In Friedman and colleagues' study (22), abnormal serum creatinine and blood urea nitrogen values were uncovered in 3.3% and 3.4% of screened patients, respectively. Although the sensitivity of these tests for mild to moderate degrees of renal insufficiency is not high (31-33), the value of detecting asymptomatic patients rests on increasing evidence that antihypertensive treatment and possibly dietary protein or phosphorus restriction are effective in retarding the progression of chronic renal insufficiency (34-36). The results of this therapy are not so compelling, however, as to warrant a recommendation that more accurate (but more cumbersome and expensive) measures of renal function, such as creatinine clearance, be obtained routinely for asymptomatic persons. Instead, we concur with Beck and Kassirer's recommendation (37) that measurement of serum creatinine levels, either alone or with blood urea nitrogen levels, represents a reasonable compromise in the ambulatory setting. When abnormal creatinine values are obtained, creatinine clearance should be measured to assess the need for further diagnostic evaluation or therapy.

5. Screening for abnormalities of serum calcium concentrations is controversial. Elevations may occur in various malignant, inflammatory, bony and endocrinologic conditions. For most of these conditions, the post-test probability of disease after abnormal calcium results is not sufficiently high to warrant the inclusion of calcium determinations in a screening profile. Some authors have challenged this view, citing the value of detecting clinically silent primary hyperparathyroidism (38-40). Boonstra and Jackson (41) reported 50 new cases of hyperparathy-

roidism among 50 000 persons screened for serum calcium levels in a general diagnostic clinic over a 10-year period. In another study, investigators at the Mayo Clinic (42) reported a vast increase in the diagnosis of primary hyperparathyroidism since the start of biochemical screening in their area in 1974. After screening was initiated, the average age-adjusted incidence of primary hyperparathyroidism was $27.7 \pm 5.8/100\ 000$. Although economic arguments were raised to support screening practices, the authors did not emphasize that more than half of their patients had clinical findings suggesting the diagnosis (42). Not reported also were the total number of abnormal calcium values obtained and the cost of repeated and follow-up tests performed among disease-free persons. On the basis of other studies, we would expect these costs to be quite high in the screening setting. Finally, there are no established criteria for operative treatment of asymptomatic or mild primary hyperparathyroidism, and medical therapy (for example, with phosphate salts) may cause more harm than benefit. Until parathyroidectomy can be shown to be beneficial in asymptomatic patients with primary hyperparathyroidism, or until other acceptable therapies are discovered and shown to improve the disease's natural history, screening to detect this disorder does not appear to be warranted.

6. New diagnoses are made with reasonable frequency by screening for increased concentrations of alkaline phosphatase (primarily Paget's disease) and uric acid (primarily gout). The prognostic and therapeutic implications of asymptomatic Paget's disease or asymptomatic elevations in uric acid levels are unclear, however. Paget's disease may remain clinically asymptomatic throughout normal adult life; currently, most therapy is directed at relieving symptomatic disease, and therapeutic efforts to alleviate progression of disease involve potentially toxic drugs. Screening for this disease therefore is not warranted. Likewise, in the absence of arthritic symptoms, hypertension, or renal dysfunction, the benefits of treating asymptomatic hyperuricemia are probably exceeded by the associated costs and risks (43). Thus, screening for abnormalities of uric acid is not warranted.

7. On the basis of low diagnostic yield and lack of safe and effective therapy, we believe that screening also is not

warranted for the following components of the sample biochemical profile: sodium, potassium, chloride, aspartate aminotransferase, lactate dehydrogenase, total protein, and albumin.

PREADMISSION TESTING

Biochemical profile testing on admission to the hospital has been studied in several investigations (44-50). The focus of these studies has been to determine the effect of routine preadmission screening on the following five variables: new diagnoses uncovered in screened populations as compared with control groups that did not undergo such screening; the total number of diagnostic investigations performed and their temporal sequence (early or late during hospitalization); the number of consultations obtained during hospitalization; the total cost of hospitalization; and the average length of hospitalization.

Early studies (44, 45) tended to focus on new diagnoses discovered from routine on-admission testing with biochemical profiles. In an uncontrolled study, biochemical tests were done routinely on admission for 2204 patients admitted to two North Carolina hospitals (44). Unexpected and "medically significant" diagnoses were ascribed to profile testing for approximately 5% and 10% of patients at the respective hospitals. In a second study of routine profile screening for 1046 consecutive patients admitted to the medical and surgical services of a community hospital in Massachusetts, Belliveau and coworkers (45) retrospectively surveyed the physician responsible for each patient to determine whether abnormal test results had been expected and whether the results indicated new and unexpected diagnoses. Altogether, 43.2% of the 18-component profiles had 1 or more abnormal results, and the authors ascribed to the program a 4% yield of new or alternative diagnoses. The 42 patients with additional or alternative diagnoses included 21 with new diabetes mellitus, 9 with gout, 6 with hepatic cirrhosis, 5 with hypercholesterolemia, and 1 with multiple myeloma. A higher proportion of unexpectedly abnormal test results were ascribed to patients on the medical service than on the surgical service.

Later investigations tended to evaluate more globally the impact of preadmission testing with biochemical profiles. In two similar controlled trials in Great Britain (46, 48, 49), investigators studied the effect of such testing on diagnostic yield, total number of diagnostic investigations, total hospital costs, length of stay, and rapidity of the initiation of treatment. On the positive side, Whitehead and Wootton (46) reported that the admissions testing program decreased the number of diagnostic tests performed during the patients' first week of hospitalization, as compared with a control group. Nevertheless, the total number of tests performed during the hospital stay were equivalent in the two groups, and the average length of hospital stay was longer (nonsignificantly) in the screened group. More than 40% of the screened patients had at least one biochemical abnormality; 33.5% of these abnormal tests were found to have normal results when repeated, and 80% of the remainder were left unexplained by the time of hospital discharge. Whereas no adverse effect on the patient due to follow-up of these abnormalities was detected, the authors noted a potential adverse psychological impact on the physician as a result of "information overload."

Durbridge and coworkers (48, 49) did a randomized clinical study of preadmission testing, including a biochemical profile among a large battery of other tests, for 1000 patients. No significant differences were found in various indices of inpatient progress, including the rapidity with which therapy was initiated. The screened group had 25% more consultations and 32% more repeated tests than did the control groups. Average lengths of stay were the same for both groups. Finally, because of an estimated 64% increase in the cost of studying patients who had extensive admission testing, the total cost of hospital care was increased by about 5%.

Evidence from these and other studies (45, 48, 51) shows that routine preadmission use of biochemical profiles uncovers abnormalities in about 40% of patients, that these abnormalities lead to new diagnoses in a small proportion (between 4% and 10%) of patients, and that overall resource use in the hospital appears to be largely unaffected by such testing programs. The value of biochemical profiles in terms of changes in patient management, potential complications averted, overall hospital discharge status, or specialty-specific yields has been less well studied.

Two reports are noteworthy with regard to routine biochemical testing before elective surgical admissions. In a review of the literature, Robbins and Mushlin (51) analyzed several components of the usual biochemical profile and recommended three that "might be considered but are of uncertain value": the serum creatinine or blood urea nitrogen determination, which the authors estimated would detect 3 cases of renal insufficiency among 10 000 surgical patients in whom this disorder was not previously known to exist; aspartate aminotransferase activity, which would detect 2.5 cases of occult hepatitis among 10 000 patients; and a 2-hour postprandial glucose determination, which would detect 29 cases of asymptomatic diabetes mellitus per 10 000 patients. In a retrospective audit of 2000 patients having elective surgery at the University of California at San Francisco, Kaplan and coworkers (52) classified routine preoperative tests as clinically indicated or unindicated and further characterized test results either as potentially relevant or not relevant to perioperative care. Of 514 six-factor profiles ordered, 1 of 176 unindicated batteries yielded an abnormal creatinine value (1.8 mg/dL), which the authors reported had no effect on patient care. By similar analysis, 4 of 361 unindicated glucose determinations gave abnormal values, and 2 of these were considered potentially significant for perioperative management.

RECOMMENDATIONS FOR PREADMISSION TESTING

1. On the basis of the evidence described, we conclude that routine preadmission testing with existing biochemical profiles is not warranted. The expectations that such testing would have a favorable net impact on patient care, hospital costs, and lengths of stay have not been met.

2. Certain components of the sample biochemical profile may be useful if done on a routine basis, at least for selected patient groups. On the basis of current evidence, however, we cannot make specific recommendations about these tests or patient groups. Certain groups of patients having nonmedical elective hospitalizations might be targeted for more intensive future investigation. Among the important groups to study are patients who have no apparent medical illnesses but are admitted for elective surgical, gynecologic, or psychiatric care. These patients might not be seen in consultation by the internist

before elective hospitalization and, if no complication occurs during the hospital stay, might escape comprehensive medical evaluation altogether. Without some routine testing in these patient groups, clinically important conditions may remain undetected and adversely affect the patients' health status during or after hospitalization. Other considerations include the identification of risk factors for infection of health care personnel in the hospital; for example, this consideration influenced the recommendation of Robbins and Mushlin (49) regarding preoperative testing for hepatitis.

Conclusion

Detecting disease in patients who have no known or clinically apparent medical illness is a vexing clinical problem. The reasons for selecting an entire battery of biochemical tests in these patients are myriad and apparently persuasive on superficial analysis. The direct charges to the patient or payer often are lower when profile testing is done than when a selected smaller group of tests is ordered. Other reasons for profile testing include the promise of more information and the increased convenience to the laboratory, physician (who has only to check one box on the laboratory slip), and patient (who need not be subjected to multiple blood samplings).

On closer inspection, however, some of these rationales for biochemical profile testing are more apparent than real. In populations with low disease prevalence, theory and empirical evidence converge on the same conclusions: that abnormal test results are much more likely than not to be falsely abnormal, and that the proportion of false-positive results increases with an increase in the number of component tests in the profile. Because of this evidence, arguments favoring the use of profiles because of their cost or convenience appear inordinately simplistic. Faced with an unexpectedly abnormal test result, the clinician has the choice of ignoring it, repeating the test, or doing further tests for the disease implied by the finding. The induced costs, inconvenience, and potential risk of further investigations may more than offset the initial benefits ascribed to profile testing. On the other hand, whereas clinicians often state that they should follow up the abnormality (53), in practice they most often do not (54, 55). Why, then, it may be argued, was the profile requested in the first place?

Table 5. Recommendations for Use of Biochemical Profiles in Ambulatory Screening and Preadmission Testing of Adults

Ambulatory screening
1. General biochemical profiles are not indicated for routine screening of asymptomatic adults.
2. Selected components of biochemical profiles that may be indicated for screening asymptomatic adults include:
   a. The blood glucose test (either fasting or after an oral glucose challenge), to identify diabetes mellitus
   b. The serum cholesterol determination, to identify hypercholesterolemia
   c. The serum creatinine test with or without the blood urea nitrogen test, to identify renal dysfunction

Preadmission testing
1. General biochemical profiles are not indicated routinely before elective admission to the hospital.
2. Further research is needed to determine whether specific components of profiles are warranted routinely before elective admission of selected patient groups.

Explanations related to financial incentives and "defensive medicine" aside, it appears that biochemical profiles are requested in asymptomatic persons primarily to detect important and clinically inapparent disease. The evidence is reasonably consistent in documenting a yield of treatable conditions ranging from 0% to 15% in the two testing settings described in this article, with most component tests yielding fewer than 5% unanticipated and potentially important findings.

Ultimately, the focus of debate involves considerations of the trade-offs among the costs, risks, and clinical benefits of early disease detection. In other terms, the issue becomes the determination of the optimal ratio between the costs and risks of false-positive as compared with false-negative findings in populations with low disease prevalence (56). As stated succinctly by Kaplan and colleagues (52) in regard to preoperative laboratory screening: "The different conclusions seem to depend on whether, for example, the authors consider an expenditure of $50,000 to find one patient who might later become jaundiced reasonable [57] or not [58]."

In recommending that biochemical profiles be abandoned for screening and routine preadmission testing purposes, we side with those who find their yield too low and their related costs and risks too high (Table 5). In analyzing the specific component tests, however, we find that some warrant consideration for routine ambulatory screening. Specifically, we believe that periodic screening is warranted for serum glucose, cholesterol, and, perhaps, blood urea nitrogen and creatinine abnormalities, although the optimal frequency of such screening is less clear. Similarly, we believe that formal evaluation of selected patient groups may uncover specific components of the biochemical profile that would be useful in routine preadmission testing. Precisely which tests would be most useful for which patient groups should be the subject of study by those interested in the costs and quality of medical care in the hospital setting.

ACKNOWLEDGMENTS: The authors thank Dr. Laurence Beck for his review of earlier drafts of this manuscript, and Linda Gary for manuscript preparation.

Grant support: Dr. Cebul is a Henry J. Kaiser Family Foundation Faculty Scholar in General Medicine. Dr. Beck is the recipient of Research Career Development Award LM00086 from the National Library of Medicine.

References

1. CANADIAN TASK FORCE ON THE PERIODIC HEALTH EXAMINATION. The periodic health examination. CAN MED ASSOC J. 1979;**121**:1193-254.
2. BRESLOW L. An historical review of multiphasic screening. *Prev Med.* 1973;**2**:177-96.
3. COLLEN MF. Periodic health examinations using an automated multi-test laboratory. *JAMA.* 1966;**195**:142-5.
4. GARFIELD SR. Multiphasic health testing and medical care as a right. *N Engl J Med.* 1970;**283**:1087-9.
5. BENSON ES. Research and operational strategies: an overview. In: CONNELLY DP, BENSON ES, BURKE MD, FENDERSON D, eds. *Clinical Decisions and Laboratory Use.* Minneapolis, Minnesota: University of Minnesota Press; 1982:275.
6. SACKETT DL. The usefulness of laboratory tests in health-screening programs. *Clin Chem.* 1973;**19**:366-72.
7. WILLIAMS SV, EISENBERG JM, PASCALE LA, KITZ DS. Physicians' perceptions about unnecessary diagnostic testing. *Inquiry.* 1982;**19**:363-70.
8. SPECIAL TASK FORCE ON PROFESSIONAL LIABILITY AND INSURANCE, AMERICAN MEDICAL ASSOCIATION. *Professional Liability in the '80s.* Chicago: American Medical Association; 1984.
9. EISENBERG JM. *Doctors' Decisions and the Cost of Medical Care: The Reasons for Doctors' Practice Patterns and Ways to Change Them.* Ann Arbor, Michigan: Health Administration Press; 1986:15-8, 57-8.
10. RUBENSTEIN LV, WARD NC, GREENFIELD S. In pursuit of the abnormal serum alkaline phosphatase: a clinical dilemma. *J Gen Intern Med.* 1986;**1**:38-43.
11. SCHROEDER SA, SHOWSTACK JA. Financial incentives to perform medical procedures and laboratory tests: illustrative models of office practice. *Med Care.* 1978;**16**:289-98.

12. DAVIS JE. Automation. In: KAPLAN LA, PESCE AJ, eds. *Clinical Chemistry: Theory, Analysis, and Correlation.* St. Louis: C.V. Mosby; 1984:261-72.

13. SKENDZEL LP, BARNETT RN, PLATT R. Medically useful criteria for analytic performance of laboratory tests. *Am J Clin Pathol.* 1985;**83:**200-5.

14. KAPLAN LA, PESCE AJ, eds. *Clinical Chemistry: Theory, Analysis, and Correlation.* St. Louis: C.V. Mosby; 1984.

15. CHARAP MH. The periodic health examination: genesis of a myth. *Ann Intern Med.* 1981;**95:**733-5.

16. MEDICAL PRACTICE COMMITTEE, *American College of Physicians.* Periodic health examination: a guide for designing individualized preventive health care in the asymptomatic patient. *Ann Intern Med.* 1981;**95:**729-32.

17. FRAME PS, CARLSON SJ. A critical review of periodic health screening using specific screening criteria: 3. Selective diseases of the genitourinary system. *J Fam Pract.* 1975;**2:**189-94.

18. PETERSON J, MANCHESTER D, TOAN A. *Enhancing Hospital Efficiency: A Guide to Expanding Beds Without Bricks: A Study of Fifteen Hospitals.* Ann Arbor, Michigan: AVPHA Press; 1980:59.

19. Appendix 1. In: AMERICAN COLLEGE OF PHYSICIANS. *Medical Necessity Project Recommendations: Summary, 1978-1981.* [Available from Department of Health and Public Policy, American College of Physicians, 4200 Pine Street, Philadelphia, PA 19104.]

20. ALLER RD. Interpretive reporting. *Clin Lab Med.* 1983;**3:**205-17.

21. STATLAND BE, WINKEL P. Physiologic variation of the concentration values of selected analytes in healthy young adults. In: ELEVITCH FR, ed. *Proceedings of the 1976 Aspen Conference on Analytical Goals in Clinical Chemistry.* Chicago: College of American Pathologists; 1977:94-101.

22. FRIEDMAN GD, GOLDBERG M, AHUJA JN, SIEGELAUB AB, BASSIS ML, COLLEN MF. Biochemical screening tests: effect of panel size on medical care. *Arch Intern Med.* 1972;**129:**91-7.

23. BATES B, YELLEN JA. The yield of multiphasic screening. *JAMA.* 1972;**222:**74-8.

24. GREGERMAN RI. Diabetes mellitus. In: BARKER LR, BURTON JR, ZIEVE PD, eds. *Principles of Ambulatory Medicine.* Baltimore: Williams & Wilkins; 1982:683-5.

25. KERN DE, BLACKMAN MR. Plasma lipids and hyperlipidemia. In: BARKER LR, BURTON JR, ZIEVE PD, eds. *Principles of Ambulatory Medicine.* Baltimore: Williams & Wilkins; 1982:754-69.

26. Lowering blood cholesterol to prevent heart disease [Consensus Conference]. *JAMA.* 1985;**253:**2080-6.

27. WYNDER EL, FIELD F, HALEY NJ. Population screening for cholesterol determination: a pilot study. *JAMA.* 1986;**256:**2839-42.

28. The Lipid Research Clinics Coronary Primary Prevention Trial results: I. Reduction in incidence of coronary heart disease. *JAMA.* 1984;**251:**351-64.

29. NEATON JD, KULLER LH, WENTWORTH D, et al. Total and cardiovascular mortality in relation to cigarette smoking, serum cholesterol concentration and diastolic blood pressure among black and white males followed up for five years. *Am Heart J.* 1984;**108:**759-70.

30. STAMLER J, WENTWORTH D, NEATON JD. Is the relationship between serum cholesterol and risk of premature death from coronary heart disease continuous and graded? *JAMA.* 1986;**256:**2823-8.

31. WILSON RF, SOULLIER G, ANTONENKO D. Creatinine clearance in critically ill surgical patients. *Arch Surg.* 1979;**114:**461-7.

32. PRICE M, KOTTKE FJ. Comparison of glomerular filtration rate, blood urea nitrogen and serum creatinine in patients with chronic urinary tract disease. *Minn Med.* 1980;**63:**781-2.

33. LUKE RG. Uremia and the BUN [Editorial]. *N Engl J Med.* 1981;**305**:1213-5.
34. MOGENSEN CE. Diabetes mellitus and the kidney. *Kidney Int.* 1982;**21**:673-5.
35. ROSMAN JB, TER WEE PM, MEIJER S, et al. Prospective randomised trial of early dietary protein restriction in chronic renal failure. *Lancet.* 1984;**2**:1291-6.
36. MASCHIO G, OLDRIZZI L, TESSITORE N, et al. Effects of dietary protein and phosphorus restriction on the progression of early renal failure. *Kidney Int.* 1982;**22**:371-6.
37. BECK LH, KASSIRER JP. Serum electrolytes, serum osmolality, blood urea nitrogen, and serum creatinine. In: SOX HC JR, ed. *Common Diagnostic Tests: Use and Interpretation.* Philadelphia: American College of Physicians; 1987. (In press).
38. Detecting disease by biochemistry of blood. *Stat Bull Metropol Life Insur Co.* 1971;**52**:5-7.
39. WALDENSTRÖM JG. Systematic serum calcium screening—will it be necessary? *Acta Med Scand.* 1973;**193**:145-6.
40. WILLIAMSON E, VAN PEENAN HJ. Patient benefit in discovering occult hyperparathyroidism. *Arch Intern Med.* 1974;**133**:430-1.
41. BOONSTRA CE, JACKSON CE. Serum calcium survey for hyperparathyroidism: results in 50,000 clinic patients. *Am J Clin Pathol.* 1971;**55**:523-6.
42. HEATH H III, HODGSON SF, KENNEDY MA. Primary hyperparathyroidism: incidence, morbidity, and potential economic impact in a community. *N Engl J Med.* 1980;**302**:189-93.
43. SCOTT JT. Gout. In: SCOTT JT, ed. *Copeman's Textbook of the Rheumatic Diseases.* London: Churchill Livingstone; 1978:683.
44. BRYAN DJ, WEARNE JL, VIAU A, MUSSER AW, SCHOONMAKER FW, THIERS RE. Profile of admission chemical data by multichannel automation: an evaluative experiment. *Clin Chem.* 1966;**12**:137-43.
45. BELLIVEAU RE, FITZGERALD JE, NICKERSON DA. Evaluation of routine profile chemistry screening of all patients admitted to a community hospital. *Am J Clin Pathol.* 1970;**53**:447-51.
46. WHITEHEAD TP, WOOTTON IDP. Biochemical profiles for hospital patients. *Lancet.* 1974;**2**:1439-43.
47. LEONARD JV, CLAYTON BE, COLLEY JRT. Use of biochemical profile in children's hospital: results of two controlled trials. *Br Med J.* 1975;**2**:662-5.
48. DURBRIDGE TC, EDWARDS F, EDWARDS RG, ATKINSON M. Evaluation of benefits of screening tests done immediately on admission to hospital. *Clin Chem.* 1975;**22**:968-71.
49. DURBRIDGE TC, EDWARDS F, EDWARDS RG, ATKINSON M. An evaluation of multiphasic screening on admission to hospital: precis of a report to the National Health and Medical Research Council. *Med J Aust.* 1976;**1**:703-5.
50. KORVIN CC, PEARCE RH, STANLEY J. Admissions screening: clinical benefits. *Ann Intern Med.* 1975;**83**:197-203.
51. ROBBINS JA, MUSHLIN AI. Preoperative evaluation of the healthy patient. *Med Clin North Am.* 1979;**63**:1145-56.
52. KAPLAN EB, SHEINER LB, BOECKMANN AJ, et al. The usefulness of preoperative laboratory screening. *JAMA.* 1985;**253**:3576-81.
53. CASSCELLS W, SCHOENBERGER A, GRABOYS TB. Interpretation by physicians of clinical laboratory results. *N Engl J Med.* 1978;**299**:999-1001.
54. BATES B, MULINARE J. Physicians' use and opinions of screening tests in ambulatory practice. *JAMA.* 1970;**214**:2173-80.
55. LINK K, CENTOR R, BUCHSBAUM D, WITHERSPOON J. Why physicians don't pursue abnormal laboratory tests: an investigation of hypercalcemia and the follow-up of abnormal test results. *Hum Pathol.* 1984;**15**:75-8.

56. McNeil BJ, Keeler E, Adelstein SJ. Primer on certain elements of medical decision making. *N Engl J Med.* 1975;**293:**211-5.
57. Schemel WH. Unexpected hepatic dysfunction found by multiple laboratory screening. *Anesth Analg.* 1976;**55:**810-2.
58. Crider EF. Is routine laboratory (SMA) screening justified [Letter]? *Anesth Analg.* 1977;**56:**470-2.

Serum Electrolytes, Serum Osmolality, Blood Urea Nitrogen, and Serum Creatinine

LAURENCE H. BECK, M.D.; and JEROME P. KASSIRER, M.D.

FEW PATIENTS complete a hospital admission on a medical or surgical service without measurement of serum electrolyte, blood urea nitrogen, and creatinine concentrations at least once. Many patients, particularly the sicker ones, have these determinations carried out daily or even more frequently. Similarly, the routine biochemical profile obtained by many physicians in the evaluation of ambulatory patients almost always includes these tests. Abnormalities in these tests are common in patients with severe disease. Fluid and solute administration, as well as dietary management in such patients, is appropriately guided by serial measurement of these values.

Despite widespread usage of these tests, their clinical value has not been systematically reviewed nor recommendations made for their optimal use in different clinical settings. In this article, we review the individual utilities of the serum sodium, potassium, and chloride concentration, CO_2 content, blood urea nitrogen, and serum creatinine concentrations. Because serum osmolality has many physiologic similarities to the serum sodium concentration, its utility is also evaluated. Recommendations for each of these tests are provided.

Serum Electrolytes

Serum electrolyte measurements are among the most frequently ordered blood chemistry tests. Despite this high usage, little information has been published on the test characteristics of electrolytes or on the clinical utility of tests in specific conditions. Most of the following recommendations are based on assessments of the minimal data available and on our extensive clinical experience.

Most published studies of the value of electrolyte tests as a group have assessed a panel of 10 to 20 biochemical tests, including electrolytes. As expected, no careful studies of biochemical screening, including electrolytes, have shown such screening to be beneficial in an unselected population. When routine on-admission screening packages included electrolyte measurements, studies showed few additional disorders were discovered that required a change in patient management (1-5).

On the other hand, in selected populations, tests for individual electrolytes (or for the group) may be beneficial in case-finding and in management. Such usage is stressed in the following sections, although there is little support in the literature either for or against such recommendations.

POTASSIUM

Although most of the body's potassium is inside cells (where the concentration is greater than 100 mmol/L), total body potassium content is difficult to measure. The potassium concentration in extracellular fluid, however, is easily measured (in serum or plasma) and is an important determinant of all neuromuscular activity, particularly cardiac conduction and function.

The serum (or plasma) potassium concentration, although often obtained as part of the set of electrolyte tests, is probably the commonest single electrolyte test ordered. Serum levels usually parallel changes in total body potassium, although the correlation is weak because of several factors that alter potassium distribution between intracellular fluid and extracellular fluid. Nevertheless, the most important determinants of serum potassium levels are those that determine overall potassium balance: potassium intake and excretion, especially renal excretion. Therefore, abnormalities of the serum concentration occur most often in patients with renal impairment, patients on diuretic therapy or with large gastrointestinal fluid losses, and patients with unusually high (or low) potassium intakes.

Most laboratories measure serum potassium concentrations with automated flame photometry or with ion-selective electrodes. The normal concentration ranges from 3.5 to 5.0 meq/L (6).

Most errors in serum potassium determination result in false elevation of the value. Hemolysis of the blood during venipuncture or during clotting can release intracellular (erythrocyte) potassium into the serum and produce a falsely high value. This error is often suspected when pink serum is noted. A less common event, "pseudohyperkalemia," occurs when serum is from blood with extremely high platelet or leukocyte counts. During clotting, the usually abnormal leukocytes or platelets release potassium, which results in an artifactual elevation. The "true" value can be determined by inhibiting clotting with heparin and measuring the plasma potassium concentration.

Use in Screening Unselected Populations: Measuring serum potassium levels does not appear useful for general screening. Studies indicate that such abnormalities rarely, if ever, occur in inpatients who do not have a clinical history or manifestations that would predict the abnormality (1-5). Belliveau and associates' (2) study of biochemical screening of 1046 consecutive nonobstetric patients admitted to a community hospital showed that the serum potassium concentration was abnormal (> 3 SD from the mean of normals) in almost 1% of samples tested, yet no new diagnosis was made in any patient with an abnormal value.

Similarly, Korvin and coworkers (4) analyzed the clinical benefit of admission screening in 1000 consecutive patients admitted to a general hospital. The frequency of abnormal serum potassium concentrations was identical to that in Belliveau and associates' survey. Of the nine abnormal values found, most were anticipated, and in only two patients was the finding considered to be of probable benefit (both had diuretic-induced hypokalemia). Similar studies of routine screening of outpatients are not available, but the yield would probably be even lower because of the lower disease prevalence in ambulatory populations.

In contrast to the preceding studies, admission screening of 50 consecutive elderly patients (mean age, 81) admitted to the hospital for acute illness showed hypokalemia in 12 (24%), including 8 in whom an abnormal potassium concentration was not clinically expected (7).

Use in Screening Selected Outpatients: In selected groups of patients, measuring the serum potassium concentration is valuable in case-finding. One disorder that can be detected is hyperkalemia in renal disease. Patients with mild interstitial renal disease may have abnormal potassium excretion, sometimes manifested by serious hyperkalemia requiring specific therapy. This abnormal serum potassium excretion may occur in up to 50% of diabetics with mild renal insufficiency (8). In persons with nondiabetic renal disease, the prevalence is unknown but is probably much lower. If hyperkalemia is not present at the initial diagnosis, the serum potassium concentration should be measured once or twice a year to detect any trend toward hyperkalemia.

Serum potassium measurements are also useful in detecting hypertension due to primary hyperaldosteronism. Although an uncommon cause of hypertension (0.5% to 1%) (9), primary hyperaldosteronism is potentially curable, so screening for disease, at least in hypertensive patients, seems reasonable. Because most patients with primary hyperaldosteronism have moderate to mild hypokalemia (sensitivity is 73% for a serum potassium concentration of less than 3.5 meq/L [10]) and because unprovoked hypokalemia is uncommon in other hypertensive patients not taking diuretics, the probability of hyperaldosteronism is high when hypokalemia is present. Thus, the serum potassium level is an appropriate case-finding test.

Some authors (11) have suggested that diuretic-induced hypokalemia in the hypertensive patient should stimulate an investigation for primary hyperaldosteronism. However, the yield may be low. Because 7% of diuretic-treated hypertensive patients develop serum potassium concentrations below 3.0 meq/L (12) and because the prevalence of primary hyperaldosteronism is at most 1% in the hypertensive population, the probability of this abnormality given a low potassium value would be no higher than 13%; therefore, further evaluations of false-positive results would be required in about seven patients for every one patient found to have this condition.

A third disorder for which serum potassium determinations are valuable is renal tubular acidosis. Because early intervention benefits patients with this disorder, at least children, early diagnosis is desirable. Hypokalemia occurs in virtually all patients with classic renal tubular acidosis. Therefore, serum potassium determination is indicated in children with poor growth, muscle weakness, kidney stones, or other suggestive symptoms.

Indications for Outpatient Management: Certain symptoms or signs should prompt the clinician to test for serum potassium concentration, especially in patients with conditions known to be associated with altered potassium metabolism (gastrointestinal disease, renal tubular acidosis, diuretic therapy). Such indicators include generalized weakness or proximal muscle weakness, new atrial tachyarrhythmias, nocturia, polyuria, or ileus.

Whether serum potassium values should be measured in hypertensive patients on chronic diuretic therapy is less certain. Most nonedematous patients begun on diuretic therapy have an average fall in serum potassium concentration of 0.5 to 0.7 meq/L (12). Despite this fall, total body potassium content is unchanged or decreased only minimally (13). Only a few patients develop serum concentrations of 3.0 meq/L or less; most clinicians agree that this small subgroup should be given potassium replacement therapy or potassium-sparing diuretics (14).

Some investigators have reported an increased frequency of ventricular ectopy and tachycardia (with some deaths) in patients with serum potassium concentrations of 3.1 to 3.5 meq/L who are taking diuretics without potassium replacement (15). Others have pointed out methodologic inadequacies in these studies and have warned against the hazards of serious (and fatal) hyperkalemia in potassium-supplemented patients (14).

A physician's interpretation of these observations will influence the decision about measuring serum potassium concentrations in diuretic-treated patients. Nevertheless, most studies agree that the concentration falls promptly after diuretic therapy is initiated, reaching its nadir at 6 to 12 weeks (16), and that it remains relatively stable thereafter. Therefore, a reasonable recommendation in the hypertensive patient is to measure the serum potassium concentration before initiation of treatment, again after 6 to 12 weeks, and then yearly (or not at all thereafter) in the absence of other important clinical changes. Concentrations should be measured more frequently (every 6 months) in patients receiving diuretics and concurrent digitalis preparations, because hypokalemia increases the incidence of serious arrhythmias in such patients (17).

Indications for Inpatient Management: Severe hyperkalemia or hypokalemia has dramatic effects, particularly on cardiac rhythm and function. Therefore, prompt therapy for abnormal serum potassium concentrations in ill patients is essential. Many factors (pH, catecholamines, osmolality, insulin, mineralocorticoids) affect the serum potassium concentration, so their summative effect in a given clinical situation, particularly in acutely ill patients, is not always predictable. Serum potassium concentration should be measured on admission in every acutely ill patient and again whenever there is an important change in clinical status.

Daily measurements are sometimes indicated, especially in patients with changing renal function (as in acute renal failure), patients treated for cardiac arrhythmias (particularly those receiving digitalis), and patients with persistent gastrointestinal losses. In a few patients, serum potassium should be measured every several hours until levels are stable. This group includes patients on intensive fluid replacement therapy, particularly when accompanied by carbohydrate loads or insulin, and patients being treated for severe hyperkalemia or hypokalemia, severe metabolic acidosis (for example, diabetic ketoacidosis), or on intensive diuretic therapy (for example, for correction of severe hyponatremia).

SODIUM

The status of water balance throughout body fluids is reflected by the serum sodium concentration. Because sodium is the major extracellular cation, and because osmolality is the same in almost all body fluids, the serum sodium concentration can be used to estimate body fluid osmolality, which is usually about twice the serum sodium concentration (see following discussion for exceptions and for a more precise formula for estimating plasma osmolality). The normal range for serum sodium concentration is 135 to 145 meq/L, representing the mean $\pm$ 2 SD (6).

The serum sodium concentration is not an index of total body sodium and should never be used (alone) to assess sodium balance or to predict a patient's need for more or less sodium. (In the absence of edema, hyponatremia usually indicates total body sodium depletion; an example is the patient receiving diuretics for a nonedematous disorder who develops hyponatremia.) Nor can the serum sodium concentration be used alone to assess the status of the extracellular fluid volume, which must be determined by clinical examination.

Use in Osmolality Calculations: Serum sodium concentration may not reflect fluid osmolality in two general circumstances. The first is when another solute relatively restricted to the extracellular fluid space is present in excess in that space, as in hyperglycemia. As glucose accumulates in the extracellular fluid, it causes osmotic movement of intracellular water into the extracellular fluid, diluting it and thereby lowering the serum sodium concentration. In such a case, the osmolality of body fluids must be assessed by estimating (or measuring) plasma osmolality.

In hyperglycemia, the magnitude of the drop in serum sodium concentration can be estimated with a formula (18):

$$\Delta \text{ (serum Na)} = -1.6 \times \Delta \text{ (glucose/100)}$$

where serum sodium is expressed in milliequivalents per liter, and glucose is expressed in milligrams per deciliter. This theoretic formula is widely used, although it has never been validated clinically.

The second situation is when large quantities of lipids or proteins occupy a higher than normal fraction of plasma, thereby falsely lowering the serum sodium concentration (pseudohyponatremia). Theoretic formulae (19, 20) to estimate the degree of this false lowering have not been validated, and their results are method dependent (21). Laboratories that use automated ion-selective electrodes for serum sodium determinations are not affected by this error, unless the specimen is diluted before reading. Plasma osmolality can be used in these instances to confirm that such hyponatremia is false.

Use in Screening Unselected Populations: Alterations of serum sodium concentration are rare in ambulatory patients in the absence of other clinical manifestations of organ failure or serious illness. The only important exception is the syndrome of inappropriate secretion of antidiuretic hormone (SIADH), in which chronic hyponatremia may be clinically silent. The serum sodium concentration is a highly sensitive marker for this condition (in fact, hyponatremia is one requirement for diagnosis). However, because the prevalence of this syndrome is so low, screening in an unselected ambulatory population is not recommended.

Indications for Outpatient Management: The serum sodium concentration may be useful in case-finding in more selected populations. Among patients with hypertension, for example, identification of primary hyperaldosteronism is important because of the disorder's potential curability. The serum sodium concentration is often mildly elevated in patients with primary aldosteronism, but there is not a sharp cutoff value that separates primary hyperaldosteronism from other forms of hypertension. Thus, the serum sodium concentration alone is not useful in case-finding (22).

In patients with polyuria and polydipsia not due to diabetes mellitus, the serum sodium concentration has been suggested to distinguish between diabetes insipidus and primary polydipsia. Although patients with diabetes insipidus tend to be hypernatremic and those with primary polydipsia hyponatremic, assessment of the serum sodium concentration is of little value compared with a standard water deprivation test (23) or measurement of plasma vasopressin levels (24). (See Serum Osmolality for further discussion of diabetes insipidus.)

Measurement of the serum sodium concentration is appropriate in the management of patients receiving chronic lithium therapy for bipolar affective disorders. In many patients, lithium causes nephrogenic diabetes insipidus, with renal water-wasting (25) that predisposes patients to dehydration and hypernatremia. Elderly patients especially may have defective thirst regulation (26) and be unable to protect themselves from dehydration. Therefore, serum sodium concentration can be used as an index of hydration in patients after initiation of lithium therapy.

Hyponatremia in congestive heart failure, cirrhosis, and nephrotic syndrome occurs as a consequence of impaired water excretion that develops as the underlying disease process worsens. Although hyponatremia may cause no symptoms of its own, its recognition should alter management. Thus serum sodium measurement is indicated in these disorders when manifestations of the underlying disease change. Similarly, patients with chronic renal insufficiency have a limited ability to excrete free water. The reduced capacity for excretion becomes important as the glomerular filtration rate falls to 10% to 15% of normal, even when fluid intake is normal, because hyponatremia may develop insidiously. Therefore, when the serum creatinine level reaches 7 to 8 mg/dL, serum sodium concentration should be measured at regular intervals, perhaps every 2 to 3 months. Other indications for measurement in outpatients include rapid changes in weight, fluid balance (severe vomiting, diarrhea, polyuria), or mental status, and clinical evidence of dehydration or volume depletion.

Indications for Inpatient Management: Because abnormalities of water balance are common in acutely and chronically ill inpatients, serum sodium determination is appropriate and indicated for most patients on admission to the hospital or when there is a change in clinical status (especially in mental or neurologic status or in any of the conditions listed in the preceding paragraph). Even so, the utility of on-admission testing is low. The studies by Belliveau and colleagues (2) and by Korvin and coworkers (4) mentioned newly detected serum sodium abnormalities in only 0.7% and 1.5% of admission screening studies, but few, if any, new or unexpected diagnoses were detected. Serum sodium concentration need not be determined in otherwise healthy patients admitted for elective surgery or diagnostic procedures.

Repeated serum sodium measurements are indicated in any hospitalized patient who has an initially abnormal value, rapid change in weight or fluid balance, or serious cardiac, renal, or hepatic disorders. The prevalence of hyponatremia in a general hospitalized population is 2.5%; two thirds of cases are hospital acquired (27). Recognition of this abnormality may be important because the mortality of these patients in one study was 60 times that of patients without documented hyponatremia (although correction of the hyponatremia did not appear to influence the poor outcome) (27). The appropriate frequency of serum sodium determinations should be based on the rate of anticipated changes. Patients receiving parenteral fluids require determination once daily, but some patients receiving intensive corrective fluid therapy (for example, for diabetic ketoacidosis, intensive diuresis, correction of severe hyponatremia) require measurements every few hours.

CHLORIDE

Determination of the plasma or serum chloride concentration alone is never indicated. Nevertheless, the chloride concentration is helpful, when available as part of an electrolyte panel, for proper interpretation of the bicarbonate concentration (total CO_2) and for calculation of the anion gap.

BICARBONATE (TOTAL CO_2)

Most laboratories measure the total CO_2 content with the standard electrolytes. The total CO_2 content represents the sum of the bicarbonate concentration plus carbonic acid concentration plus dissolved CO_2. Because bicarbonate makes up 90% to 95% of the total CO_2 content, total CO_2 content is usually a useful surrogate for bicarbonate concentration.

In most laboratories, total CO_2 content is measured automatically by a process that liberates the gas from plasma by acidification, with CO_2 measured by one of several methods. The normal range in venous blood is 24 to 30 mmol/L (6).

Because acid-base abnormalities rarely occur until well into the clinical course of chronic pulmonary, cardiac, renal, or gastrointestinal disease, the total CO_2 content is a poor screening test for these conditions in ambulatory patients without other signs. On the other hand, it is useful in determining the nature and severity of those diseases, and therefore its measurement is indicated in the initial assessment of patients with chronic diarrhea, chronic renal failure, renal tubular acidosis, and severe cardiopulmonary disease, particularly those on diuretic therapy. In patients who have initial abnormalities or who are undergoing therapy to correct or diminish the acid-base disorder, measurement of total CO_2 content should be repeated until therapy has had the desired effect.

Admission screening studies (2, 4) have not shown a clinical benefit from measuring total CO_2 content. However, because unexpected and clinically important derangements of acid-base status often complicate serious illnesses, total CO_2 determination is indicated in all seriously ill patients, both at admission and when important clinical deterioration occurs. Abnormal values often should be pursued with repeated arterial blood gas determination (for instance, in patients with chronic pulmonary disease and acute respiratory failure). If arterial blood gas determinations are made frequently, daily (or more frequent) total CO_2 determinations are redundant. However, patients with serious metabolic acid-base disorders undergoing therapy may need repeated (and frequent) determinations of total CO_2 content. Patients with diabetic ketoacidosis or other types of severe metabolic acidosis may need a full set of electrolytes every 2 to 4 hours during the first several hours of therapy.

Serum Osmolality

Estimates of serum osmolality can be derived from serum electrolyte, blood glucose, and blood urea nitrogen (BUN) concentrations. Serum osmolality can be measured very accurately with several methods, but the one used most frequently relies on the depression in freezing point of a serum sample (28). Normal osmolality ranges from 285 to 295 mosmol/kg of water in serum. Few data are available on how often this value should be measured, but it is done almost exclusively in hospitalized patients. Undoubtedly, serum osmolality is measured excessively, because the indications for its use are few.

Patients with diabetes insipidus lose large quantities of water in urine and develop slight hyperosmolality, which in turn increases their thirst. By contrast, patients with psychogenic polydipsia drink large quantities of water, develop slight hypoosmolality, and excrete large quantities of water. At times distinguishing between these two clinical states is difficult, because in both the patients are thirsty and drink large quantities of water. Measurement of plasma electrolyte concentrations alone is not sensitive enough to detect the small difference in plasma osmolality between the two groups, but measurement of serum osmolality may be. Patients with psychogenic polydipsia tend to have serum osmolalities below 285 mosmol/kg, and those with diabetes insipidus, greater than 285 mosmol/kg. In such patients several measurements are required while the patient's water intake is uninhibited. In most patients, a consistent pattern emerges, and a diagnosis can be made with confidence. However, a standard water deprivation test, with measurement of urine and serum osmolalities, should be carried out in patients in whom the diagnosis remains unclear. Data from Zerbe and Robertson (24) indicate that this standard test can classify correctly about 87% of patients with either central diabetes insipidus or psychogenic polydipsia (when plasma vasopressin levels are used as the reference standard for classification).

Several substances increase the osmolality of the serum but are not measured in usual laboratory testing procedures: mannitol, glycerol, alcohol, and certain toxic chemicals ingested most often by alcoholics (methanol and ethylene glycol). Measurement of serum osmolality can confirm whether one of these substances exists in the serum. When one of these materials is suspected, the measured osmolality can be subtracted from the estimated osmolality (calculated from serum concentrations of sodium, glucose, and BUN) to obtain an "osmolar gap." This method of recognizing unusual intoxications is particularly useful in emergency services (29). Unfortunately, few validation studies have been carried out. In one large study of traumatized patients with concurrent ethanol intoxication, serum osmolality and measured blood alcohol levels correlated highly, but the osmolar gap was consistently greater than the contribution expected from ethanol, suggesting that other endogenous osmoles may be released in traumatized patients (30).

Despite these inconsistencies, measurement of plasma osmolality and calculation of the osmolar gap has been found to be clinically useful in three circumstances: estimating the level of mannitol in a patient with renal failure and mannitol intoxication (31); managing increased intracranial pressure with glycerol therapy in children (32) or dimethyl sulfoxide therapy in adults (33); and recognizing propylene glycol intoxication in patients treated with topical preparations for extensive burns (34). On the basis of our experience and these few studies, we recommend measurement of serum osmolality in patients who are receiving mannitol and who develop either unexplained symptoms or a substantial change in serum sodium concentration; alcoholic patients who develop unexplained, disordered central nervous system function; and patients brought to the emergency room with unexplained metabolic acidosis (usually severe) and an increase in the anion gap.

Most patients with hyponatremia have hypoosmolality and require no measurement of serum osmolality. In the hyponatremic patient with lipemic plasma or in the patient with serum globulin levels in excess of 8 g/dL, a single measurement of serum osmolality is often useful in ensuring that the serum sodium reduction does not represent true hypoosmolality (*see* Sodium).

When blood glucose and blood urea nitrogen concentrations are normal and when no extraneous substances are present, the serum osmolality can be estimated for clinical purposes by doubling the serum sodium concentration. More complicated formulae have been offered that include other plasma solutes. Dorwart and Chalmers (35) used 13 published equations to compare measured and estimated osmolality in 715 hospital samples. Although several equations gave reasonable accuracy and precision, the best fit was achieved with the following formula:

$$\text{osmolality} = [1.86 \, (\text{serum Na})] + (\text{glucose}/18) + (\text{BUN}/2.8) + 9$$

where serum sodium is expressed in milliequivalents per liter, and glucose is expressed in milligrams per deciliter. When blood glucose, BUN, or both are increased, this formula should be used.

Many incorrectly believe that the syndrome of inappropriate secretion of antidiuretic hormone (SIADH) can be diagnosed with certainty only if serum osmolality is measured. The serum sodium concentration in such patients, in the absence of extraneous substances, hyperlipidemia, hyperproteinemia, and hyperglycemia, is an excellent surrogate measurement for serum osmolality.

Blood Urea Nitrogen and Serum Creatinine

The BUN and serum creatinine concentrations are the two clinical tests most often employed to assess kidney function, where they are surrogates for measurements of urea or creatinine clearance, respectively (both of which are indices of the glomerular filtration rate). When the glomerular filtration rate is constant, serum creatinine levels vary little from hour to hour and day to day (36, 37) and thus this test is highly useful for assessing kidney function. Creatinine is released from muscle at a fairly constant rate and is excreted unchanged in urine, so few clinical disturbances not accompanied by changing kidney function affect its concentration.

By contrast, the BUN concentration is affected by factors other than change in glomerular filtration rate, including the nitrogen load and the rate of urine flow. An increase in either protein intake or breakdown yields an increase in nitrogen load and thus an increase in the BUN; the reverse is also true. Water intake and urine flow rate also may influence the BUN because the excretion of urea is closely associated with the excretion of water. High urine flow rates are accompanied by low rates of urea reabsorption and low levels of BUN; low urine flow rates are associated with high rates of urea reabsorption and higher levels of BUN. From these observations, it is apparent that the BUN reflects considerably more than the glomerular filtration rate alone. It can be used to assess the rate of urine flow (and thus the hydration of the patient) and the nitrogen load (and thus catabolism).

In practice, BUN and serum creatinine concentrations are frequently measured simultaneously. Indeed, automated laboratory equipment that measures one often measures the other as well. Both are measured colorimetrically, and probably little savings are realized by measuring only one.

The BUN concentration usually is measured by one of two colorimetric methods, each of which yields the same normal range, 10 to 18 mg/dL. Serum creatinine is usually measured with one of several modifications of the Jaffe picrate method, which detects not only true creatinine but also noncreatinine chromogens (28). The normal range is 0.6 to 1.2 mg/dL. Men generally have higher values than women due to their larger muscle mass. Most of the assays based on the Jaffe reaction give falsely elevated values in the presence of ketone bodies (38) or cephalosporins, especially cefoxitin (39).

Methods that measure true creatinine concentrations are not interfered with by ketone bodies and cephalosporins, but these methods are more time consuming because of the need to absorb the noncreatinine chromogens in a separate step. Many hospital laboratories are beginning to use the recently developed automated enzymatic methods for measurement of true creatinine levels (40). The normal range with this method is approximately 0.4 to 1.0 mg/dL.

USE IN ESTIMATING GLOMERULAR FILTRATION RATE

As a screening test for kidney function in ostensibly normal persons or patients with various medical or surgical conditions, the serum creatinine is preferred to the BUN because it is more closely correlated with the glomerular filtration rate than is the BUN. In fact, creatinine clearance (as a surrogate of the glomerular filtration rate) can be predicted reasonably accurately from the serum creatinine concentration alone, factored for age and weight (41):

$$\text{creatinine clearance} = [(140 - \text{age}) \times \text{weight}] / (72 \times S_{Cr})$$

where weight is expressed in kilograms and serum creatinine (S_{Cr}) in milligrams per deciliter.

Although the creatinine clearance is assumed to be a reasonable approximation of the glomerular filtration rate, the correlation between this rate and creatinine clearances calculated with creatinine values measured by the Jaffe picrate method is somewhat fortuitous. Throughout the range of normal to moderately decreased values for glomerular filtration rate, the serum noncreatinine chromogen level measured by the Jaffe method is approximately balanced by the small tubular secretion of creatinine, and these two factors cancel each other out to make the creatinine clearance a reasonable estimate of glomerular filtration rate. At low levels of glomerular filtration, however, the secretory component becomes proportionately increased, leading to as much as a 50% overestimation of the glomerular filtration rate by creatinine clearance measurements (42-44). The increase in tubular secretion, with resultant overestimation of glomerular filtration rate, occurs particularly in patients with nephrotic syndrome (45). (Certain drugs, especially cimetidine and trimethoprim-sulfamethoxazole, inhibit tubular secretion of creatinine and may lead to an elevated serum creatinine concentration in the absence of a decrease in glomerular filtration rate [39].) Creatinine clearances measured with a true creatinine method appear to give a much closer approximation of the actual glomerular filtration rate (as measured by inulin clearance) than those calculated from a picrate method (42, 43), but there has not been wide clinical experience with the newer method.

The geometric relationship between serum creatinine concentration and creatinine clearance means that a clinically important fall in creatinine clearance can occur before the serum creatinine concentration rises out of the "normal" range (Figure 1). In many laboratories, such a rise in serum creatinine concentration is within the error of measurement. Therefore, serum creatinine concentra-

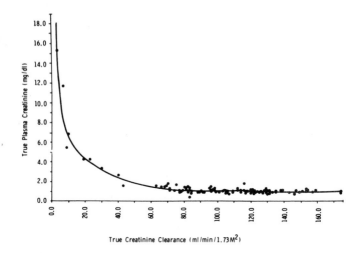

True Creatinine Clearance (ml/min/1.73M^2)

Figure 1. Relation between true plasma creatinine and true creatinine clearance (duplicate points have been omitted for clarity). From Bauer and colleagues (42); reproduced with permission of the *American Journal of Kidney Diseases*.

tion is not a highly sensitive index of early renal insufficiency.

TEST SENSITIVITY AND SPECIFICITY

The few studies that assess the sensitivity of serum creatinine and BUN concentrations for detecting decreased glomerular filtration rate indicate that these tests are not highly sensitive. Wilson and colleagues (46) evaluated 131 critically ill surgical patients in the intensive care unit of their institution, using 2-hour and 24-hour creatinine clearances as an estimate of glomerular filtration rate. When a lower limit of normal of 80 mL/min was used, only 37 (28%) of these patients had a normal creatinine clearance, whereas the rest had mild to severe reduction. Of the 94 with reduced creatinine clearances, 56 had an elevated BUN concentration, giving the BUN test a sensitivity of only 67%. Conversely, the specificity was 68%. The sensitivity of the serum creatinine concentration (cutoff value, 1.4 mg/dL) was only 47%, although specificity was 95%.

The low sensitivity of the serum creatinine measurement in acutely ill patients is not surprising, because a fall in glomerular filtration rate is not accompanied by an instant rise in BUN and serum creatinine concentrations. Instead, urea and creatinine accumulate gradually over hours to days until new steady-state serum concentrations are achieved, at which time production rates of urea and creatinine equal the excretion rates. Measurement of BUN or serum creatinine values before this new steady-state concentration is reached underestimates the change in glomerular filtration rate.

In clinically stable patients, serum creatinine and BUN measurements also lack sensitivity for decreased glomerular filtration. Inulin clearances were measured in 1418 patients with spinal cord injury and compared with simultaneous serum creatinine and BUN measurements (47). In 114 (8%), inulin clearance was abnormal (> 2 SD below the normal mean, corrected for body surface area). In those patients with mild decreases in glomerular filtration rate (46 to 72 mL/min · 1.73 m^2 body surface area), BUN and creatinine tests had sensitivities of only 14% and 19%, respectively. At greater degrees of dysfunction (20 to 45 mL/min), sensitivity of BUN was 34% and that of creatinine was 84%. Only at very low glomerular filtration rates (< 20 mL/min) did their sensitivities approach 100%; specificities in these patients were approximately 99% for BUN and 90% for creatinine.

USE IN SCREENING AND MANAGEMENT

Most authors recommend the creatinine measurement as superior to the BUN test for detection of renal insufficiency (48). If the findings noted in the preceding section can be generalized to other populations, this recommendation is appropriate. However, in screening or case-finding in populations with low disease prevalence, the yield of serum creatinine testing may be low. Although most clinicians do measure BUN and serum creatinine concentration as screening tests in ambulatory patients, none of the recent recommendations for routine health screening suggests such measurements, in part because of the low prevalence of chronic renal failure and the unavailability of specific therapy (49, 50). Despite the low sensitivity of the serum creatinine test, we nevertheless recommend it in screening for renal insufficiency in most ambulatory patients, because antihypertensive treatment and, perhaps, dietary protein or phosphorus restriction appear to be effective in slowing progression of established chronic renal disease (51-53).

Although creatinine clearance measurement might be the preferred screening test because of its sensitivity, such a recommendation is impractical for an unselected patient population due to logistics and cost.

Instead, we recommend the serum creatinine test as a reasonable compromise for case-finding. In patients in whom a high-normal or elevated value is detected, the creatinine clearance should be measured to determine the need for further diagnostic studies or therapy. Needless to say, other clinical (hypertension, long-standing diabetes mellitus) and laboratory findings (proteinuria on urinalysis) are complementary information that should trigger the measurement of serum creatinine levels or creatinine clearance. Once a baseline creatinine clearance has been determined in a given patient, the serum creatinine concentration can be used subsequently to assess renal function; any rise in the serum creatinine concentration should reflect a proportionate fall in creatinine clearance.

The serum creatinine concentration can be used to assess changes in kidney function from day to day (for example, in the patient with acute renal failure, with suspected transplant rejection, or on aminoglycoside therapy) or over longer periods (for example, the patient with gradually progressive renal damage over several years). Although the relation of serum creatinine concentration with time is curvilinear in most patients with chronic renal failure, the reciprocal of the serum creatinine concentration tends to change linearly with time, allowing prediction of a change in creatinine clearance over time in an individual patient (54) (Figure 2).

The type of renal disease is the prime determinant of how frequently the serum creatinine concentration should be measured. Except in rapidly progressive renal disease, chronic renal insufficiency usually develops over several years. Because uremic symptoms are rarely present and because dialysis usually is not needed before the glomerular filtration rate falls below 10% of normal, measurement two to three times per year is usually sufficient once serial measurements have established the pace of disease.

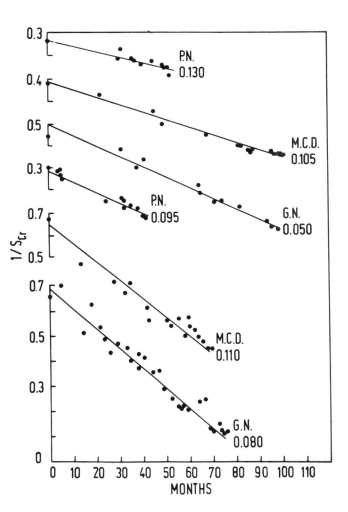

Figure 2. Composite plot of reciprocal serum creatinine concentrations (S_{Cr}) (expressed in milligrams per deciliter) in relation to months of observation in six patients with chronic renal failure. The final value for the reciprocal of serum creatinine concentration is shown for each patient. The ordinate has uniform divisions of 0.1 dL/mg. Diagnoses in these patients are indicated (P.N. = pyelonephritis; M.C.D. = medullary cystic disease; G.N. = glomerulonephritis). From Mitch and colleagues (54); reproduced with permission of *The Lancet*.

Table 1. Recommended Uses for Electrolytes, Blood Urea Nitrogen and Serum Creatinine Measurements

Test and Setting	Indications (Frequency of Testing)
Potassium	
Screening unselected populations	Not recommended
Screening selected outpatients	Chronic renal disease, especially diabetes (at diagnosis, then 1 to 2 times a year)
	Hypertension, for diagnosis of hyperaldosteronism (at diagnosis of hypertension before therapy)
Outpatient management	Diuretic treatment of hypertension (before therapy, then at 6 to 12 weeks)
	Concurrent diuretic and digitalis treatments (every 6 months)
Inpatient management	Acutely ill patients (on admission)
	Change in clinical status (as indicated, *see* text)
Sodium	
Screening unselected populations	Not recommended
Outpatient management	Edematous states, chronic renal failure (at time of clinical change; or when serum creatinine reaches 7 to 8 mg/dL, then every 2 to 3 months)
	Lithium treatment (after initiation of therapy)
Inpatient management	Acutely ill patients (on admission; and at time of clinical change)
Chloride	
Screening unselected populations	Not recommended
Inpatient management	Acutely ill patients (whenever total CO_2 measurement is indicated, to calculate anion gap)
Total CO_2	
Screening unselected patients	Not recommended
Outpatient management	Patients with chronic pulmonary, cardiac, renal, and gastrointestinal disease (at diagnosis, then at time of clinical change)

Table 1. (Continued)

Test and Setting	Indications (Frequency of Testing)
Inpatient management	Seriously ill patients (on admission; at time of clinical change; or to follow therapy of acid-base disorder)
Serum osmolality	See text
Serum creatinine/BUN*	
Screening unselected populations	Recommended (*see* text for limitations)
Screening selected populations	Hypertension (at diagnosis, followed by creatinine clearance measurement if abnormal)
Outpatient management	Hypertension (every 1 to 2 years)
	Chronic renal disease (every 4 to 6 months, depending on underlying renal disease)
Inpatient management	Aminoglycoside therapy (2 to 3 times a week)
	Oliguria, acute renal failure (every 1 to 2 days)
	Seriously ill patients (once a week, more often if indicated)

* Serum creatinine and blood urea nitrogen (BUN) are usually measured together or creatinine is measured alone. CNS = central nervous system.

During assessment of kidney function in a patient with an unusually high or low nitrogen load or in a patient with an unusually high or low rate of urine flow, the serum creatinine concentration is preferred to the BUN. It is difficult to imagine a clinical situation in which only a BUN test is indicated, because any BUN value has to be compared with a simultaneous serum creatinine value to assess whether an abnormality can be attributed to a change in kidney function. There are many situations in which the BUN is dramatically elevated despite a normal serum creatinine concentration (55) or is low despite an elevated serum creatinine concentration. Reliance on BUN measurements alone in such instances would give a false impression of kidney function. The ratio between the BUN and serum creatinine is approximately 10 in certain conditions (56): ingestion of a "normal" protein intake (approximately 1 g/kg body weight · day), ingestion of a "normal" amount of fluid, and excretion of "normal" quantities of urine (approximately 1 mL/min). The ratio can be higher than 10 when the nitrogen load is high or when urine flow is low, and the converse is also true. Such a disproportion between BUN and creatinine therefore can provide valuable diagnostic clues (56). On the basis of these physiologic principles, some conditions that warrant simultaneous measurement of BUN and serum creatinine concentrations include acute renal insufficiency (in which the differential diagnosis includes volume contraction), gastrointestinal bleeding complicated by some degree of renal insufficiency, and advanced renal insufficiency (serum creatinine of 7 mg/dL or above). In advanced renal insufficiency, the serum creatinine value is likely to be a reasonably accurate guide to the severity of renal damage, whereas the BUN is likely to be a more accurate reflector of the patient's risk for "uremic" symptoms (43, 48). The BUN in such patients is also a valuable guide to the effectiveness of dietary protein restriction. Disproportionately low BUN levels imply that the nitrogen load has been reduced successfully and that the risk of uremic symptoms has been reduced; disproportionately high levels connote the opposite.

Simultaneous measurements of BUN and serum creatinine concentrations may be useful in supporting a diagnosis of water intoxication or syndrome of inappropriate secretion of antidiuretic hormone (SIADH). In such patients the serum creatinine value tends to be slightly low, but the BUN level typically is unmistakably low; serum creatinine values of 0.7 to 0.8 mg/dL are often associated with BUN values of 4 to 8 mg/dL (57).

Recommendations

Table 1 summarizes the recommendations made in the review regarding measurement of electrolyte concentrations, and blood urea nitrogen and serum creatinine concentrations in various situations.

References

1. DAUGHADAY WH, ERICKSON MM, WHITE W, SELIGMAN A. Evaluation of routine 12-channel chemical profiles on patients admitted to a university general hospital. In: BENSON ES, STRANDJORD PE, eds. *Multiple Laboratory Screening*. New York: Academic Press; 1969.

2. BELLIVEAU RE, FITZGERALD JE, NICKERSON DA. Evaluation of routine profile chemistry screening of all patients admitted to a community hospital. *Am J Clin Pathol.* 1970;**53**:447-51.
3. WHITEHEAD TP, WOOTTON IDP. Biochemical profiles for hospital patients. *Lancet.* 1974;**2**:1439-43.
4. KORVIN CC, PEARCE RH, STANLEY J. Admissions screening: clinical benefits. *Ann Intern Med.* 1975;**83**:197-203.
5. DURBRIDGE TC, EDWARDS F, EDWARDS RG. An evaluation of multiphasic screening on admission to hospital: precis of a report to the National Health and Medical Research Council. *Med J Aust.* 1976;**1**:703-5.
6. SCULLY RE, MCNEELY BU, GALDABINI JJ. Case records of the Massachusetts General Hospital: normal reference laboratory values. *N Engl J Med.* 1980;**302**:37-48.
7. SEWELL JMA, SPOONER LLR, DIXON AK, RUBENSTEIN D. Screening investigations in the elderly. *Age Ageing.* 1981;**10**:165-8.
8. DEFRONZO RA. Hyperkalemia and hyporeninemic hypoaldosteronism. *Kidney Int.* 1980;**17**:118-34.
9. MELBY JC. Primary aldosteronism. *Kidney Int.* 1984;**26**:769-78.
10. BRAVO EL, TARAZI RC, DUSTAN HP, et al. The changing clinical spectrum of primary aldosteronism. *Am J Med.* 1983;**74**:641-51.
11. CONN JW, COHEN EL, ROVNER DR, NESBIT RM. Normokalemic primary aldosteronism. *JAMA.* 1965;**193**:100-6.
12. MORGAN DB, DAVIDSON C. Hypokalaemia and diuretics: an analysis of publications. *Br Med J.* 1980;**280**:905-8.
13. KOHVAKKA A, EISALO A, MANNINEN V. Maintenance of potassium balance during diuretic therapy. *Acta Med Scand.* 1979;**205**:319-24.
14. HARRINGTON JT, ISNER JM, KASSIRER JP. Our national obsession with potassium. *Am J Med.* 1982;**73**:155-9.
15. HOLLAND OB, NIXON JV, KUHNERT L. Diuretic-induced ventricular ectopic activity. *Am J Med.* 1981;**70**:762-8.
16. SANDOR FF, PICKENS PT, CRALLAN J. Variations of plasma potassium concentrations during long-term treatment of hypertension with diuretics without potassium supplements. *Br Med J [Clin Res].* 1982;**284**:711-5.
17. SMITH TW. Digitalis glycosides. *N Engl J Med.* 1973;**288**:719-22, 942-6.
18. KATZ MA. Hyperglycemia-induced hyponatremia—calculation of expected serum sodium depression. *N Engl J Med.* 1973;**289**:843-4.
19. WAUGH WH. Utility of expressing serum sodium per unit of water in assessing hyponatremia. *Metabolism.* 1969;**18**:706-12.
20. NARINS RG, JONES ER, STOM MC, RUDNICK MR, BASTL CP. Diagnostic strategies in disorders of fluid, electrolyte and acid-base homeostasis. *Am J Med.* 1982;**72**:496-520.
21. LADENSON JH, APPLE FS, KOCH DD. Misleading hyponatremia due to hyperlipemia: a method-dependent error. *Ann Intern Med.* 1981;**95**:707-8.
22. STREETEN DHP, TOMYCZ N, ANDERSON GH. Reliability of screening methods for the diagnosis of primary aldosteronism. *Am J Med.* 1979;**67**:403-13.
23. LEAF A. Neurogenic diabetes insipidus. *Kidney Int.* 1979;**15**:572-80.
24. ZERBE RL, ROBERTSON GL. A comparison of plasma vasopressin measurements with a standard indirect test in the differential diagnosis of polyuria. *N Engl J Med.* 1981;**305**:1539-46.
25. COX M, SINGER I. Lithium and water metabolism. *Am J Med.* 1975;**59**:153-7.
26. PHILLIPS PA, ROLLS BJ, LEDINGHAM JGG, et al. Reduced thirst after water deprivation in healthy elderly man. *N Engl J Med.* 1984;**311**:753-59.
27. ANDERSON RJ, CHUNG HM, KLUGE R, SCHRIER RW. Hyponatremia: a prospective analysis of its epidemiology and the pathogenetic role of vasopressin. *Ann Intern Med.* 1985;**102**:164-8.

28. BAUER JD, ed. *Clinical Laboratory Methods.* 9th ed. St. Louis: C.V. Mosby Co.; 1982.
29. PAPPAS AA, GADSDEN RH JR, GADSDEN RH SR, GROVES WE. Computerized calculation with osmolality and its automatic comparison with observed serum ethanol concentration. *Am J Clin Pathol.* 1982;**77**:449-51.
30. BRITTEN JS, MYERS RA, BENNER C, CARSON S, COWLEY RA. Blood ethanol and serum osmolality in the trauma patient. *Am Surg.* 1982;**48**:451-5.
31. BORGES HF, HOCKS J, KJELLSTRAND CM. Mannitol intoxication in patients with renal failure. *Arch Intern Med.* 1982;**142**:63-6.
32. PITLICK WH, PIRIKITAKUHLR P, PAINTER MJ, WESSEL HB. Effect of glycerol and hyperosmolality on intracranial pressure. *Clin Pharmacol Ther.* 1982;**31**:466-71.
33. RUNCKEL DN, SWANSON JR. Effect of dimethyl sulfoxide on serum osmolality. *Clin Chem.* 1980;**26**:1745-7.
34. BEKERIS L, BAKER C, FENTON J, KIMBALL D, BERMES E. Propylene glycol as a cause of an elevated serum osmolality. *Am J Clin Pathol.* 1979;**72**:633-6.
35. DORWART WV, CHALMERS L. Comparison of methods for calculating serum osmolality from chemical concentrations, and the prognostic value of such calculations. *Clin Chem.* 1975;**21**:190-4.
36. DOOLAN PD, ALPEN EL, THEIL GB. A clinical appraisal of the plasma concentration and endogenous clearance of creatinine. *Am J Med.* 1962;**32**:65-79.
37. RAPOPORT A, HUSDAN H. Endogenous creatinine clearance and serum creatinine in the clinical assessment of kidney function. *Can Med Assoc J.* 1968;**98**:149-56.
38. MOLITCH ME, RODMAN E, HIRSCH CA, DUBINSKY E. Spurious serum creatinine elevations in ketoacidosis. *Ann Intern Med.* 1980;**93**:280-1.
39. MUTHER RS. Drug interference with renal function tests. *Am J Kidney Dis.* 1983;**3**:118-20.
40. FOSSATI P, PRENCIPE L, BERTI G. Enzymic creatinine assay: a new colorimetric method based on hydrogen peroxide measurement. *Clin Chem.* 1983;**29**:1494-6.
41. COCKCROFT DW, GAULT MH. Prediction of creatinine clearance from serum creatinine. *Nephron.* 1976;**16**:31-41.
42. BAUER JH, BROOKS CS, BURCH RN. Clinical appraisal of creatinine clearance as a measurement of glomerular filtration rate. *Am J Kidney Dis.* 1982;**2**:337-46.
43. KASSIRER JP, GENNARI FJ. Laboratory evaluation of renal function. In: EARLEY LE, GOTTSCHALK CW, eds. *Strauss and Welt's Diseases of the Kidney.* 3rd ed. Boston: Little, Brown & Company; 1979:46-8.
44. ROLIN HA III, HALL PM, WEI R. Inaccuracy of estimated creatinine clearance for prediction of iothalamate glomerular filtration rate. *Am J Kidney Dis.* 1984;**4**:48-54.
45. CARRIE BJ, GOLBETZ HV, MICHAELS AS, MYERS BD. Creatinine: an inadequate filtration marker in glomerular diseases. *Am J Med.* 1980;**69**:177-82.
46. WILSON RF, SOULLIER G, ANTONENKO D. Creatinine clearance in critically ill surgical patients. *Arch Surg.* 1979;**114**:461-7.
47. PRICE M, KOTTKE FJ. Comparison of glomerular filtration rate, blood urea nitrogen and serum creatinine in patients with chronic urinary tract disease. *Minn Med.* 1980;**63**:781-2.
48. LUKE RG. Uremia and the BUN [Editorial]. *N Engl J Med.* 1981;**305**:1213-5.
49. FRAME PS, CARLSON SJ. A critical review of periodic health screening using specific screening criteria: 3. Selected diseases of the genitourinary system. *J Fam Pract.* 1975;**2**:189-94.

50. CANADIAN TASK FORCE ON THE PERIODIC HEALTH EXAMINATION. The periodic health examination. *Can Med Assoc J.* 1979;**121:**1193-254.

51. MOGENSEN CE. Diabetes mellitus and the kidney. *Kidney Int.* 1982;**21:**673-5.

52. ROSMAN JB, TER WEE PM, MEIJER S, PIERS-BECHT TP, SLUITER WJ, DONKER AJM. Prospective randomised trial of early dietary protein restriction in chronic renal failure. *Lancet.* 1984;**2:**1291-6.

53. MASCHIO G, OLDRIZZI L, TESSITORE N, et al. Effect of dietary protein and phosphorus restriction on the progression of early renal failure. *Kidney Int.* 1982;**22:**371-6.

54. MITCH WE, WALSER M, BUFFINGTON GA, LEMANN J JR. A simple method of estimating progression of chronic renal failure. *Lancet.* 1976;**2:**1326-8.

55. KUMAR R, STEEN P, MCGEOWN MG. Chronic renal failure or simple starvation?: a case-report. *Lancet.* 1972;**2:**1005.

56. DOSSETOR JB. Creatininemia versus uremia: The relative significance of blood urea nitrogen and serum creatinine concentration in azotemia. *Ann Intern Med.* 1966;**65:**1287-99.

57. DECAUX G, GENETTE F, MOCKEL J. Hypouremia in the syndrome of inappropriate secretion of antidiuretic hormone. *Ann Intern Med.* 1980;**93:**716-7.

APPENDIXES

Introduction to the Blue Cross and Blue Shield Association Guidelines

LAWRENCE C. MORRIS, Senior Vice President, Health Benefits Management, Blue Cross and Blue Shield Association

THE BLUE CROSS AND BLUE SHIELD Association began the Medical Necessity Project in 1976, with the cooperation of the American College of Physicians, the American College of Radiology, and the American College of Surgeons. Originally, the project dealt with new procedures of unproven value; established procedures of dubious current usefulness; procedures that tended to be redundant when done in combination with other procedures; and procedures unlikely to yield additional information through repetition. The project first entered the more sophisticated arena of patterns of care in 1979 with admission battery policies. These policies reflected the view of the American College of Physicians and the American College of Surgeons that tests for hospitalized patients should be ordered on an individualized basis, and not simply as parts of pre-established batteries, indiscriminately applied.

The program's work since that point has recognized that the more complex questions are more important. The cooperating medical organizations and the Association have increasingly focused on perfectly valid procedures that, through habit, collateral application with more modern procedures, or simply through authoritative definition of indications have tended to be overused. Thus, the emphasis has shifted from procedures of fundamentally dubious usefulness to proper utilization of fundamentally useful procedures.

The basic principles upon which the program was established remain. Quality of care is considered no less important than cost; no approach to cost-effectiveness can ignore the need to maintain quality.

The Blue Cross and Blue Shield Association continues to believe that knowledge of what constitutes good medical practice resides within the medical community. Identifying and conveying that information, and support through the attention-arresting effects of payment policy, are the Association's contributions. The program is not an effort to deny claims. The authoritativeness of the investigations underlying the guidelines, and their endorsement by medical organizations with acknowledged leadership, will diminish over-utilization and thus unnecessary claims.

The imponderables of medical practice are such that payment policy can never anticipate all contingencies. There will always be circumstances in which nearly any procedure might be medically justifiable. The carrier should provide exception processes through which those circumstances can be recognized and accommodated.

The guidelines in this appendix address the effective use of common laboratory procedures, preoperative x-rays, and electrocardiograms. They have been developed not only from commissioned reviews of the literature, but also from amplified and modified conclusions based on those reviews in a multispecialty clinical conference sponsored by the Association and, most importantly, from rigorous review of the papers before their publication in *Annals of Internal Medicine*. The peer-review processes of *Annals* have affected both the papers and the conclusions based on them.

In addition to their implications for quality of care, which we cannot overemphasize, the guidelines should have a useful economic effect. Complex, capital-intensive technologies command a great deal of public attention. But simpler, less dramatic, and noninvasive procedures such as clinical laboratory tests, radiographs, and electrocardiograms are a greater source of health care expenditure. This effort to assess the actual or comparative clinical utility of diagnostic and therapeutic procedures may address outmoded habits, lack of awareness of current knowledge, and perhaps unnecessary use in defensive medicine. Much of the vulnerability to defensive practice arises from the lack of definitive information about what it is generally *not* useful to do.

The emergence of prospective payment systems, not only in traditional public and private programs but in such alternative delivery systems as HMOs, generates increased interest in knowing what is cost-effective. This trend is in pleasant contrast to the traditional bias in favor of overutilization in the name of quality. It forces a more proper definition: the use of the right procedures in the right time on the right patient.

The guidelines tend to be phrased in the affirmative. They are to help in determining appropriate care and are not—and not intended to be—a series of proscriptions.

They reflect a view of what constitutes good practice, with the hope that this will be helpful as we all strive to get the most from available resources. The guidelines also may counter the potential for underutilization under the pressures of prospective payment.

The Blue Cross and Blue Shield Association intends to give these guidelines wide public dissemination. The purpose is not only to achieve the widest possible currency within the medical community, but to discourage unfounded expectations on the part of those who confuse more utilization with higher quality.

We want particularly to thank Harold C. Sox, Jr., M.D., for coordinating the development of the review articles that are the basis for the guidelines. We thank each of the authors responsible for the review articles and the staffs of the American College of Physicians and *Annals of Internal Medicine* for their consultation and assistance. The guidelines represent the combination of a major cooperative effort that should benefit not only Blue Cross and Blue Shield subscribers, but the public and provider communities in general by promoting quality care through appropriate use of technology. We are pleased to be a part of this effort, and to incorporate the guidelines in the Association's Medical Necessity Program.

Serum Enzyme Assays in the Diagnosis of Myocardial Infarction

Definition

Serum enzymes and isoenzymes useful in the diagnosis of myocardial infarction (MI) include creatine kinase (CK), CK isoenzyme (CK-MB), lactate dehydrogenase (LDH), and LDH isoenzymes (LDH1 and LDH2).

Rationale

When myocardial cells are damaged, enzymes present in large quantities in heart muscle are released into the bloodstream. Abnormal levels of these enzymes, detected with serum enzyme assays, are among the diagnostic criteria for myocardial infarction. Although enzyme levels can also be used to make qualitative estimates of infarct size, these estimates should not be used to predict mortality or long-term prognosis for individual patients; other factors, including how much myocardium has been lost in the past and how much myocardium is in jeopardy, are better predictors of long-term prognosis.

Recommendations

1. Diagnosis of Myocardial Infarction
   1.1 The use of enzyme assays other than CK, CK-MB, LDH, and LDH isoenzymes is not indicated.
   1.2 A single set of cardiac enzymes is not sufficiently sensitive to exclude a diagnosis of myocardial infarction.
   1.3 If myocardial infarction is suspected, CK and CK-MB are indicated on admission and approximately 12 and 24 hours later.
   1.4 If more than 24 hours has elapsed since onset of chest pain and if CK and CK-MB are not diagnostic, a total LDH is indicated.
       1.4.1 If total LDH is elevated, LDH isoenzymes (LDH1 and LDH2) are indicated.
       1.4.2 If the initial LDH1:LDH2 ratio is only slightly less than 1.0, a second assay is indicated to confirm the diagnosis.

1.5 If chest pain recurs after admission, CK and CK-MB assays are indicated at 0, 12, and 24 hours.

    1.5.1 "Surveillance" enzyme levels, or routine daily CK and CK-MB levels, are not indicated in asymptomatic postinfarct patients without ECG changes.

2. Diagnosis of Myocardial Infarction in Cardiac Procedures

2.1 In suspected myocardial infarction coincidental to cardiac surgery, CK-MB is indicated at 0, 12, and 24 hours.

2.2 In cardiac surgery, several factors are considered suggestive of infarction, including:

    2.2.1 CK-MB elevation persisting more than 12 hours;

    2.2.2 New Q waves on ECG;

    2.2.3 Regional defect on technetium pyrophosphate scintigraphy.

2.3 In suspected myocardial infarction coincidental to nonoperative cardiac procedures, including cardiac catheterization, percutaneous transluminal angioplasty, and electrical countershock, CK-MB is indicated at 0, 12, and 24 hours.

3. Diagnosis of Myocardial Infarction in Noncardiac Procedures

3.1 In suspected myocardial infarction coincidental to non-cardiac surgery, CK-MB is indicated at 0, 12, and 24 hours. The isoenzyme pattern of CK elevation should be evaluated to distinguish myocardial infarction from noncardiac muscle trauma associated with surgery.

4. General Considerations

4.1 Conditions other than myocardial infarction may be responsible for an elevated CK-MB (myocarditis, renal failure, neuromuscular diseases, or trauma), but the pattern of elevation usually differs from the typical rise and fall of CK and CK-MB, and other evidence associated with infarction is usually absent.

4.2 Some persons have variant CKs that will resemble CK-MB on chromatographic assays but can be distinguished by electrophoretic assay. Such variants should be suspected if the clinical setting or the pattern of rise and fall is atypical for myocardial infarction.

Preoperative and General Hospital Admission Electrocardiograms

Definition

Routine preoperative or general admission electrocardiogram (ECG) in patients without evidence of heart disease refers to the 12-lead ECG taken at rest in patients scheduled for surgery with either general anesthesia or regional anesthesia and sedation or patients admitted to medical and other specialty services; it does not include patients admitted to intensive care units.

Rationale

Routine use of preoperative or general admission ECGs may provide the primary or sole evidence of conditions that increase the risks associated with surgery, systemic diseases, arrhythmias, or recent unrecognized myocardial infarction. However, an ECG may not always reveal evidence of a recent infarction and may reveal abnormalities in the absence of myocardial disease. Preoperative ECGs are, therefore, of limited value in deciding whether a patient should proceed with surgery. An ECG should be ordered judiciously, based on clinical judgment, and in selected populations at increased risk of heart disease and at increased preoperative risk. The following guidelines attempt to identify such patients.

Recommendations

1. Screening/Case-finding
    1.1 An ECG is not routinely indicated solely because of general hospital admission.
    1.2 An ECG is not routinely indicated before noncardiac surgery.
    1.3 An ECG may be indicated in patients at increased risk for occult heart disease.
        1.3.1 An ECG may be useful in men aged 35 to 40 years and older and in postmenopausal women aged 50 and older.
            1.3.1.1 The prevalence of ECG abnormalities that predict cardiac complications increases with advancing age.

        1.3.1.2 The incidence of previously unrecognized recent myocardial infarction increases with advancing age.

1.3.2. An ECG may be useful in detecting certain arrhythmias associated with perioperative risk that are not apparent on physical examination ("silent" arrhythmias).

        1.3.2.1 A rhythm other than sinus or premature atrial contractions on the last preoperative ECG or ventricular ectopy with five or more premature ventricular beats per minute documented at any time before surgery is associated with increased perioperative cardiac morbidity and mortality.

        1.3.2.2 Patients at increased risk of "silent" arrhythmias include those with a history or physical findings suggestive of cardiovascular disease and asymptomatic older patients.

1.3.3 An ECG may be useful in patients with systemic diseases or other conditions that may be associated with clinically important but previously unrecognized cardiac abnormalities.

        1.3.3.1 Diseases that may be associated with unrecognized coronary atherosclerosis include hypertension, atherosclerotic peripheral vascular disease, and diabetes mellitus.

        1.3.3.2 Diseases that may be associated with unrecognized cardiac involvement include certain malignancies, collagen vascular diseases, infectious diseases, and electrolyte abnormalities.

1.3.4 An ECG may be useful in patients prescribed certain noncardiac medications.

        1.3.4.1 Medications that may be associated with cardiac toxicity or ECG alterations include phenothiazines, tricyclic antidepressants, doxorubicin and related drugs, and others.

    1.4 An ECG may be indicated in patients with cardiac signs or symptoms.

        1.4.1 An ECG may be useful in patients with a history of or physical findings suggesting clinically important heart disease, including arrhythmias.

2. General Considerations

    2.1 The value of a preoperative ECG has not been ascertained but may be useful for certain surgical procedures.

        2.1.1 Patients having intrathoracic, intraperitoneal, or aortic surgery or emergency operations under general or regional anesthesia are at increased risk of cardiac complications.

        2.1.2 Patients undergoing intracranial and other major neurological operations may be at increased risk of ECG alterations.

        2.1.3 Patients at any age who have had prior surgery with documented dysarrhythmias during surgery or postoperatively.

Routine Chest Radiographs

Definition

Routine chest radiographs refer to the radiographic examination routinely performed on hospital admission or prior to surgery.

Rationale

Although admission and preoperative chest radiographs are able to detect unexpected or occult abnormalities in a patient otherwise asymptomatic for chest disease, the findings of a routine chest radiograph rarely affect patient management or enhance patient care. In addition, the false-positive or false-negative results that may arise from routine chest radiographs may lead to unnecessary diagnostic tests or unwarranted reassurance. The history and physical examination and the clinical judgment of the physician will determine the need for a chest radiograph.

Recommendations

1. Screening/Case-finding
   1.1 A chest radiograph is not routinely indicated solely because of hospital admission.
   1.2 A chest radiograph is not routinely indicated as part of a preoperative evaluation, prior to anesthetic administration, or for a baseline assessment.
   1.3 A chest radiograph is not indicated solely because of advanced age.
       1.3.1 Because of the high prevalence of symptoms and signs of chest disease in this age group, many elderly patients will require a chest radiograph.
   1.4 A routine preoperative chest radiograph is generally indicated for patients scheduled for intrathoracic surgical procedures.
2. Evaluation of Suspected Disease
   2.1 An admission or preoperative chest radiograph is indicated in patients with signs or symptoms of active chest disease.
       2.1.1 A history and physical examination will identify most patients in whom there is chest disease.
       2.1.2 A chest radiograph in a patient with clinical evidence of chest disease provides a basis for subsequent diagnostic procedures and possible diagnoses.

Arterial Blood Gas Analysis

Definition

Arterial blood gas analysis refers to the evaluation of oxygen and carbon dioxide gas exchange and acid-base status, specifically pH, P_{CO_2}, P_{O_2}, and calculated bicarbonate.

Rationale

Traditionally, arterial blood gas analysis has been used to evaluate suspected significant aberrations in blood gas exchange or acid-base balance. Many clinicians believe arterial blood gas analysis is done too frequently. However, the utility and appropriate frequency of blood gas analysis in diagnosis and clinical management have not been thoroughly studied. The recommendations for the use of arterial blood gas analysis should be interpreted within this context.

Recommendations

1. Diagnosis
   1.1 Arterial blood gas analysis may be indicated in adult patients who are severely ill due to conditions that produce gas exchange abnormalities or acid-base disturbances.
   1.2 Arterial blood gas analysis may be indicated when patients undergo resting pulmonary function tests, exercise pulmonary function tests, shunt studies, sleep disorder studies, or respiratory control sensitivity studies.
2. Monitoring
   2.1 Arterial blood gas analysis may be indicated in chronically ill patients when a change in clinical status occurs or when a change in patient management is being considered.
   2.2 Arterial blood gas analysis may be indicated in patients with life-threatening cardiovascular conditions in the intensive care unit when a change in clinical status occurs or when a change in patient management is being considered.
      2.2.1 Serial arterial blood gas analyses may be useful in monitoring patient progress, adjusting oxygen and other medication regi-

mens, and making management decisions concerning mechanical ventilation, positive end-expiratory pressure, and weaning from ventilatory support.

2.2.2 Patients with life-threatening cardiovascular conditions in intensive care units frequently have significant fluctuation in Po_2; repeat arterial blood gas analyses may not be necessary when changes in arterial blood gases are not accompanied by changes in clinical status.

2.3 Arterial blood gas analysis may be indicated for acutely ill asthmatic patients.

2.3.1 Arterial blood gas tensions are moderately correlated with severity of asthma.

2.3.1.1 Spirometry (peak expiratory flow rates [PEFR] or forced expiratory volume in 1 second [FEV_1]) can identify patients at increased risk for hypercarbia or respiratory failure and identify patients who may require arterial blood gas analysis.

2.4 Arterial blood gas analysis is indicated in patients requiring mechanical ventilation.

2.4.1 Standardized weaning protocols and safe techniques for limiting mechanical ventilation time can decrease the need for repeated arterial blood gas measurements. Use of arterial blood gas analysis is an important tool for evaluating weaning success.

2.5 Arterial blood gas analysis is indicated to identify patients requiring long-term oxygen therapy.

2.6 Arterial blood gas analysis is not routinely indicated in the following contexts:

2.6.1 Patients receiving prophylactic, low-flow oxygen in the hospital—for example, patients with suspected myocardial infarction receiving nasal oxygen.

2.6.2 Patients with acute uncomplicated myocardial infarction before, during, or at the discontinuation of low- or moderate-flow supplemental nasal oxygen.

3. General Considerations

3.1 Noninvasive arterial blood gas analysis using finger or ear oximetry or transcutaneous electrodes in critically ill adults requires further clinical study.

3.1.1 Finger or ear oximetry may be useful for evaluating oxygen gas exchange in patients who are candidates for long-term supplemental oxygen therapy or patients who are undergoing sleep or exercise studies.

3.1.2 Oximetry may be considered as an alternative to arterial blood gas analysis in chronically ill patients when oxygenation rather than Pco_2 or acid-base disturbances is of concern.

4. The preceding guidelines should be applied when using arterial blood gas analysis to evaluate the following conditions.

  4.1 Gas exchange abnormalities (Po_2, Pco_2)

    4.1.1 Actue and chronic pulmonary disease

      4.1.1.1 Obstructive (bronchitis, emphysema, chronic obstructive pulmonary disease, asthma)

      4.1.1.2 Restrictive (pneumonia, atelectasis, pulmonary edema, acute or chronic infiltrative lung disease)

      4.1.1.3 Pulmonary vascular (pulmonary embolism, vasculitis)

      4.1.1.4 Ventilatory control (sleep apnea syndromes, hyperventilation syndrome, central nervous system disease)

    4.1.2 Acute respiratory failure

      4.1.2.1 Any obstructive disease (bronchitis, emphysema, chronic obstructive disease, asthma)

      4.1.2.2 Adult respiratory distress syndrome

      4.1.2.3 Trauma

      4.1.2.4 Drugs and toxins

    4.1.3 Cardiovascular diseases

      4.1.3.1 Congestive heart failure

      4.1.3.2 Shock (with pulmonary shunt)

      4.1.3.3 Assessment of intracardiac shunt.

    4.1.4 Rest and exercise pulmonary function tests

    4.1.5 Monitoring acute high-flow or long-term oxygen therapy

    4.1.6 Sleep disorder studies

  4.2 Acid-base disturbances

    4.2.1 Metabolic acidosis

      4.2.1.1 Lactic acidosis

      4.2.1.2 Renal failure

Erythrocyte Sedimentation Rate

Definition

The erythrocyte sedimentation rate (ESR) refers to the rate at which red blood cells settle in anticoagulated blood. Although several methods of measuring ESR are acceptable, the Westergren or modified Westergren methods are recommended because of the increased accuracy associated with either of these techniques.

Rationale

The ESR may be useful in diagnosing and monitoring a variety of diseases. However, the ESR should be ordered with the following caveats:

1. An increased ESR is seldom the sole manifestation of disease. A careful history and physical examination will usually disclose the cause of an elevated ESR and suggest a more specific diagnostic evaluation. In patients without complaints and abnormalities on physical examination, an elevated ESR is usually transient and will normalize within several months.
2. A normal ESR in a patient with vague, unexplained symptoms does not exclude occult malignancy or other serious disease.

Recommendations

1. Screening/Case-finding
   1.1 The ESR is not indicated in asymptomatic persons.
   1.2 An ESR should be used selectively and interpreted with caution in patients with symptoms that are not explained by results of a careful history and physical examination.
2. Diagnosis
   2.1 The ESR is indicated for the diagnosis of temporal arteritis (giant cell arteritis) and polymyalgia rheumatica.
      2.1.1 A normal ESR virtually excludes the diagnosis of temporal arteritis in most patients who are suspected of having the disease.
      2.1.2 When there is strong clinical evidence for temporal arteritis and the ESR is normal,

further efforts to diagnose temporal arteritis are required.

 2.1.3 A normal ESR virtually excludes the diagnosis of polymyalgia rheumatica.

2.2 A careful history and physical examination are the most reliable means of making a diagnosis of rheumatoid arthritis. In patients with an equivocal examination, an ESR may be indicated, and an abnormal result is a clue to the presence of this disease.

3. Monitoring

 3.1 The ESR is indicated for monitoring temporal arteritis and polymyalgia rheumatica.

  3.1.1 The ESR is one indicator of disease activity in temporal arteritis and polymyalgia rheumatica. Clinical status should be the principal indication for adjusting the dosage of corticosteroids.

 3.2 Routine repetitive use of the ESR is not recommended for monitoring disease activity in rheumatoid arthritis. Judicious use of the ESR combined with other clinical observations may be of value in some patients with rheumatoid arthritis.

 3.3 The ESR may be indicated for monitoring patients with treated Hodgkin's disease.

 3.4 The ESR may be indicated for monitoring patients with acute rheumatic fever.

4. General Considerations

 4.1 Although the ESR is used by physicians and may be of value in a variety of other clinical situations, there have been no studies that confirm or disprove its role in these situations.

Complete Blood Count and Leukocyte Differential Count

Definition

The complete blood count (CBC) includes the measurement of hemoglobin, hematocrit, total leukocyte count, and computer-derived red cell indices. The CBC does not include platelet count, reticulocyte count, or leukocyte differential count.

The leukocyte differential count (LDC) involves the estimation (based on counting 100 cells) of the percentages of leukocytes that are mature polymorphonuclear neutrophils, band neutrophils, lymphocytes, monocytes, eosinophils, basophils, or other cell types.

The definition of CBC or LDC does not include the systematic review of the blood smear by visual examination. Reasons to examine the blood smear visually are not addressed in these guidelines.

Rationale

The CBC and LDC are two of the most commonly used clinical laboratory tests for purposes of screening, diagnosis, and monitoring. However, routine use of CBCs and LDCs in populations of low disease prevalence have a low yield. In addition, there may be little benefit from detection of mild asymptomatic abnormalities. The CBC and LDC should be ordered selectively, in situations where there is demonstrable benefit to patients. Only specific components of the CBC should be chosen according to clinical need.

Recommendations: Complete Blood Count (CBC)

1. Outpatient Screening/Case-finding
   *1.1 The CBC is appropriate at initial outpatient evaluation; repeat CBCs are not indicated in patients in whom no abnormality is suspected.

---

* The recommendation in this paragraph of the guidelines is not the opinion of the authors of the foregoing paper.

1.2 In specific subsets of the population with higher prevalences of anemia, the CBC may be useful to identify those who are significantly anemic because of poor nutrition or undiagnosed chronic illness, including the following:

    1.2.1 Pregnant women in whom there is a suspicion that iron supplementation or nutrition has not been adequate;

    1.2.2 The institutionalized elderly (75 years old or more);

    1.2.3 Recent immigrants from third world countries, especially persons at increased risk of malnourishment.

2. Hospital Admission Screening/Case-finding

2.1 The CBC is indicated in patients admitted to the hospital for surgery that may involve substantial blood loss.

2.2 The CBC is not routinely indicated on hospital admission in patients in whom no abnormality is suspected, including the following:

    2.2.1 Patients undergoing elective minor surgery in which substantial blood loss is not anticipated;

    2.2.2 Patients undergoing minor diagnostic procedures, such as gastrointestinal endoscopy, who have not been bleeding;

    2.2.3 Patients admitted for exacerbation of dermatological disease when infection is not suspected.

3. Diagnosis of Suspected Abnormality

3.1 The CBC is indicated in the diagnosis of infection or primary hematological disorders.

    3.1.1 The CBC is indicated in patients in whom there are clinical findings suggestive of anemia, including fatigue, mucous membrane pallor, or peripheral neuropathy, abnormal bleeding, or findings suggestive of polycythemia.

3.2 The CBC may be useful in conditions that may be associated with severe anemia, including renal insufficiency and malignancy.

3.3 The CBC may be useful when infection is suspected, especially when other confirming findings are absent.

4. Monitoring

4.1 Repeat CBCs may be useful in the following:

    4.1.1 Patients in whom there is concern that treatment has not been effective;

4.1.1.1 When looking for evidence of response to treatment for anemia, repeat hemoglobins and hematocrits may be useful after 1 to 2 weeks of iron therapy.

4.1.2 Anemic or bleeding patients in whom transfusions are anticipated;

4.1.3 Patients in whom significant changes in CBC that might affect patient management are anticipated—for example, chemotherapy. The appropriate frequency for repeat testing when looking for evidence of response in hospitalized patients has not been determined, but is unlikely to be less than every 2 days unless clinically important changes in the results are anticipated.

4.2 Repeat CBCs are not indicated in patients in whom no abnormality is suspected.

Recommendations: Leukocyte Count and Leukocyte Differential Count (LDC)

1. Outpatient Screening/Case-finding
   1.1 The LDC is not routinely indicated in ambulatory asymptomatic patients.
2. Hospital Admission Screening/Case-finding
   2.1 The LDC is not indicated in patients in whom there is no reason to expect an abnormality.
   2.2 The LDC may be useful on hospital admission to confirm a suspected infection or to detect patients at risk of infection due to granulocytopenia caused by treatment or known disease.
   2.3 The LDC is not routinely indicated in patients admitted for elective surgery.
3. Diagnosis of Suspected Abnormality
   3.1 The LDC may be useful, regardless of the total leukocyte count, in the diagnostic evaluation of the following:
      3.1.1 Newly suspected infection;
      3.1.2 New fever;
      3.1.3 Suspicion of primary hematological disorder—for example, anemia, leukemia;
      3.1.4 Suspicion of disease associated with secondary abnormalities of LDCs—for example, lymphoma, lymphocytopenia;
   3.2 The LDC may be indicated in the diagnostic evaluation of patients with an abnormal leukocyte count if there is uncertainty about the

cause of abnormality or when management may be affected—for example, isolation of leukopenic patients.

    3.2.1 The LDC is generally not indicated when bacterial infection is known and when leukocytosis is present.

4. Monitoring
   4.1 The leukocyte count is useful in patients at risk of leukopenia due to chemotherapy or bone marrow disease.
       4.1.1 If the leukocyte count is greater than 4500, repeat LDC is not necessary to screen for granulocytopenia.
   4.2 Repeat leukocyte count and LDC may be useful in patients in whom it is unclear if treatment is effective or in whom the course of disease is difficult to discern.
   4.3 The appropriate interval for repeat LDC testing needs further study but is unlikely to be less then every 2 days in 7 in leukopenic patients.
   4.4 The LDC may be indicated in monitoring the following:
       4.4.1 Patients with infection not improving clinically;
       4.4.2 Patients with new symptoms to suggest infection or hematologic disorder;
       4.4.3 Patients with leukopenia;
       4.4.4 Patients on cytotoxic therapy if leukopenia is developing;
       4.4.5 Patients whose current illness is associated with previous abnormalities to assure their resolution.
   4.5 An LDC is not indicated in patients who are improving clinically.

Activated Partial Thromboplastin Time and Prothrombin Time

Definition

The activated partial thromboplastin time (APTT) and prothrombin time (PT) are tests used to assess blood coagulation.

Rationale

The APTT and PT assess the time required for various stages of the coagulation process to occur. The results yield information on the adequacy of a patient's coagulation system.

Recommendations

1. Screening/Case-finding
   1.1 Preoperative evaluation
       1.1.1 Preoperative evaluation with APTT or PT is not indicated for patients without clinical findings suggestive of increased bleeding risk.
       1.1.2 Preoperative evaluation with both the APTT and PT is indicated for the following:
           1.1.2.1 Patients with abnormal clinical findings (active bleeding, history of abnormal bleeding, evidence of liver disease, malabsorption or malnutrition, or recent use of anticoagulants);
           1.1.2.2 Patients in whom adequate clinical assessment is not possible (history is unavailable);
           1.1.2.3 Patients whose normal coagulation may be disrupted by the operative procedure (insertion of a peritoneovenous shunt and procedures involving extracorporeal circulation).
       1.1.3 If results of an APTT or PT are abnormal, the test should be repeated. If the results are still abnormal, additional studies are indicated.

1.2 Nonsurgical evaluation

    1.2.1 The APTT and PT are not indicated for evaluation of asymptomatic patients who are not undergoing invasive procedures.

2. Evaluation of Abnormal Bleeding

    2.1 The APTT and PT are indicated as initial studies in all patients who experience spontaneous bleeding or prolonged bleeding after an injury or surgical procedure.

        2.1.1 If results of both tests are normal, no additional coagulation studies are indicated. However, a platelet count and studies of platelet function may be indicated.

        2.1.2 If results of one or both tests are abnormal, additional coagulation studies are indicated.

3. Monitoring Anticoagulation Therapy

    3.1 Daily APTTs are indicated to monitor heparin therapy.

        3.1.1 More frequent measurements may be indicated initially while titrating therapeutic dosages of heparin.

    3.2 The PT is indicated at the following intervals to monitor warfarin therapy:

        3.2.1 Daily during the first week of therapy;

        3.2.2 Weekly for the next few weeks;

        3.2.3 Monthly when stable.

        3.2.4 More frequent determinations may be indicated when starting a new drug that may interact with warfarin.

    3.3 Both the APTT and PT are indicated simultaneously only if monitoring a change from one type of anticoagulation therapy (heparin, warfarin) to the other.

    3.4 Monitoring is not indicated when using prophylactic, low-dose, subcutaneous injections of heparin.

Blood Cultures

Definition

Blood cultures used for detecting clinically significant bacteremia entail sampling and incubation in culture medium of a patient's blood one or more times. A variety of blood culture techniques are available for detecting bacterial growth, identifying specific organism(s), and testing antimicrobial susceptibility.

Rationale

Blood cultures are the only tests available to diagnose bacteremia definitively and often provide the only information on the causative organism. However, the utility of blood cultures, based on the sensitivity and specificity of the tests, depends on a variety or factors, including the timing of the cultures, number of samplings, volume of blood sampled, growth characteristics of the culture medium, system for detecting growth in the culture, and the clinician's ability to interpret results.

Both the sensitivity and specificity of blood cultures are increased by obtaining additional cultures; the maximum diagnostic certainty is usually attained within a series of three cultures.

Recommendations

1. Clinical Utility
   1.1 Blood cultures are useful in establishing a diagnosis of bacteremia in high-risk populations— for example, febrile hospitalized patients, febrile neutropenic patients, and patients with nosocomial infections and patients with known valvular heart disease.
   1.2 Blood cultures are useful in identifying the organisms responsible for serious bacteremia—for example, infective endocarditis and spontaneous pneumococcal bacteremia.
       1.2.1 Blood cultures may be useful in identifying organisms responsible for infections that may be difficult to diagnose directly—for example, osteomyelitis.

1.3 Blood cultures are useful in providing prognostic information and identifying potential complications of infections—for example, osteomyelitis and meningitis.
1.4 Blood cultures are useful in monitoring therapy.
1.5 Certain conditions may affect the interpretation and, therefore, the utility of blood culture results, including the following:
  1.5.1 Infective endocarditis in patients with prosthetic rather than natural valves;
  1.5.2 Patients with drug addiction;
  1.5.3 Transient bacteremia.
2. Test Performance
  2.1 The sensitivity and specificity of blood cultures in patients with bacteremia may be altered by the following factors:
    2.1.1 Small inoculum of blood;
    2.1.2 Prior use of antibiotics;
    2.1.3 Lack of anaerobic cultures;
    2.1.4 Contamination of sample;
    2.1.5 Timing.
3. Number of Required Tests
  3.1 One set of blood cultures is rarely if ever indicated. (A set is defined as one sample of blood.)
  3.2 Two sets of blood cultures may be sufficient in patients in whom the probability of bacteremia is low to moderate and when the anticipated pathogen is different from the usual contaminating flora.
    3.2.1 If both sets of cultures are negative, the probability of bacteremia is extremely low.
  3.3 Three sets of blood cultures are usually indicated in patients in whom the probability of bacteremia is high or in the diagnosis of suspected continuous bacteremia—for example, infective endocarditis.
  3.4 Four to six blood culture sets may be indicated to exclude bacteremia when the pretest probability of bacteremia is high and one of the following conditions exists:
    3.4.1 The anticipated pathogens are also common contaminants—for example, prosthetic valve infective endocarditis;
    3.4.2 The patient with suspected infective endocarditis has received antimicrobials within the prior 2 weeks.

Syphilis Tests

Definition

Diagnostic tests for syphilis include the direct identification of the infectious agent, *Treponema pallidum*, in the exudate of lesions or the demonstration of antibodies in blood or cerebrospinal fluid (CSF). Direct methods include the darkfield test or direct fluorescent antibody treponemal test; indirect, or serological, methods include nontreponemal and treponemal tests. Nontreponemal tests include the Venereal Disease Research Laboratory (VDRL) test; treponemal tests include the fluorescent treponemal antibody absorption test (FTA-ABS) and microhemagglutination tests for syphilis (MHA-TP).

Rationale

Selection of the appropriate test is determined by stage of disease, which can be categorized as primary, secondary, early latent, late latent, late, or congenital and the purpose of the test, including screening, diagnosis, or monitoring.

Recommendations

1. Screening/Case-finding
   1.1 Routine testing for syphilis as part of a preoperative or hospital admission evaluation is not indicated.
   1.2 The VDRL is indicated in select populations, including:
      1.2.1 Pregnant women;
      1.2.2 Sexual contacts of persons with known, infectious syphilis;
      1.2.3 Other high-risk groups.
   1.3 The MHA-TP or FTA-ABS is indicated to confirm a positive VDRL (in an otherwise asymptomatic person).
2. Diagnosis
   2.1 The darkfield test (for genital lesions) or direct fluorescent antibody test (for oral lesions) is indicated in the diagnosis of primary syphilis.
   2.2 The VDRL or darkfield test (on exudate from moist or scarified dry lesions) is indicated in the diagnosis of secondary syphilis.
   2.3 The VDRL is indicated in the diagnosis of early latent syphilis.
   2.4 The CSF-VDRL and CSF cell count are indicated only in serum-positive persons at high

risk of developing neurosyphilis, including the following:

   2.4.1 Patients with syphilis and neurological abnormalities;

   2.4.2 Before retreatment of syphilis patients who have relapses;

   2.4.3 Before treatment with nonpenicillin regimens.

3. Monitoring

  3.1 The VDRL is indicated after treatment of known or suspected syphilis, including:

   3.1.1 Treated women with newly diagnosed serum-positive syphilis late in pregnancy;

   3.1.2 Treated contacts of persons with known syphilis.

  3.2 The CSF cell count is indicated after treatment to monitor effectiveness of treatment of neurosyphilis.

4. Known or suspected syphilis in infants

  4.1 Infants born to mothers who have been adequately treated with penicillin require surveillance; the VDRL is indicated monthly for 3 months.

  4.2 Infants born to mothers inadequately treated for syphilis should be treated immediately for early syphilis, as diagnostic confirmation with VDRL is not indicated prior to treatment. The VDRL is indicated 1, 3, and 6 months after treatment.

  4.3 The CSF-VDRL and CSF cell count are indicated in infants suspected of congenital syphilis.

5. General Considerations

  5.1 A positive VDRL should always be titered to provide maximum information.

  5.2 A VDRL that is either nonreactive or has a stable titer in association with a positive treponemal test (FTA-ABS or MHA-TP) may be diagnostic of late latent syphilis, but these laboratory findings may also be due to the following:

   5.2.1 Nonsyphilitic treponemal disease;

   5.2.2 False-positive treponemal test;

   5.2.3 Adequately treated syphilis.

  5.3 The MHA-TP and FTA-ABS are highly sensitive in symptomatic late syphilis.

  5.4 Indirect tests have decreased specificity in the elderly or in individuals with certain other diseases.

  5.5 Indirect tests have low sensitivity in the incubating stage of syphilis.

Throat Cultures and Rapid Tests for Diagnosis of Group A Streptococcal Pharyngitis

Definition

Tests useful in the diagnosis of adult sore throat due to group A beta-hemolytic streptococci include throat cultures and non-culture-based rapid antigen detection tests.

Rationale

The diagnosis and treatment of group A streptococcal pharyngitis depend on several factors, including the pretest probability of disease, the benefits and risks of treatment, the availability of diagnostic tests, and the speed with which the results of these tests become available.

The probability of disease is positively correlated with the prevalence of group A streptococcal pharyngitis in the population and the number of signs and symptoms of disease manifested by the patient. The following signs and symptoms have been identified as independent predictors of disease and are the basis for these recommendations: *tonsillar exudates, swollen tender anterior cervical nodes, history of fever, and the lack of a cough.*

Benefits associated with the antibiotic treatment of group A streptococcal pharyngitis include the following: a decrease in the morbidity and duration of disease; reduction in the spread of the disease in the population; prevention or reduction in suppurative complications of pharyngitis; and a decrease in the incidence of post-streptococcal rheumatic fever. Risks associated with antibiotic therapy include allergic reactions, especially to penicillin, and undesirable side effects—for example, nausea from erythromycin.

The methods for diagnosing group A beta-hemolytic streptococcal pharyngitis include throat cultures and non-culture-based rapid antigen detection tests. The accuracy of the tests varies with the method used, as does the length of time necessary to achieve results. Sensitivity estimates have been reported as low as 29%

for office cultures, between 76% and 90% for laboratory cultures, and between 80% and 96% for rapid tests. A specificity of 99% has been achieved for office and laboratory cultures and rapid tests, with greater variability reported for office cultures (ranging from 76% to 99%). The time required to achieve results ranges from 7 to 70 minutes for rapid tests and from 24 to 48 hours for throat cultures.

The recommendations in these guidelines are based on a model of disease probability as a function of clinical presentation and assume a 10% prevalence of group A streptococcal pharyngitis in the population. The decision to treat immediately or to culture will vary with disease prevalence; lower disease prevalence favors testing before treatment, whereas higher disease prevalence favors immediate treatment.

Recommendations

1. Throat Culture
   1.1 A throat culture is not routinely indicated to confirm the diagnosis of group A streptococcal pharyngitis in adult patients presenting with sore throats who have a high clinical probability of disease.
      1.1.1 Patients manifesting three or more of the following signs or symptoms of group A streptococcal pharyngitis are at increased risk of disease: tonsillar exudates; swollen anterior cervical nodes; history of fever; lack of cough. Based on prevalences of group A streptococcal pharyngitis in most adult populations, it may be appropriate to begin treating these patients immediately. If other clinical findings reduce the physician's estimate of disease probability, testing may be indicated.
   1.2 A throat culture is indicated to confirm the diagnosis of group A streptococcal pharyngitis before treatment of adult patients presenting with sore throats who have less than three signs or symptoms of disease. If other findings raise the estimated probability of disease, treatment without testing may be indicated.
      1.2.1 If patient compliance to follow-up is not expected, it may be appropriate to begin treating these patients immediately.

2. Rapid Antigen Detection Tests

  2.1 Based on prevalences of group A streptococcal pharyngitis in most adult populations, rapid tests may be indicated to diagnose group A streptococcal pharyngitis before treatment in most adult patients presenting with sore throats, regardless of the number of signs and symptoms of disease and provided that test results become available during the initial visit. [This recommendation is based on the decision analysis presented by Centor, Meier and Dalton (1986). Others suggest that the threshold for using the rapid antigen detection test (the number of symptoms) should be the same as the throat culture test.]

  2.2 Based on the limited experience with rapid tests done in physician offices, the significance of the rapid test results should be interpreted cautiously.

    2.2.1 These guidelines apply to clinical setting where the tests are done by trained personnel and where appropriate quality control is maintained.

3. General Considerations

  3.1 Office cultures and rapid antigen detection tests should be routinely monitored by quality control protocols to ensure their accuracy.

Urinalysis and Urine Culture (and Other Tests) in Women with Acute Dysuria

Definition

Tests useful in evaluating women with different suspected causes of acute dysuria include urinalysis; urine culture; Gram stain (urine or discharge); Thayer-Martin and New York City culture; vaginal examination; and microscopic examination of abnormal discharge.

Rationale

The patient with acute dysuria may have one of a number of clinical conditions, each diagnosed and managed differently. The roles of urinalysis, urine culture, and other tests are different in each of these conditions. There is also a role for urinalysis and urine culture in diagnosing patients at significant risk of infection but without symptoms.

These guidelines are limited to urinary tract and vaginal infections in symptomatic women or women suspected of having asymptomatic bacteriuria. They do not apply to other populations or disorders, including children of either sex; adult men; or patients with indwelling urinary catheters, noninfectious urinary tract disorders, or various systemic diseases. In addition, the recommendations in these guidelines are based on the assumption that clean specimens have been obtained for urinalysis and urine cultures; contaminated specimens may lead to misdiagnoses.

Recommendations (categorized by suspected cause)

1. Asymptomatic Women
   1.1 Urinalysis and urine culture are not routinely indicated to screen for asymptomatic bacteriuria, except perhaps in pregnant women, where diagnosis and treatment of asymptomatic bacteriuria may reduce the likelihood of subsequent clinically overt urinary infection.
2. Acute Pyelonephritis
   2.1 Acute pyelonephritis is a clinical condition suggested by fever, flank pain, nausea and vomiting, rigors, costovertebral angle tenderness, and other findings in association with dysuria, frequency, and urgency (although these symptoms sometimes may be absent).

2.2 The following diagnostic tests are indicated in any patient suspected of having acute pyelonephritis

	Test	Expected Results
2.2.1	Urinalysis	Pyuria and bacteriuria
2.2.2	Urine culture	100 000 bacteria/mL*
2.2.3	Urine Gram stain	Gram-negative bacilli or gram-positive cocci

* Occasionally, the criterion for positive urine culture (100 000 bacteria/mL) is not present in acute or subclinical pyelonephritis.

2.3 Urine culture is indicated shortly after completion of therapy to confirm bacteriologic cure.

3. Subclinical Pyelonephritis

3.1 Subclinical pyelonephritis is a clinical condition that presents with symptoms of a lower urinary tract bacterial infection, including dysuria, frequency, and urgency, without fever or other symptoms or signs of acute pyelonephritis; however, the patient has upper tract infection. Several clinical factors increase the likelihood that these patients have subclinical pyelonephritis, including: known underlying urinary tract disorders; diabetes mellitus or other conditions or therapies producing an immunocompromised state; a history of urinary infections in childhood; documented relapsing infection with the same bacterium at any time in the past; symptoms for 7 to 10 days before seeking care; three or more urinary infections in the past year; acute pyelonephritis in the past year; and lower socioeconomic status.

3.2 The following diagnostic tests are indicated in any patient suspected of having subclinical pyelonephritis

	Test	Expected Results
3.2.1	Urinalysis	Pyuria and bacteriuria
3.2.2	Urine culture	100 000 bacteria/mL*
3.2.3	Urine Gram stain	Gram-negative bacilli or gram-positive cocci

* Occasionally, the criterion for positive urine culture (100 000 bacteria/mL) is not present in acute or subclinical pyelonephritis.

3.3 Urine culture and urinalysis, or urine culture alone, are indicated shortly after completion of treatment.

4. Chlamydial Urethritis

4.1 Chlamydial urethritis is a clinical condition suggested by prolonged dysuria (and frequency or urgency) when a patient has a sexual partner with recent urethritis or has a new sexual partner, when hematuria is absent, or when mucopurulent cervical discharge with an edematous exocervix is noted.

4.2 The following diagnostic test is indicated in any patient suspected of having chlamydial urethritis:

Test	Expected Results
4.2.1 Urinalysis	Pyuria without bacteriuria

4.3 Urine culture is not necessary in a patient suspected of having chlamydial urethritis.

5. Gonococcal Urethritis

5.1 Gonococcal urethritis is a clinical condition suggested by a recent history of documented gonorrhea in the patient or her sexual partner, or having a sexual partner with recent urethritis.

5.2 The following diagnostic tests are indicated in any patient suspected of having gonococcal urethritis:

Test	Expected Results
5.2.1 Urinalysis	Pyuria without bacteriuria
5.2.2 Gram stain of purulent discharge from urethral or cervical os	Gram-negative intracellular diplococci
5.2.3 Culture on Thayer-Martin or New York City media	*Neisseria gonorrhoeae*

6. Vaginitis

6.1 Vaginitis is a clinical condition suggested by dysuria, vaginal discharge, itch, or irritation.

6.2 The following diagnostic tests are indicated in

any patient suspected of having vaginitis:

Test	Expected Results
6.2.1 Vaginal examination	Abnormal discharge
6.2.2 Microscopic examination of abnormal discharge	Budding yeast and pseudohyphae, trichomonads, "clue cells"

6.3 Urinalysis and urine culture are not routinely indicated in a patient suspected of having vaginitis.

7. Lower Urinary Tract Bacterial Infection
    7.1 Lower urinary tract bacterial infection is a clinical condition suggested by dysuria, frequency, and urgency without fever and in which the clinical features suggesting other causes of acute dysuria are absent.
    7.2 The following diagnostic test is indicated in any patient suspected of having a lower urinary tract bacterial infection:

	Test	Expected Results
7.2.1	Urinalysis	Pyuria and bacteriuria

    7.3 Urine culture may not be routinely indicated in a patient suspected of having a lower urinary tract bacterial infection.
        7.3.1 In recurrent lower urinary tract infection, urine culture may be useful to guide subsequent therapy.
    7.4 Urine culture following treatment is not routinely indicated in a patient suspected of having a lower urinary tract bacterial infection.
        7.4.1 In treatment failure, urine culture may be useful in patient management.

8. Dysuria with no apparent infectious pathogen
    8.1 Dysuria without pyuria and that does not respond to antimicrobial treatment suggests that an infectious pathogen will not be identified.
    8.2 The following diagnostic test is indicated in any patient presenting with dysuria and no other clinical findings.

	Test	Expected Results
8.2.1	Urinalysis	No pyuria, no bacteriuria

Carcinoembryonic Antigen

Definition

Carcinoembryonic antigen (CEA) is one of a class of oncofetal antigens normally present in fetal life. The antigen occurs at low concentrations in adults and circulates in high concentrations in patients with certain malignancies, particularly epithelial tumors.

Rationale

Extreme elevations of CEA are unusual in apparently healthy people. Although CEA levels are increased in the presence of a variety of cancers and benign diseases, its primary value is in the management of colorectal cancer.

Recommendations

1. Screening/Case-finding
    1.1 The CEA test is not indicated for detecting early-stage colorectal cancer in asymptomatic patients.
2. Diagnosis
    2.1 The CEA test has limited value in the initial diagnosis of colorectal cancer.
        2.1.1 The CEA level cannot, in itself, establish the diagnosis of colorectal cancer. However, CEA may be useful, in conjunction with other noninvasive tests, in deciding how actively to pursue a diagnostic work-up for colorectal cancer.
        2.1.2 The CEA test does not replace the following methods of diagnosing colorectal cancer, if cancer is suspected: barium enema; sigmoidoscopy or colonoscopy, with biopsy of abnormal appearing lesions.
        2.1.3 The CEA test is not indicated for distinguishing locally invasive polyps from benign polyps.
3. Prognosis
    3.1 Although CEA levels can predict recurrence of colorectal cancer at time of diagnosis (prior to treatment), this information is of limited value in patient management.

4. Monitoring
   4.1 Although CEA tests can detect recurrence of colorectal cancer after surgery, earlier than other methods, this information is of limited value in patient management.
   4.2 The CEA test may be useful for monitoring a patient's response to treatment.
       4.2.1 The CEA test may be useful only if selection of therapy is contingent on test results (certain chemotherapy regimens when there is no alternative method to assess disease progression).
5. General Considerations
   5.1 The CEA test is of limited value in the management of patients with colorectal cancer. It is even less useful in the management of cancer at various other sites, including gastrointestinal, breast, and lung tumors.

Biochemical Profiles in Ambulatory Screening and Preadmission Testing of Adults

Definition

A biochemical profile is a general battery of biochemical tests measured on large volume, automated instruments; these guidelines do not address batteries of tests directed primarily at individual organ systems. Screening refers to efforts to detect disease in asymptomatic individuals or other persons without risk factors or other reasons to suggest higher probability of disease. Preadmission testing in these guidelines refers to routine use of biochemical profiles prior to, or at the time of, hospital admission; that is, testing that is conducted without regard to clinical evidence in an individual patient.

Rationale

Biochemical profiles have been performed in order to detect important but clinically inapparent disorders in asymptomatic patients. However, statistical and epidemiologic principles predict that the routine use of biochemical profiles in populations with low disease prevalence may yield high rates of false-positive results. In addition, the greater the number of component tests in a profile, the greater the likelihood of false-positive findings. Based on the prevalence of disease and the availability of treatment, specific components of biochemical profiles may be useful.

Recommendations

1. Ambulatory Screening
    1.1 Biochemical profiles are not routinely indicated for screening asymptomatic adults.
        1.1.1 Specific components of biochemical profiles that are not indicated for screening include the following.
            1.1.1.1 Serum calcium;
            1.1.1.2 Alkaline phosphatase;
            1.1.1.3 Uric acid;
            1.1.1.4 Sodium;
            1.1.1.5 Potassium;
            1.1.1.6 Chloride;

        1.1.1.7 Aspartate aminotransferase (AST);
        1.1.1.8 Lactate dehydrogenase (LDH);
        1.1.1.9 Total protein and albumin.

1.2 Selected components of biochemical profiles may be indicated for screening asymptomatic adults.

    1.2.1 Serum glucose may be indicated to identify diabetes mellitus.

    1.2.2 Serum cholesterol may be indicated to identify hypercholesterolemia.

    1.2.3 Serum creatinine, with or without blood urea nitrogen, may be useful to identify renal dysfunction.

2. Preadmission Testing

    2.1 Biochemical profiles are not routinely indicated prior to elective admission to the hospital.

3. In many cases current technology will not permit selective test ordering as recommended above.

Serum Electrolytes and Serum Osmolality

Definition

Serum electrolyte tests include the measurement of the concentrations of serum potassium, serum sodium, chloride, and total CO_2.

Rationale

Although serum electrolyte tests are among the most frequently used blood chemistries, there is a paucity of evidence in the literature to support their clinical utility. The recommendations for the use of serum electrolytes should be interpreted within this context.

Recommendations: Potassium

Rationale
Serum potassium concentration usually parallels total body potassium content and is an important determinant of neuromuscular activity throughout the body, especially cardiac conduction and function. Abnormalities of serum potassium concentration occur most in patients with renal impairment, patients on diuretics, patients with large gastrointestinal fluid losses, and in patients with unusually high or low intakes of potassium.

1. Screening
   1.1 Serum potassium measurement is not indicated in unselected populations.
      1.1.1 Potassium abnormalities rarely occur in patients who do not have a clinical history or manifestations of disease associated with potassium abnormality.
2. Case-finding/Diagnosis in Selected Populations
   2.1 Serum potassium measurement is indicated in patients with chronic renal disease, including diabetic renal insufficiency.
   2.2 Serum potassium measurement is indicated in patients with hypertension to detect primary hyperaldosteronism.
      2.2.1 Serum potassium measurement is indicated at the time of diagnosis of hypertension, before initiation of therapy.
   2.3 Serum potassium measurement is indicated in

patients with symptoms or signs suggestive of renal tubular acidosis.

2.4 Serum potassium measurement is indicated in patients with signs and symptoms suggestive of altered serum potassium concentration, including generalized or proximal muscle weakness, new atrial tachyarrhythmias, nocturia, polyuria, or ileus.

3. Patient Management

3.1 Serum potassium measurement is indicated in hypertensive patients receiving diuretic therapy.

   3.1.1 Serum potassium measurement is indicated in hypertensive patients receiving diuretic therapy prior to initiation of treatment, at 6 to 12 weeks, and at appropriate intervals thereafter, in the absence of other important clinical changes.

   3.1.2 Serum potassium measurement may be useful to monitor patient compliance with drug regimens.

3.2 Serum potassium measurement may be useful every 6 months in diuretic-treated patients concurrently receiving digitalis.

3.3 Serum potassium measurement may be useful on hospital admission for every acutely ill patient.

3.4 Serum potassium measurement may be useful in hospitalized patients in whom there is a change in clinical status.

   3.4.1 Daily measurements of serum potassium may be useful in the following:

      3.4.1.1 Patients with changing renal function, as in acute renal failure;

      3.4.1.2 Patients being treated for cardiac arrhythmias, especially those on digitalis;

      3.4.1.3 Patients with persistent gastrointestinal losses.

   3.4.2 Serum potassium measurements may be useful every several hours until the patient is stable in the following conditions:

      3.4.2.1 Patients undergoing intensive fluid replacement therapy, particularly when accompanied by carbohydrate loads or insulin;

      3.4.2.2 Patients treated for severe hyperkalemia or hypokalemia;

      3.4.2.3 Patients treated for severe metabolic acidosis—for example, diabetic ketoacidosis;

3.4.2.4 Patients treated with intensive diuretic therapy—for example for correction of severe hyponatremia.

3.5 If hyperkalemia is not present at the time of initial diagnosis of renal disease, serum potassium measurements may be useful to monitor a trend toward hyperkalemia.

Recommendations: Sodium

Rationale

Serum sodium concentration reflects the status of water balance throughout body fluids and can frequently be used to estimate body fluid osmolality.

Serum sodium concentration may not reflect fluid osmolality in certain situations (hyperglycemia, pseudohyponatremia). Serum sodium concentration is not an index of total body sodium. Serum sodium concentration should never be used alone to assess sodium balance or to predict patient need for sodium, nor to assess status of extracellular fluid volume.

1. Screening
   1.1 Serum sodium measurement is not indicated in unselected ambulatory patients in the absence of other clinical manifestations of disease.
2. Case-finding/Diagnosis in Selected Populations
   2.1 Serum sodium concentration is not indicated in hypertensive patients to identify primary aldosteronism.
      2.1.1 Serum sodium concentration elevation does not distinguish primary aldosteronism from other forms of hypertension.
   2.2 Serum sodium measurement is not indicated in otherwise healthy patients admitted for elective surgery or diagnostic procedures.
   2.3 Serum sodium measurement may be indicated in patients with the following signs or symptoms:
      2.3.1 Rapid change in weight;
      2.3.2 Rapid change in fluid balance (severe vomiting, diarrhea, polyuria);
      2.3.3 Rapid change in mental status;
      2.3.4 Clinical evidence of dehydration or volume depletion.

3. Patient Management

    3.1 Serum sodium measurement may be useful as an index of hydration in patients treated with lithium, especially in elderly persons or others who may fail to ingest adequate quantities of water to maintain water balance.

    3.2 Serum sodium measurement may be useful in patients with chronic renal insufficiency at the following frequencies:

        3.2.1 At the time of change in clinical status;

        3.2.2 When serum creatinine reaches 7 to 8 mg/dL, thereafter every 2 to 3 months.

    3.3 Serum sodium measurement may be indicated in most acutely or chronically ill patients on hospital admission or at the time of change in clinical status, especially change in mental or neurologic status, fluid balance, weight, or dehydration or volume depletion—for example, patients with congestive heart failure, cirrhosis, or nephrotic syndrome.

        3.3.1 Repeat measurements of serum sodium are indicated in any hospitalized patient who has an initially abnormal value.

        3.3.2 The frequency of serum sodium determinations should be based on the rate of anticipated changes.

            3.3.2.1 Serum sodium measurements no more than once a day may be sufficient in patients receiving parenteral fluids.

            3.3.2.2 Serum sodium measurement may be useful every few hours in some patients undergoing intensive corrective fluid therapy, for diabetic ketoacidosis, intensive diuresis, or correction of severe hyponatremia.

Recommendations: Chloride

Rationale

Chloride losses, which usually follow those of sodium, may be compensated for by increases in serum bicarbonate. In addition, chloride deficiency is closely associated with a deficit in potassium. A measurement of serum or plasma chloride concentration alone is never indicated.

1. Screening

    1.1 Chloride measurement is not indicated in unselected populations.

2. Patient Management
    2.1 Chloride measurement, as part of a set of elec-
    trolytes tests, is indicated in acutely ill patients
    for proper interpretation of bicarbonate concen-
    tration (total CO_2) and for calculation of anion
    gap.
        2.1.1 Chloride measurement is indicated when
        a total CO_2 test is indicated.

Recommendation: Bicarbonate: Total CO_2

Rationale
    Total CO_2 concentration represents the sum of bi-
    carbonate concentration plus carbonic acid concen-
    tration plus dissolved CO_2 gas and is often used as a
    surrogate for bicarbonate concentration, which com-
    prises 90% to 95% of the total CO_2.
1. Screening
    1.1 Total CO_2 measurement, is not indicated in am-
    bulatory patients in whom there are no signs or
    symptoms of disease.
        1.1.1 Acid-base abnormalities usually do not
        occur until well into the course of chronic
        pulmonary, cardiac, renal, or gastrointes-
        tinal disease.
2. Patient Management
    2.1 Total CO_2 measurement may be useful at the
    following frequencies when determining the na-
    ture and severity of disease in patients with
    chronic diarrhea, chronic renal failure, renal tu-
    bular acidosis, and severe cardiopulmonary dis-
    ease, especially those on diuretics:
        2.1.1 At initial signs and symptoms of disease;
        2.1.2 At change in clinical status.
    2.2 Total CO_2 measurement may be useful at the
    following frequencies in seriously ill patients:
        2.2.1 On hospital admission;
        2.2.2 At change in clinical status;
        2.2.3 To follow therapy for an acid-base disor-
        der.
            2.2.3.1 In patients with severe ketoacido-
            sis or other types of servere meta-
            bolic acidosis, a complete set of
            electrolyte tests may be useful ev-
            ery 2 to 4 hours during the first
            several hours of therapy.

Recommendations: Serum Osmolality

Rationale

Indications for measuring serum osmolality are few and almost exclusively in hospitalized patients.

1. Patient Management

    1.1 In the absence of increased osmotically active compounds, the measurement of serum osmolality may not be indicated in hyponatremic patients.

        1.1.1 Measurement of serum osmolality may be indicated in hyponatremic patients with lipemic plasma or in patients with serum globulins in excess of 8 g/dL in order to provide reassurance that reduction in serum sodium does not represent true hypo-osmolality.

    1.2 Measurement of serum osmolality may be useful to detemine if one of the following substances exists in serum that is not otherwise being measured: mannitol, glycerol, alcohol, methanol, ethylene glycol, or other toxic chemicals ingested by alcoholics.

    1.3 Serum osmolality is more useful than plasma electrolytes in distinguishing between diabetes insipidus and psychogenic polydipsia.

        1.3.1 Serum osmolality must be determined several times under conditions of water deprivation to distinguish the pattern of disease when establishing a diagnosis.

Blood Urea Nitrogen Concentration and Serum Creatinine Concentration

Definition

Blood urea nitrogen concentration (BUN) and serum creatinine concentration are used to assess kidney function.

Rationale

The BUN and serum creatinine tests reflect urea or creatinine clearance respectively, both of which are indices of glomerular filtration rate (GFR). The BUN, in addition to reflecting GFR, can be used to assess the rate of urine flow and thus the hydration of the patient, and the nitrogen load, and thus can be used as an index of catabolism. As a screening test for kidney function, serum creatinine is preferred to BUN because it is more closely correlated with GFR than BUN. A BUN test alone is rarely indicated, but must be compared to a simultaneous serum creatinine measurement to assess whether an abnormal value can be attributed to a change in kidney function.

Recommendations

1. Screening
    1.1 Serum creatinine measurement, with or without BUN, may be useful in unselected ambulatory persons without signs or symptoms of disease.
2. Case-finding/Diagnosis in Selected Populations
    2.1 Measuring BUN and serum creatinine concentration, or creatinine alone, may be useful in hypertensive or diabetic patients.
        2.1.1 Measuring BUN and serum creatinine concentration is indicated initially, followed by creatinine clearance measurement if results are abnormal.
3. Patient Management
    3.1 Measuring BUN and serum creatinine concentration, or creatinine alone, may be useful for the following conditions and at the following frequencies:
        3.1.1 Uncomplicated hypertensive patients, every 1 to 2 years;

       3.1.2 Chronic renal disease, every 4 to 6 months;

       3.1.3 Patients receiving aminoglycoside treatment, two to three times per week;

       3.1.4 Oliguric patients in acute renal failure, every 1 to 2 days;

       3.1.5 Seriously ill patients, at least once a week.

3.2 A BUN test alone is rarely indicated.

       3.2.1 A BUN test must be compared to measuring simultaneous serum creatinine to assess whether an abnormal BUN value can be attributed to a change in kidney function.

3.3 Conditions in which both the BUN and serum creatinine concentration may be indicated include the following:

       3.3.1 Acute renal insufficiency with suspected volume contraction;

       3.3.2 Gastrointestinal bleeding complicated by some degree of renal insufficiency;

       3.3.3 Advanced renal insufficiency: serum creatinine 7 or above;

       3.3.4 A suspected diagnosis of water intoxication;

       3.3.5 Syndrome of inappropriate antidiuretic hormone secretion.

NOTES

NOTES